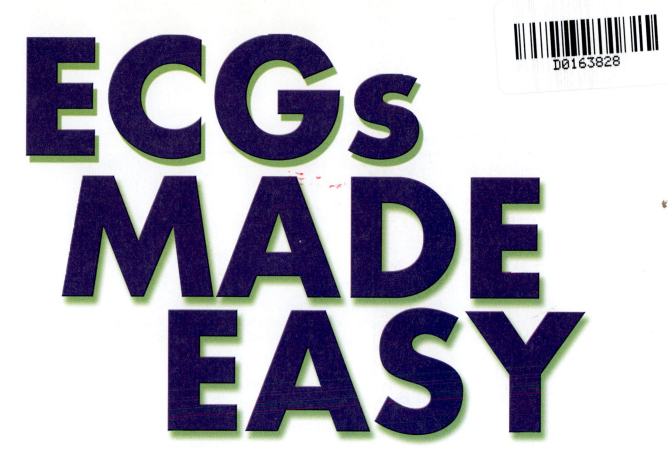

ECGs MADE EASY

SECOND EDITION

BARBARA AEHLERT, RN, BSPA

Southwest EMS Education, Inc.
Glendale, Arizona

Illustrations (except ECGs and those
otherwise noted) by Kimberly Battista

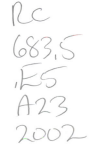 Mosby

A Harcourt Health Sciences Company

St. Louis   London   Philadelphia   Sydney   Toronto

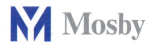

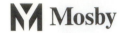

A Harcourt Health Sciences Company

Editor-in-Chief: *Andrew Allen*
Executive Editor: *Claire Merrick*
Developmental Editor: *Laura Bayless*
Project Manager: *John Rogers*
Senior Production Editor: *Helen Hudlin*
Designer: *Kathi Gosche*

Mosby, Inc.
A Harcourt Health Sciences Company
11830 Westline Industrial Drive
St. Louis, Missouri 63146

Printed in the United States of America

ISBN 0-323-01432-1

01 02 03 04 05 TG/KPT 9 8 7 6 5 4 3 2 1

PREFACE

This book is designed for use by paramedics, nursing, and medical students and ECG monitor technicians, nurses, and other allied health personnel working in emergency departments, critical care units, post-anesthesia care units, operating rooms, and telemetry units wishing to master the skill of basic ECG recognition. This book may be used alone or as part of a formal course of instruction in basic dysrhythmia recognition.

The material in this text focuses on the essential information needed to interpret basic dysrhythmias and understand their significance. A description of each dysrhythmia is provided with possible patient signs and symptoms related to the dysrhythmia. Where appropriate, current recommended treatment for the dysrhythmia is discussed.

After discussion of each dysrhythmia, a sample rhythm strip is displayed. Additional rhythm strips are provided for practice at the conclusion of each chapter. Answers for each rhythm strip are provided in the appendix. All rhythm strips shown in this text were recorded in lead II unless otherwise noted.

Features new to the second edition include:

- **Expanded anatomy and physiology and basic electrophysiology chapters.** Chapters 1 and 2 of the text have been expanded to include a more in-depth discussion of the coronary blood supply, conduction system, waveforms, and lead placement.
- **ECG facts.** Interesting ECG facts have been added to enhance the reader's understanding of the material.
- **Stop and review.** A matching self-assessment exercise has been added to each chapter. A comprehensive post-test consisting of multiple choice, true/false, fill-in questions, and rhythm strips is also included.
- **12-lead ECG chapter.** A new chapter has been added providing an introduction to 12-lead ECG recognition. This chapter presents information including lead placement; bundle branch blocks; recognizing ECG signs of ischemia, injury, and infarction; chamber enlargement; and ECG changes associated with electrolyte disturbances and medications.

Every attempt has been made to provide information that is consistent with current literature, including current resuscitation guidelines; however, the reader is advised to learn and follow local protocols as defined by his/her medical advisors.

I hope you find this text of assistance and welcome your comments and suggestions.

Barbara Aehlert, RN

For my best friend,
Maryalice Witzel, RN
Thank you for always being there for me.

ACKNOWLEDGMENTS

I would like to thank:

- Patty Seneski, RN; Bill Loughran, RN; James Bratcher, CEP; Timothy Klatt, RN; Holly Button, CEP; Gretchen Chalmers, CEP; Thomas Cole, CEP; Brent Haines, CEP; Joe Martinez, CEP; Stephanos Orphanidis, CEP; Steve Ruehs, CEP; Dionne Socie, CEP; Kristina Tellez, CEP; and Fran Wojculewicz, RN, for providing many of the rhythm strips used in this text.
- Claire Merrick for her direction and support of this project. It is a pleasure working with you and your team.
- The Southwest EMS Education "team"—James Bratcher, CEP; Lynn Browne-Wagner, RN; Ken Bruck, CEP; Randy Budd, CEP; Thomas Cole, CEP; Bill Loughran, RN; Captain Garret Olson, CEP; Jeff Pennington, CEP; Captain Greg Ruiz, CEP; and Maryalice Witzel, RN, for the hours spent in the classroom and on the telephone discussing many topics that ultimately affect what we teach and how we deliver the information to our students.
- My family—Dean, Andrea, Sherri, Sean, and Tony. Thanks for your patience and taking care of things on a daily basis as I worked to complete this project.
- The reviewers of this text. Your thorough review, comments, and suggestions were sincerely appreciated. Areas of this text were rewritten, reorganized, and clarified because of your efforts. Thank you.

ABOUT THE AUTHOR

Barbara Aehlert, RN, is the President/CEO of Southwest EMS Education, Inc. in Arizona. She has been a registered nurse for more than 20 years with clinical experience in medical/surgical and critical care nursing and, for the past 15 years, in prehospital education. As an active instructor, Barbara regularly teaches courses related to the care of the adult cardiac patient and takes a special interest in teaching basic dysrhythmia recognition to nurses and paramedics.

In addition to this text and the accompanying *ECGs Made Easy Pocket Reference*, Barbara is the author of the following Mosby publications: *ACLS Quick Review Study Guide, ACLS Quick Review Study Cards, ACLS Quick Review Slide Set, Mosby's ACLS Test Generator,* and *Pediatric Advanced Life Support Study Guide.* Barbara has also acted as a consultant on other Mosby educational materials, as a reviewer of several texts, and has contributed to several Mosby CD-ROM projects.

CONTENTS

9 INTRODUCTION TO THE 12-LEAD ECG, 192

CHAPTER 1

Anatomy and Physiology

OBJECTIVES

On completion of this chapter, you will be able to:

1. Describe the location of the heart.
2. Distinguish between the apex and base of the heart.
3. Identify and describe the chambers of the heart and the vessels that enter or leave each.
4. Define the term *atrial kick.*
5. Describe the structure and location of the pericardium, epicardium, myocardium, and endocardium.
6. Name and identify the location of the atrioventricular (AV) and semilunar (SL) valves.
7. Explain how heart sounds are created and the clinical significance of the first and second heart sounds.
8. Beginning with the right atrium, describe the flow of blood through the normal heart and lungs to the systemic circulation.
9. Identify the phases of the cardiac cycle.
10. Name the primary branches of the right and left coronary arteries.
11. Identify the portions of the myocardium and conduction system supplied by the right and left coronary arteries.
12. Describe the role of baroreceptors in controlling heart rate.
13. Define the terms *chronotropy* and *inotropy.*
14. Compare and contrast the effects of sympathetic and parasympathetic stimulation of the heart.
15. Name the primary neurotransmitter of the parasympathetic division of the autonomic nervous system and describe its effects on the heart.
16. Name the primary neurotransmitter of the sympathetic division of the autonomic nervous system and describe its effects on the heart.
17. Describe the effects of stimulation of alpha-receptors, beta-1-receptors, beta-2-receptors, and dopaminergic receptors.
18. Identify the factors affecting venous return.
19. Identify and define the components of cardiac output.
20. Define the terms *preload* and *afterload.*

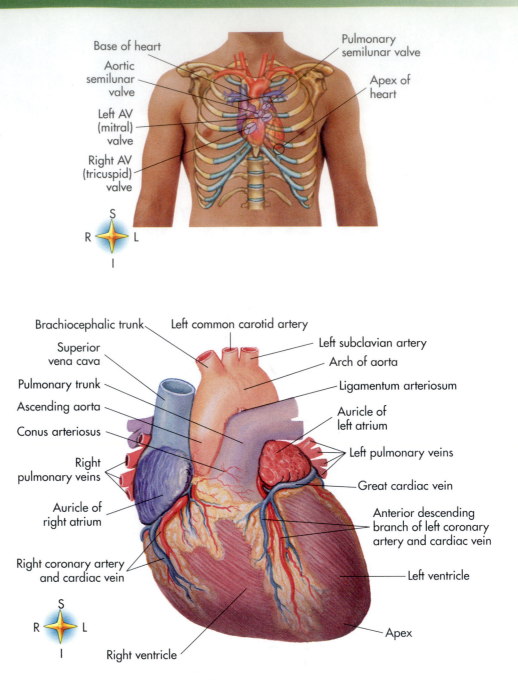

FIGURE 1-1 Location of the heart. The heart lies in the middle of the thoracic cavity (mediastinum) behind the sternum and between the lungs.

FIGURE 1-2 Anterior view of the heart and great vessels.

LOCATION OF THE HEART

Mediastinum: Located in the middle of the thoracic cavity; contains the heart, great vessels, trachea, and esophagus, among other structures; extends from the sternum to the vertebral column.

Great vessels: Pulmonary arteries, and veins, aorta, superior and inferior vena cavae.

The heart is a hollow muscular organ that lies in the middle of the thoracic cavity **(mediastinum)** behind the sternum, between the lungs, and just above the diaphragm. It is surrounded by a protective sac (pericardium) and is attached to the thorax through the **great vessels** (pulmonary arteries and veins, aorta, superior and inferior vena cavae) (Figure 1-1).

The **apex** (bottom) of the heart is formed by the tip of the left ventricle. It is positioned just above the diaphragm to the left in an anterior position, at the fifth intercostal space, midclavicular line. The **base** (top) of the heart is at approximately the level of the second intercostal space. The anterior surface of the heart consists primarily of the right ventricle. The inferior (diaphragmatic) surface is formed by the right and left ventricles (predominantly the left) (Figure 1-2).

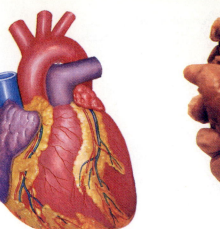 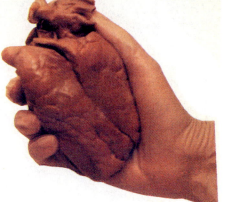

FIGURE **1-3**
The adult heart is cone shaped and is approximately 5 inches long, 3½ inches wide, and 2½ inches thick. It weighs approximately 250 to 350 g and is about the size of a fist.

Size and Shape of the Heart

The adult heart is cone shaped and is approximately 5 inches (12 cm) long, 3½ inches (9 cm) wide, and 2½ inches (6 cm) thick. It typically weighs between 250 and 350 g (approximately 11 oz) and is about the size of a man's fist (Figure 1-3). Heart size and weight are influenced by age, body weight and build, frequency of physical exercise, and heart disease.

The weight of the heart is approximately 0.45% of a man's body weight and about 0.40% of a woman's.

HEART CHAMBERS

The heart is divided into four cavities or chambers but functions as a two-sided pump. The two upper chambers are the right and left atria, and the two lower chambers are the right and left ventricles.

The right side of the heart is a low-pressure system that pumps venous blood to the lungs. The left side is a high-pressure system that pumps arterial blood to the systemic circulation.

The heart pumps approximately 4300 gallons of blood every day.

The surface of the heart has grooves that indicate the positions of the **septa,** which separate the heart chambers. The coronary arteries and their major branches lie in these grooves. The septa are muscular partitions that separate the heart into two functional pumps: the right atrium and right ventricle (low-pressure pump) and the left atrium and left ventricle (high-pressure pump).

Septum: Partition (plural form = septa).

Atria

The **atria** are thin-walled, low-pressure chambers that *receive* blood. An internal wall of connective tissue called the *interatrial septum* separates the right and left atria. Externally, the coronary **sulcus** (groove) encircles the heart and separates the atria from the ventricles. It contains the coronary blood vessels and epicardial fat.

Atria: Upper chambers of the heart.

Sulcus: Groove.

Think of the atria as "holding tanks" or "reservoirs" for blood.

The right atrium receives deoxygenated blood from the superior vena cava (which carries blood from the head and upper extremities), the inferior vena cava (which carries blood from the lower body), and the coronary sinus (which receives blood from the intracardiac circulation). The left atrium receives oxygenated blood from the lungs via the right and left pulmonary veins.

The right atrium is approximately 2 mm thick; the left atrium is approximately 3 mm thick.

There is normally a continuous flow of blood from the superior and inferior vena cavae into the atria. Approximately 70% of this blood flows directly through the atria and into the ventricles before the atria contract. With atrial contraction, an additional 30% is

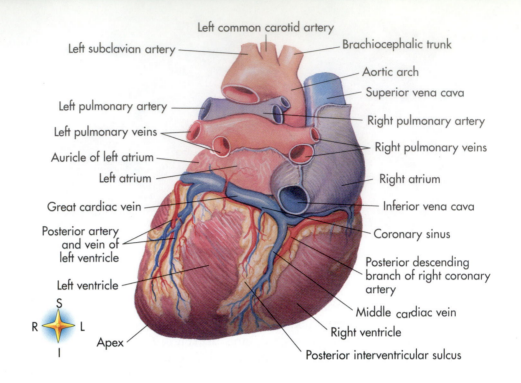

Left common carotid artery
Left subclavian artery
Brachiocephalic trunk
Aortic arch
Superior vena cava
Left pulmonary artery
Right pulmonary artery
Left pulmonary veins
Right pulmonary veins
Auricle of left atrium
Left atrium
Right atrium
Great cardiac vein
Inferior vena cava
Posterior artery and vein of left ventricle
Coronary sinus
Left ventricle
Posterior descending branch of right coronary artery
Middle cardiac vein
Apex
Right ventricle
Posterior interventricular sulcus

S
R   L
I

FIGURE 1-4
Posterior view of the heart and great vessels.

Atrial kick: Blood pushed into the ventricles as a result of atrial contraction.

added to filling of the ventricles. This additional contribution of blood because of atrial contraction is called **atrial kick.**

Ventricles

Ventricles: Lower heart chambers.

The **ventricles** pump blood to the lungs and systemic circulation. An internal wall of connective tissue called the *interventricular septum* separates the right and left ventricles. Externally, the interventricular sulcus is anatomically divided into the anterior interventricular sulcus and the posterior interventricular sulcus. These grooves indicate the position of the interventricular septum (separating the right and left ventricles) and are perpendicular to the coronary sulcus (Figure 1-4).

The right ventricle is approximately 3 to 5 mm thick; the left ventricle is approximately 13 to 15 mm.

The ventricles are larger and thicker walled than the atria. The left ventricle is a high-pressure chamber that is approximately three times thicker than the right ventricle. To pump blood out of the left ventricle to the systemic circulation, the left ventricle must contract forcefully and overcome arterial pressure and resistance. Each ventricle holds about 150 mL when full and normally ejects only about half this volume (70 to 80 mL) with each contraction.

LAYERS OF THE HEART

The heart wall is made up of three tissue layers that include the endocardium, myocardium, and epicardium (Table 1-1).

Endocardium: Innermost layer of the heart that lines the inside of the myocardium and covers the heart valves.

The **endocardium** (innermost layer) is a thin, smooth layer of epithelium and connective tissue that lines the heart's inner chambers, valves, chordae tendineae, and papillary muscles. The endocardium is continuous with the innermost layer (tunica intima) of the arteries, veins, and capillaries of the body, creating a continuous, closed circulatory system (Figure 1-5).

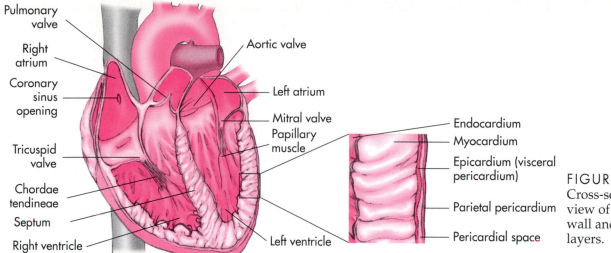

FIGURE **1-5** Cross-sectional view of the heart wall and tissue layers.

TABLE **1-1**	LAYERS OF THE HEART WALL
Epicardium	External layer of the heart
	Coronary arteries, blood capillaries, lymph capillaries, nerve fibers, and fat are found in this layer
Myocardium	Middle and thickest layer of the heart
	Responsible for contraction of the heart
Endocardium	Innermost layer of the heart
	Lines the inside of the myocardium
	Covers the heart valves

The **myocardium** (middle layer) is a thick, muscular layer that consists of cardiac muscle fibers (cells) responsible for the pumping action of the heart. The muscle fibers of the myocardium are separated by connective tissues that are richly supplied with capillaries and nerve fibers. The myocardium is firmly anchored to the fibrous skeleton of the heart.

The thickness of the myocardium varies from one heart chamber to another and is related to the amount of resistance the muscle must overcome to pump blood from the different chambers.[1] Because the atria encounter little resistance when pumping blood to the ventricles, their walls are the thinnest part of the myocardium. On the other hand, the ventricles must pump blood to either the lungs or the rest of the body. As a result the myocardium of the ventricles is thicker than that of the atria. The wall of the left ventricle is thicker than that of the right because the left ventricle propels blood to most vessels of the body, whereas the right ventricle moves blood only through the blood vessels of the lungs and back into the left atrium.

The **epicardium** (also called the *visceral layer of the serous pericardium*) is the external layer of the heart and includes blood capillaries, lymph capillaries, nerve fibers, and fat. Coronary blood vessels that supply arterial blood to the heart cross this layer before entering the myocardium.

Myocardium: Middle and thickest layer of the heart; contains the cardiac muscle fibers that cause contraction of the heart and contains the conduction system and blood supply.

Epicardium: Also known as the *visceral pericardium*; the external layer of the heart wall that covers the heart muscle.

Pericardium: Protective sac that surrounds the heart.

The **pericardium** is a double-walled sac that encloses the heart and helps protect it from trauma and infection. The rough outer layer of the pericardial sac is called the *fibrous parietal pericardium*. It is continuous with the external walls of the great vessels and blends with the fascia of the diaphragm. The inner layer, the *serous pericardium*, consists of two layers: parietal and visceral. The parietal layer lines the inside of the fibrous pericardium. The visceral layer (also called the *epicardium*) adheres to the outside of the heart and forms the outer layer of the heart muscle.

Between the visceral and parietal layers is a space (the pericardial space) that normally contains approximately 10 mL of serous fluid. This fluid acts as a lubricant, preventing friction as the heart beats. Accumulation of blood or other fluid in the pericardial space can lead to cardiac tamponade, compromising cardiac function.

CARDIAC MUSCLE

The walls of the heart are formed by cardiac muscle fibers that have striations similar to that of skeletal muscle. Cardiac muscle consists of many muscle cells (Figure 1-6, *A*).

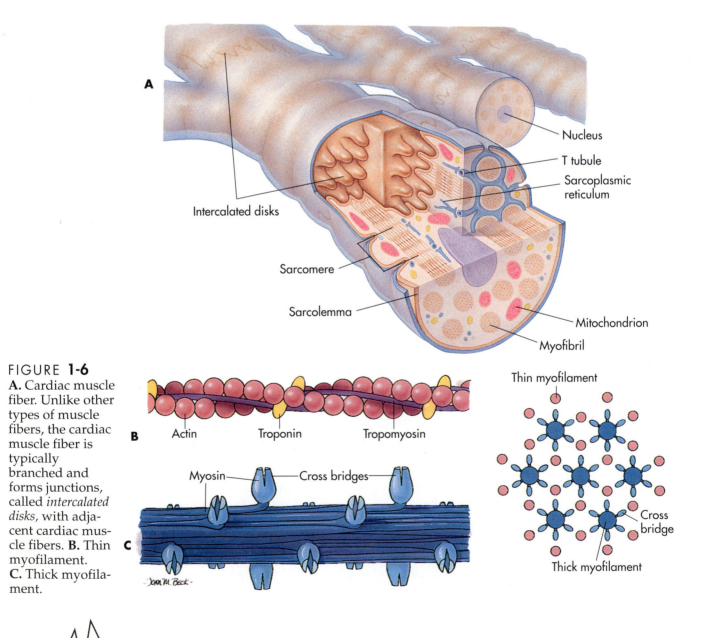

FIGURE 1-6
A. Cardiac muscle fiber. Unlike other types of muscle fibers, the cardiac muscle fiber is typically branched and forms junctions, called *intercalated disks*, with adjacent cardiac muscle fibers. **B.** Thin myofilament. **C.** Thick myofilament.

Labels in figure:
Nucleus
T tubule
Sarcoplasmic reticulum
Intercalated disks
Sarcomere
Sarcolemma
Mitochondrion
Myofibril

B Actin   Troponin   Tropomyosin

C Myosin   Cross bridges

Thin myofilament
Cross bridge
Thick myofilament

Each muscle cell is enclosed in a membrane called a **sarcolemma.** Within each cell are hundreds of long, tubelike structures called *myofibrils* (the contractile elements of myocardial muscle cells) that run parallel to each other and mitochondria (the energy-producing elements). Myofibrils consist of many **sarcomeres,** the basic protein units responsible for contraction. The process of contraction requires adenosine triphosphate (ATP) for energy. Thus the mitochondria that are interspersed between the myofibrils are important sites of ATP production.

Sarcolemma: Membrane covering smooth, striated, and cardiac muscle fibers.

Sarcomere: Smallest functional unit of a myofibril.

Each sarcomere contains two types of protein filaments: actin and myosin. Contraction occurs when the muscle is stimulated, and projections on the thin actin myofilaments (Figure 1-6, *B*) interact with the thick myosin myofilaments to form cross bridges (Figure 1-6, *C*). The cross bridges use energy (ATP) to bend, allowing the actin myofilaments to slide over the myosin myofilaments and toward the center of the sarcomere and overlap. This overlap causes shortening of the myofibrils, resulting in contraction. The actin myofilaments contain tropomyosin and troponin, two proteins that inhibit the formation of cross bridges with myosin. When cross bridge formation is inhibited, the muscle is relaxed.

Myocardial cell contracts when actin and myosin filaments slide together.

Troponin-T and I tests may be ordered for a patient experiencing a MI. If troponin-I level is elevated (positive test), myocardial necrosis (infarction) has almost certainly occurred.

Cardiac muscle fibers contain T (transverse) tubules that are extensions of the cell membrane. These tubules conduct the impulse to the center of the cell. Another system of tubules, the **sarcoplasmic reticulum,** stores calcium. During contraction, calcium is released from the sarcoplasmic reticulum. However, much of the calcium that enters the cell's cytoplasm (sarcoplasm) enters from the interstitial fluid surrounding the cardiac muscle cells through the T tubules. This is important because without the extra calcium from the T tubules, cardiac muscle contraction would be considerably reduced. Thus the strength of cardiac muscle contraction depends largely on the concentration of calcium ions in the extracellular fluid.

Sarcoplasmic reticulum: Network of tubules and sacs that plays an important role in muscle contraction and relaxation by releasing and storing calcium ions.

"Because the sarcolemma of cardiac muscle sustains each impulse longer than in skeletal muscle, calcium remains in the sarcolemma longer. This means that even though many adjacent cardiac muscle cells contract simultaneously, they exhibit a prolonged contraction rather than a rapid twitch. It also means that impulses cannot come rapidly enough to produce tetanus. Because it cannot sustain long tetanic contractions, cardiac muscle does not normally run low on ATP and thus does not experience fatigue."[3]

The sarcoplasmic reticulum of cardiac muscle is not as well developed as that of skeletal muscle and does not store enough calcium to provide full cardiac contraction.[2]

Cardiac muscle fibers are long branching cells that fit together tightly at junctions called *intercalated disks.* The anatomic arrangement of these tight-fitting junctions gives an appearance of a **syncytium,** that is, resembling a network of cells with no separation between the individual cells. The intercalated disks fit together in such a way that they form permeable gap junctions that function as electrical connections. These connections join muscle fibers into a single unit that can rapidly conduct an impulse throughout the wall of a cardiac chamber. This characteristic allows the walls of both atria (likewise, the walls of both ventricles) to contract almost simultaneously. The gap junctions present in myocardial cells allow the cells to conduct electrical impulses very rapidly.

Syncytium: Unit of combined cells.

The heart consists of two syncytiums: atrial and ventricular. The atrial syncytium consists of the walls of the right and left atria. The ventricular syncytium consists of the walls of the right and left ventricles. Normally, impulses can be conducted only from the atrial syncytium into the ventricular syncytium by means of the atrioventricular (AV) junction. This allows the atria to contract a short time before ventricular contraction.

VALVES OF THE HEART

The skeleton of the heart consists of four rings of dense fibrous connective tissue that encircle the bases of the pulmonary trunk and aorta and the heart valves. This fibrous skeleton helps form the septa that separate the atria from the ventricles and provides secure attachments for the valves and chambers of the heart (Figure 1-7).

There are four valves in the heart: two sets of atrioventricular (AV) valves and two sets of semilunar valves (Table 1-2). Their purpose is to ensure blood flow in one direction through the heart's chambers and prevent the backflow of blood.

Atrioventricular Valves

Atrioventricular (AV) valves separate the atria from the ventricles. The two AV valves consist of the following:

- Tough, fibrous rings (annuli fibrosi)
- Flaps (leaflets or cusps) of endocardium
- Chordae tendineae
- Papillary muscles

The tricuspid valve is the AV valve that lies between the right atrium and right ventricle. It consists of three separate leaflets and is larger in diameter and thinner than the mitral valve (Figure 1-8).

The pulmonary trunk begins at the pulmonary valve and divides into the right and left pulmonary arteries.

The four valves in the heart ensure blood flow in one direction.

Atrioventricular valve: Valve located between each atrium and ventricle; tricuspid separates the right atrium from the right ventricle, mitral (bicuspid) separates the left atrium from the left ventricle.

TABLE 1-2	VALVES OF THE HEART	
Valve type	**Name**	**Location**
Atrioventricular	Tricuspid	Separates right atrium and right ventricle
	Mitral (bicuspid)	Separates left atrium and left ventricle
Semilunar	Pulmonic	Between right ventricle and pulmonary artery
	Aortic	Between left ventricle and aorta

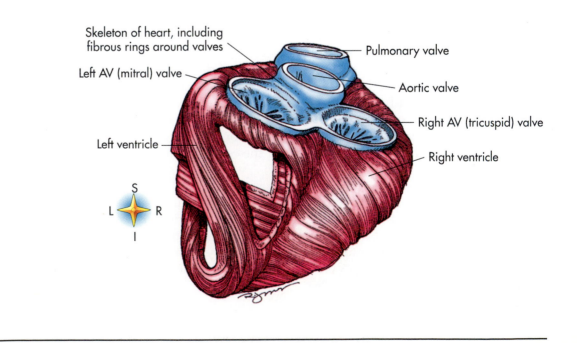

FIGURE 1-7 Posterior view of the heart. The rim of each heart valve is supported by a fibrous structure, called the *skeleton of the heart*, which encircles all four valves.

Skeleton of heart, including fibrous rings around valves

Left AV (mitral) valve

Left ventricle

Pulmonary valve

Aortic valve

Right AV (tricuspid) valve

Right ventricle

The mitral (or bicuspid) valve has only two cusps and lies between the left atrium and left ventricle (Figure 1-9).

♥ The mitral valve is so named because it is thought to resemble a mitre (bishop's hat) when open.

Pressure within the atria rises as the atria fill with blood. This forces the tricuspid and mitral valves to open and allows deoxygenated blood to empty into the right ventricle and oxygenated blood to empty into the left ventricle. After the atria contract, the pressures in the atria and ventricles equalize, and the tricuspid and mitral valves partially close. The ventricles then contract (systole), causing the pressure within the ventricles to rise sharply. The tricuspid and mitral valves close completely when the pressure within the ventricles exceeds that of the atria.

The cusps of the AV valves are attached to thin strands of fibrous connective tissue called **chordae tendineae** ("heart strings"). These structures serve as anchors and originate from small mounds of myocardium called *papillary muscles* that project inward from the ventricular walls. During ventricular contraction the papillary muscles also contract, pulling on the chordae tendineae, preventing the cusps of the AV valves from inverting into the atria.

Chordae tendineae: Thin strands of fibrous connective tissue that extend from the AV valves to the papillary muscles and prevent the AV valves from bulging back into the atria during ventricular systole (contraction).

Dysfunction of the chordae tendineae or of a papillary muscle can cause incomplete closure of an AV valve, which can result in a murmur. After an acute myocardial infarction (AMI), papillary muscles may be at risk for rupture as a result of an inadequate blood supply from the coronary circulation. For example, if a papillary muscle in the left ventricle ruptures, the leaflets of the mitral valve may not completely close and the valve leaflet may invert (prolapse). This may result in regurgitation of blood from the ventricle into the atrium and possible cardiac compromise.

Semilunar Valves

The pulmonic and aortic valves are **semilunar (SL) valves** that prevent backflow of blood from the aorta and pulmonary arteries into the ventricles during diastole (Figure 1-10). Both sets of SL valves have three cusps shaped like half-moons.

Semilunar (SL) valve: Valves shaped like half-moons that separate the ventricles from the aorta and pulmonary artery.

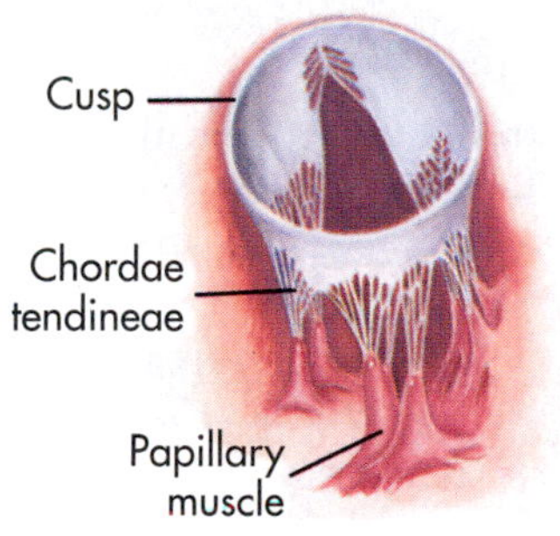

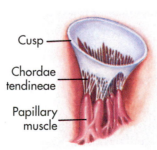

Cusp

Chordae tendineae

Papillary muscle

FIGURE **1-8**
Tricuspid valve.

Cusp

Chordae tendineae

Papillary muscle

FIGURE **1-9**
Mitral valve.

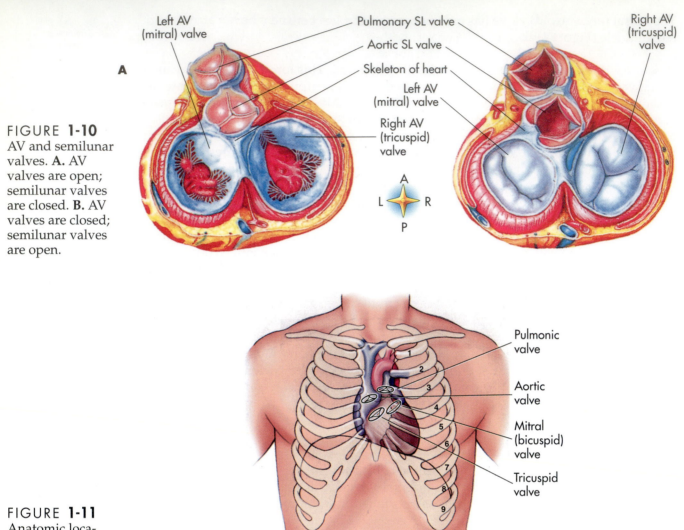

FIGURE 1-10
AV and semilunar valves. **A.** AV valves are open; semilunar valves are closed. **B.** AV valves are closed; semilunar valves are open.

FIGURE 1-11
Anatomic location of heart valves.

🦷 The sinus of Valsalva is a bulge at the base of the aorta formed by the thick leaflets of the aortic valve.

The right ventricle ejects deoxygenated blood through the pulmonic valve into the right and left pulmonary arteries. The left ventricle ejects oxygenated blood through the aortic valve to the aorta, perfusing the body's organs and tissues.

During ventricular systole, the SL valves open, allowing blood to flow out of the ventricles. The SL valves close as systole ends and the pressure in the outflow arteries exceeds that of the ventricles.

The leaflets of the SL valves are smaller and thicker than the AV valves and do not have the support of chordae tendineae. The openings of the SL valves are smaller than the openings of the AV valves. As a result the velocity of blood ejected through the aortic and pulmonary valves is much greater than that ejected through the AV valves (Figure 1-11).

HEART SOUNDS

Heart sounds occur as a result of vibrations in the tissues of the heart that are created as the blood flow is suddenly increased or slowed with the contraction and relaxation of the heart chambers and with the opening and closing of the heart's valves.

The first heart sound ("lub") occurs during ventricular contraction when the tricuspid and mitral (AV) valves are closing. The second heart sound ("dub") occurs during ventricular relaxation when the pulmonic and aortic (SL) valves are closing.

BLOOD FLOW THROUGH THE HEART

The right atrium receives blood low in oxygen and high in carbon dioxide from the superior and inferior vena cavae and the coronary sinus. Blood flows from the right atrium through the tricuspid valve into the right ventricle. When the right ventricle contracts, the tricuspid valve closes. The right ventricle expels the blood through the pulmonic valve into the pulmonary trunk. The pulmonary trunk divides into a right and left pulmonary artery, each of which carries blood to one lung (pulmonary circuit).

The coronary sinus is the largest vein that drains to the heart.

Blood flows through the pulmonary arteries to the lungs (where oxygen and carbon dioxide are exchanged in the pulmonary capillaries) and then to the pulmonary veins. Carbon dioxide is exhaled as the left atrium receives oxygenated blood from the lungs via the four pulmonary veins (two from the right lung and two from the left lung). Blood flows from the left atrium through the mitral (bicuspid) valve into the left ventricle. When the left ventricle contracts, the mitral valve closes. Blood leaves the left ventricle through the aortic valve to the aorta and its branches and is distributed throughout the body (systemic circuit). Blood from the tissues of the head and neck is emptied into the superior vena cava. Blood from the lower body is emptied into the inferior vena cava. The superior and inferior vena cavae carry their contents into the right atrium.

Deoxygenated blood passes through the pulmonary capillaries and comes in direct contact with the alveolar-capillary membrane, where oxygen and carbon dioxide are exchanged.

CARDIAC CYCLE

The cardiac cycle refers to a repetitive pumping process that includes all of the events associated with the flow of blood through the heart. The cycle has two phases for each heart chamber: systole and diastole. **Systole** is the period during which the chamber is contracting and blood is being ejected. Systole includes contraction of both atrial and ventricular muscle. **Diastole** is the period of relaxation during which the chamber is filling. Diastole includes relaxation of both atrial and ventricular muscle.

When the terms systole and diastole are used without reference to a specific chamber of the heart, the terms imply ventricular systole and diastole.

In a resting adult, each cardiac cycle lasts approximately 0.8 sec. Atrial systole requires about 0.1 sec, and ventricular systole requires about 0.3 sec. Atrial diastole lasts about 0.7 sec and ventricular diastole lasts about 0.5 sec during each cardiac cycle.

At rest, the rate of blood flow through the cardiovascular system is about 5000 mL/min.

The cardiac cycle depends on the ability of the cardiac muscle to contract and on the condition of the conduction system. The efficiency of the heart as a pump may be affected by abnormalities of cardiac muscle, the valves, or the conduction system.

During the cardiac cycle, the pressure within each chamber of the heart rises in systole and falls in diastole. The heart's valves ensure that blood flows in the proper direction. Blood flows from one heart chamber to another if the pressure in the chamber is more than the pressure in the next. These pressure relationships depend on the careful timing of contractions. The heart's conduction system provides the necessary timing of events between atrial and ventricular systole.

Atrial Systole and Diastole

During atrial diastole, blood from the superior and inferior vena cavae and the coronary sinus enters the right atrium. The right atrium fills and distends, pushing the tricuspid

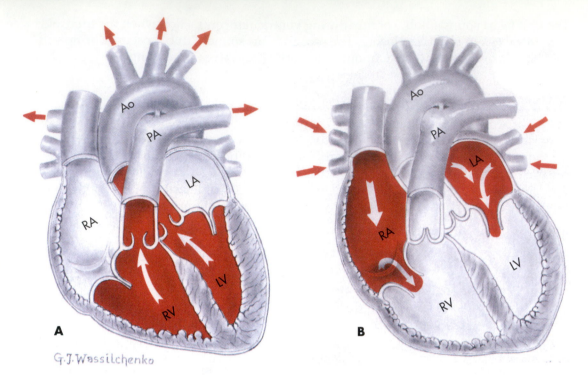

FIGURE 1-12
Blood flow during **(A)** systole and **(B)** diastole. *RA,* right atrium; *RV,* right ventricle; *LA,* left atrium; *LV,* left ventricle; *Ao,* aorta; *PA,* pulmonary artery.

valve open, and the right ventricle fills. The same sequence occurs a split second earlier in the left heart. The left atrium receives blood from the four pulmonary veins (two from the right lung and two from the left lung). The leaflets of the mitral valve open as the left atrium fills and blood flows into the left ventricle.

The ventricles are 70% filled before the atria contract. Contraction of the atria forces additional blood (approximately 30% of the ventricular capacity) into the ventricles (atrial kick). Thus the ventricles become completely filled with blood during atrial systole. During atrial systole, blood does not flow into the atria because the pressure within the atria exceeds venous pressure. The atria then enter a period of atrial diastole, which continues until the start of the next cardiac cycle.

Ventricular Systole and Diastole

Ventricular systole occurs as atrial diastole begins. As the ventricles contract, blood is propelled through the systemic and pulmonary circulation and toward the atria. The SL valves close and the heart then begins a period of ventricular diastole during which the ventricles begin to passively fill with blood, and both the atria and ventricles are relaxed. The cardiac cycle begins again with atrial systole and the completion of ventricular filling (Figure 1-12).

CORONARY CIRCULATION

At rest, coronary blood flow averages about 250 mL/min. This represents 4% to 5% of the total cardiac output.

The coronary circulation consists of coronary arteries and veins. With normal activity, 65% to 75% of the arterial oxygen content in the blood is extracted by the myocardium through the coronary arteries. This is the highest extraction rate of any tissue during normal activity and one that cannot be significantly improved. Thus the heart can improve its oxygen uptake only by increasing coronary blood flow. With strenuous activity, coronary blood flow can increase threefold to fivefold to ensure an adequate oxygen supply to the myocardium.[4] Myocardial ischemia results when the heart's demand for oxygen exceeds its supply from the coronary circulation.

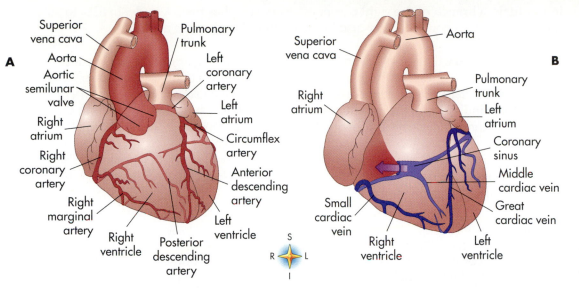

FIGURE **1-13**
Anterior views of
the coronary cir-
culation. **A.** Coro-
nary arteries.
B. Coronary
veins.

TABLE 1-3 CORONARY ARTERIES		
Coronary artery and its branches	Portion of myocardium supplied	Portion of supplied conduction system
RIGHT Posterior descending Right marginal	Right atrium Right ventricle Inferior wall of left ventricle Posterior wall of left ventricle Posterior one third of interventricular septum	SA node (50% to 60%)* AV node (85% to 90%)* Proximal portion of bundle of His Posterior-inferior fascicle of left bundle branch
LEFT Anterior descending	Anterior and part of lateral surface of left ventricle Anterior two thirds of interventricular septum	Majority of right bundle branch Anterior-superior fascicle of left bundle branch Portion of posterior-inferior fascicle of left bundle branch
Circumflex	Left atrium Anterolateral and posterolateral walls of left ventricle Posterior wall of left ventricle	SA node (40% to 50%)* AV node (10% to 15%)*

*Of population.

Coronary Arteries

Blood is supplied to the tissues of the heart during diastole by the first two branches of the aorta, the right and left coronary arteries (Table 1-3). The openings to these vessels are just beyond the cusps of the aortic SL valve (Figure 1-13). The coronary arteries cross the epicardium and branch several times. These branches enter the myocardium and endocardium and further divide to become arterioles, then capillaries.

The coronary arteries encircle the heart like a crown, or corona.

Right Coronary Artery
The right coronary artery (RCA) originates from the right side of the aorta and passes along the atrioventricular sulcus between the right atrium and right ventricle. The marginal branch of the RCA supplies the right atrium and right ventricle. In 50% to 60% of

individuals, a branch of the right coronary artery supplies the SA node. In 85% to 90% of hearts, the right coronary artery also branches into the AV node artery.[5]

Coronary artery dominance is right sided in approximately 85% of the population.[6]

The coronary artery that gives rise to the posterior descending artery is usually considered the "dominant" coronary artery. In most individuals a branch of the right coronary artery becomes the posterior descending artery. This is called a *dominant right coronary artery* system. In some individuals, the left circumflex coronary artery branches and ends at the posterior descending artery. This is described as a *dominant left coronary artery* system.

The posterior descending artery supplies blood to the walls of both ventricles. This vessel has several branches including the septal branch that supplies the posterior third of the interventricular septum.

Left Coronary Artery

Occlusion of the left main coronary artery has been referred to as the "widow maker" because of its association with sudden death.

The left coronary artery (LCA) originates from the left side of the aorta and consists of the left main coronary artery that divides into two primary branches: the left anterior descending (LAD) (also called the *anterior interventricular*) artery and the left circumflex (LC) artery. The LAD branch travels to the anterior interventricular sulcus, and its branches supply blood to the anterior surfaces of both ventricles. Branches of the LAD include the diagonal and septal arteries.

The LC artery supplies the SA node in 40% to 60% of individuals and the AV node in 10% to 15%.

The LC branch follows the coronary sulcus between the right and left ventricle and supplies blood to the left atrium and left ventricle. The left circumflex supplies the lateral wall of the left ventricle. In some patients the circumflex artery may also supply the inferior portion of the left ventricle.

When the heart contracts, blood flow to the tissues of the heart is significantly reduced because the heart's blood vessels are compressed. Thus the coronary arteries receive their blood supply during diastole or when the ventricular muscle mass is relaxing.

If the posterior wall of the left ventricle is damaged, a cardiac catheterization is usually necessary to determine which coronary artery is involved because both the RCA and LC supply blood to this area.

A myocardial infarction often begins in the subendocardial portion of the left ventricle because this area has a high demand for oxygen and a tenuous blood supply. "The reason for this is explained by following the anatomic pathway of the coronary arteries. The coronary arteries first supply the epicardium and then course deep to supply the endocardium. High intraventricular pressure or a thickened myocardium will tend to decrease blood flow to the subendocardial tissue."[7]

Coronary Veins

The coronary (cardiac) veins travel alongside the arteries. Blood that has passed through the myocardial capillaries is drained by branches of the cardiac veins that join the coronary sinus.

The great cardiac vein becomes continuous with the coronary sinus.

The coronary sinus is the largest vein that drains the heart and it lies in the coronary sulcus, which separates the atria from the ventricles. The coronary sinus receives blood from the great, middle, and small cardiac veins; the oblique vein of the left atrium; and the posterior vein of the left ventricle. The coronary sinus drains into the right atrium. The anterior cardiac veins do not join the coronary sinus but empty directly into the right atrium.

HEART RATE

The heart is innervated by both the sympathetic and parasympathetic divisions of the autonomic nervous system. The sympathetic division mobilizes the body, allowing the body to function under stress ("fight-or-flight" response). The parasympathetic division is responsible for the conservation and restoration of body resources ("feed-and-breed" response). Autonomic regulation of the cardiovascular system requires sensors, afferent pathways, an integration center, efferent pathways, and receptors.

Baroreceptors

Baroreceptors (pressoreceptors) are specialized nerve tissue (sensors) located in the internal carotid arteries and the aortic arch. These sensory receptors detect changes in blood pressure and cause a reflex response in either the sympathetic or parasympathetic divisions of the autonomic nervous system.

Baroreceptors detect changes in blood pressure.

If the systolic blood pressure decreases, the body's normal compensatory response to increase blood pressure is peripheral vasoconstriction, increased heart rate (chronotropy), and increased myocardial contractility (inotropy) (Table 1-4). In this example the compensatory responses occur because of a reflex sympathetic response (also called *adrenergic response*). If the systolic blood pressure increases, the baroreceptor reflex response decreases sympathetic stimulation and increases parasympathetic stimulation (cholinergic response).

Chronotropism: Refers to a change in heart rate.

Inotropism: Refers to a change in myocardial contractility.

Chemoreceptors

Chemoreceptors in the internal carotid arteries and aortic arch detect changes in the concentration of hydrogen ions (pH), oxygen, and carbon dioxide in the blood. The response to these changes by the autonomic nervous system can be sympathetic or parasympathetic. Decreased pH or oxygen levels in the blood or increased carbon dioxide levels cause a sympathetic response, resulting in increased heart rate, contractility, and vasoconstriction.[3] Increased pH or decreased carbon dioxide levels in the blood cause a decrease in vasoconstrictor effects, leading to a general vasodilatory effect.

Chemoreceptors detect changes in pH, O_2, and CO_2 levels in the blood.

Nerve impulses are carried from the sensory receptors to the brain by means of the vagus and glossopharyngeal nerves (afferent pathways). The medulla of the brain serves as the integration center and interprets the sensory information received. The medulla determines what body parameters need adjustment (if any) and transmits that information to the heart and blood vessels by means of motor nerves (efferent pathways).

Parasympathetic Stimulation

Parasympathetic Receptor Sites

Parasympathetic (inhibitory) nerve fibers supply the SA node, atrial muscle, and the AV junction of the heart by means of the vagus nerves. Acetylcholine, a neurotransmitter, is released when parasympathetic (cholinergic) nerve fibers are stimulated. Acetylcholine binds to parasympathetic receptors. The two main types of parasympathetic receptors

TABLE 1-4 TERMINOLOGY	
Chronotropic effect	**Inotropic effect**
Refers to a change in heart rate	Refers to a change in myocardial contractility
A positive chronotropic effect refers to an increase in heart rate	A positive inotropic effect results in an increase in myocardial contractility
A negative chronotropic effect refers to a decrease in heart rate	A negative inotropic effect results in a decrease in myocardial contractility

are nicotinic and muscarinic receptors. Nicotinic receptors are located in skeletal muscle. Muscarinic receptors are located in smooth muscle.

Parasympathetic stimulation slows the rate of discharge of the sinoatrial (SA) node, slows conduction through the AV node, decreases the strength of atrial contraction, and can cause a small decrease in the force of ventricular contraction. (There is little effect on the strength of ventricular contraction because of minimal parasympathetic innervation of these chambers). The net effect of parasympathetic stimulation is slowing of the heart rate.

Sympathetic Stimulation

Sympathetic (accelerator) nerve fibers supply the SA node, AV node, atrial muscle, and the ventricular myocardium. Stimulation of sympathetic nerve fibers results in the release of norepinephrine, a neurotransmitter, which increases the force of ventricular contraction, heart rate, blood pressure, and cardiac output (Figure 1-14).

Sympathetic Receptor Sites

Sympathetic (adrenergic) receptor sites are divided into alpha-receptors, beta-receptors, and dopaminergic receptors. Dopaminergic receptor sites are located in the coronary arteries and renal, mesenteric, and visceral blood vessels. Stimulation of dopaminergic receptor sites results in dilation.

Different body tissues have different proportions of alpha- and beta-receptors. In general, alpha-receptors are more sensitive to norepinephrine and beta-receptors are more

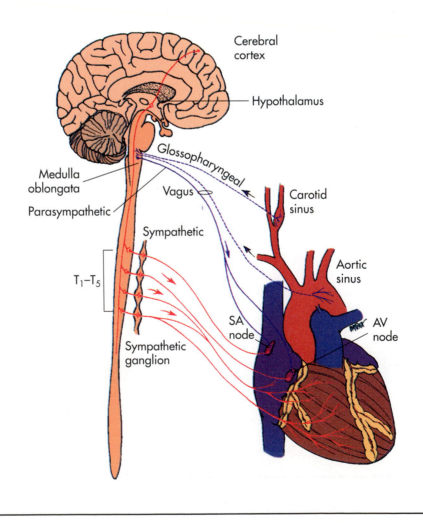

FIGURE **1-14** Autonomic nervous system innervation of the heart.

sensitive to epinephrine. Stimulation of alpha-receptor sites results in constriction of blood vessels in the skin, cerebral, and **splanchnic** circulation.

Beta-receptor sites are divided into beta-1 and beta-2. Beta-1-receptors are found in the heart. Stimulation of beta-1-receptors results in an increased heart rate, contractility, and, ultimately, irritability of cardiac cells. Beta-2-receptor sites are found in the lungs and skeletal muscle blood vessels. Stimulation of these receptor sites results in dilation of the smooth muscle of the bronchi and blood vessel dilation.

Increases in heart rate shorten all phases of the cardiac cycle, but the most important is a decrease in the length of time spent in diastole. If the length of diastole is shortened, there is less time for adequate ventricular filling. In some cases of a rapid heart rate, **vagal maneuvers** (e.g., carotid sinus pressure) may be performed to attempt to slow the rate. When vagal maneuvers are performed, baroreceptors in the carotid arteries are stimulated to slow AV conduction, resulting in slowing of the heart rate.

The concentrations of extracellular ions also affect heart rate. Excess extracellular potassium (K+) (hyperkalemia) causes the heart to become extremely dilated and flaccid and slows the heart rate. An increase in extracellular calcium (Ca++) (hypercalcemia) causes almost the exact opposite effect to those of potassium ions, causing the heart to go into spastic contraction. Decreased extracellular calcium levels (hypocalcemia) cause the heart to become flaccid, similar to the effects of increased potassium levels.

Other factors that influence heart rate include hormone levels (e.g., thyroxin, epinephrine, norepinephrine), medications, stress, anxiety, fear, and body temperature. Heart rate increases when body temperature increases and decreases when body temperature decreases.

A review of the autonomic nervous system can be found in Table 1-5.

Splanchnic: Pertaining to internal organs; visceral.

Remember: Beta-1-receptors affect the heart (you have one heart); beta-2-receptors affect the lungs (you have two lungs).

Vagal maneuvers: Methods used to stimulate the vagus nerve in an attempt to slow conduction through the AV node, resulting in slowing of the heart rate.

TABLE 1-5 REVIEW OF THE AUTONOMIC NERVOUS SYSTEM		
	Sympathetic division	**Parasympathetic division**
General effect	Fight-or-flight	Feed-and-breed
Primary neurotransmitter	Norepinephrine	Acetylcholine
Effects of Stimulation		
Abdominal blood vessels	Constriction (alpha-receptors)	No effect
Adrenal medulla	Increased secretion of epinephrine	No effect
Bronchioles	Dilation (beta-receptors)	Constriction
Blood vessels of skin	Constriction (alpha-receptors)	No effect
Blood vessels of skeletal muscle	Dilation (beta-receptors)	No effect
Cardiac muscle	Increased rate and strength of contraction (beta-receptors)	Decreased rate; decreased strength of atrial contraction, little effect on strength of ventricular contraction
Coronary blood vessels	Constriction (alpha-receptors) Dilation (beta-receptors)	Dilation

THE HEART AS A PUMP

Venous Return

Venous return: Amount of blood flowing into the right atrium each minute from the systemic circulation.

The heart functions as a pump to propel blood through the systemic and pulmonary circulations. As the heart chambers fill with blood, the heart muscle is stretched. The most important factor determining the amount of blood pumped by the heart is the amount of blood flowing into it from the systemic circulation **(venous return).**

Cardiac Output

Cardiac output: Amount of blood pumped into the aorta each minute by the heart; cardiac output = stroke volume × heart rate (CO = SV × HR).

Cardiac output is the amount of blood pumped into the aorta each minute by the heart. It is defined as the stroke volume (amount of blood ejected from a ventricle with each heartbeat) × the heart rate. In the average adult, normal cardiac output is between 4 and 8 L/min. The cardiac output at rest is approximately 5 L/min (stroke volume of 70 mL × a heart rate of 70 beats/min).

Because the cardiovascular system is a closed system, the volume of blood leaving one part of the system must equal that entering another part. For example, if the left ventricle normally pumps 5 L/min, the volume flowing through the arteries, capillaries, and veins must equal 5 L/min. Thus the cardiac output of the right ventricle (pulmonary blood flow) is normally equal to that of the left ventricle on a minute-to-minute basis.

Cardiac output may be increased by an increase in heart rate or stroke volume. An increase in myocardial contractility (and, subsequently, stroke volume) may occur because of norepinephrine and epinephrine release from the adrenal medulla, thyroxin, insulin and glucagon release from the pancreas, and medications such as calcium and digitalis. A decrease in contractility may result from severe hypoxia, decreased pH, hypercapnea (elevated carbon dioxide levels), and medications such as propranolol (Inderal).

Cardiac output varies depending on hormone balance, an individual's activity level and body size, and the body's metabolic needs. Factors that increase cardiac output include

FIGURE **1-15**
Frank-Starling law of the heart. The curve represents the relationship between stroke volume and the ventricular volume at the end of diastole. The range of values observed in a typical heart is shaded. NOTE: If the ventricle has an abnormally large volume at the end of diastole (far right portion of the curve), the stroke volume cannot compensate.

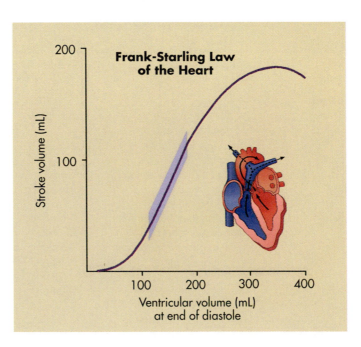

increased body metabolism, exercise, and the age and size of the body. Factors that may decrease cardiac output include shock, hypovolemia, and heart failure.

Signs and symptoms of decreased cardiac output include cold, clammy skin; color changes in the skin and mucous membranes; dyspnea, orthopnea, and crackles (rales); changes in mental status; changes in blood pressure; dysrhythmias; jugular venous distention; fatigue; and restlessness.

Blood Pressure

The mechanical activity of the heart is reflected by the pulse and blood pressure. Blood pressure is the force exerted by the circulating blood volume on the walls of the arteries. Peripheral resistance is the resistance to the flow of blood determined by blood vessel diameter and the tone of the vascular musculature. Blood pressure is equal to cardiac output × peripheral resistance. Blood pressure is affected by any condition that increases peripheral resistance or cardiac output. Thus an increase in either cardiac output or peripheral resistance will result in an increase in blood pressure. Conversely, a decrease in either will result in a decrease in blood pressure.

Tone is a term that may be used when referring to the normal state of balanced tension in body tissues.

Stroke Volume

Preload

Stroke volume is determined by the degree of ventricular filling during diastole (preload), the pressure against which the ventricle must pump (afterload), and the myocardium's contractile state. **Preload** is the force exerted on the walls of the ventricles at the end of diastole. The volume of blood returning to the heart influences preload. More blood returning to the right atrium increases preload; less blood returning decreases preload.

Preload: Force exerted by the blood on the walls of the ventricles at the end of diastole.

According to the Frank-Starling law of the heart (Figure 1-15), to a point, the greater the volume of blood in the heart during diastole, the more forceful the cardiac contraction, and the more blood the ventricle will pump (stroke volume). This is important so that the heart can adjust its pumping capacity in response to changes in venous return, such as during exercise. If, however, the ventricle is stretched beyond its physiologic limit, cardiac output may fall as a result of volume overload and overstretching of the muscle fibers.

The Frank-Starling law is named after Frank and Starling, two physiologists.

Afterload

Afterload is the pressure or resistance against which the ventricles must pump to eject blood. Afterload is influenced by arterial blood pressure, arterial distensibility (ability to become stretched), and arterial resistance. The lower the resistance (lower afterload), the more easily blood can be ejected. Increased afterload (increased resistance) results in increased cardiac workload. Conditions that contribute to increased afterload include increased blood viscosity, hypertension, and aortic stenosis.

Afterload: Pressure or resistance against which the ventricles must pump to eject blood.

REFERENCES

1. McCance KL, Huether SE: *Pathophysiology: the biologic basis for disease in adults and children,* ed 3, St Louis, 1998, Mosby.
2. Guyton AC, Hall JE: *Textbook of medical physiology,* ed 9, Philadelphia, 1996, WB Saunders.
3. Thibodeau GA, Patton KT: *Anatomy and physiology,* ed 2, St Louis, 1993, Mosby.
4. Kinney MR, editor: *Andreoli's comprehensive cardiac care,* ed 8, St Louis, 1995, Mosby.
5. Huszar RJ: *Basic dysrhythmias: interpretation and management,* ed 2, St Louis, 1994, Mosby.
6. Willerson JT, Cohn JN, editors: *Cardiovascular medicine,* New York, 1995, Churchill Livingstone.
7. Johnson R, Swartz MH: *A simplified approach to electrocardiography,* Philadelphia, 1986, WB Saunders.

BIBLIOGRAPHY

Ganong WF: *Review of medical physiology,* ed 17, Norwalk, 1995, Appleton & Lange.

Goldman L, Braunwald E: *Primary cardiology,* Philadelphia, 1998, WB Saunders.

Guyton A, Hall JE: *Textbook of medical physiology,* ed 9, Philadelphia, 1996, WB Saunders.

Kinney MR, editor: *Andreoli's comprehensive cardiac care,* ed 8, St Louis, 1995, Mosby.

Martini FH: *Fundamentals of anatomy and physiology,* ed 4, Upper Saddle River, 1998, Prentice Hall.

McCance KL, Huether SE: *Pathophysiology: the biologic basis for disease in adults and children,* ed 2, St Louis, 1994, Mosby.

Sloane E: *Anatomy and physiology: an easy learner,* Boston, 1994, Jones & Bartlett.

Spence A, Mason E: *Human anatomy and physiology,* ed 3, Menlo Park, 1987, Benjamin/Cummings.

Tartora G: *Introduction to the human body: the essentials of anatomy and physiology,* New York, 1994, HarperCollins.

Thibodeau GA, Patton KT: *Anatomy and physiology,* ed 2, St Louis, 1993, Mosby.

MATCHING

____ 1. The pressure or resistance against which the ventricles must pump to eject blood

____ 2. Occlusion of this vessel has been referred to as the "widow maker" because of its association with sudden death

____ 3. A repetitive pumping process that includes all of the events associated with the flow of blood through the heart

____ 4. Blood flows from the right atrium through the ___ valve into the right ventricle

____ 5. The amount of blood pumped into the aorta each minute by the heart

____ 6. A double-walled sac that encloses the heart and helps protect it from trauma and infection

____ 7. A positive ___ effect results in an increase in myocardial contractility

____ 8. Blood flows from the left atrium through the ___ valve into the left ventricle

____ 9. Specialized nerve tissue located in the internal carotid arteries and the aortic arch that detects changes in blood pressure

____ 10. The largest vein that drains the heart

____ 11. Coronary artery that supplies the SA node and AV node in most of the population

____ 12. This results when the heart's demand for oxygen exceeds its supply from the coronary circulation

____ 13. A negative ___ effect refers to a decrease in heart rate

____ 14. Sensors in the internal carotid arteries and aortic arch that detect changes in the concentration of hydrogen ions (pH), oxygen, and carbon dioxide in the blood

____ 15. The amount of blood flowing into the right atrium each minute from the systemic circulation

A. Cardiac output
B. Chemoreceptors
C. Venous return
D. Coronary sinus
E. Right coronary artery
F. Mitral (bicuspid)
G. Pericardium
H. Chronotropic
I. Myocardial ischemia
J. Tricuspid
K. Left main coronary artery
L. Cardiac cycle
M. Afterload
N. Baroreceptors
O. Inotropic

CHAPTER 2

Basic Electrophysiology

OBJECTIVES

On completion of this chapter, you will be able to:

1. Identify the two basic types of cardiac cells in the heart, where they are found, and the function of each.
2. List the most important ions involved in the cardiac action potential and their primary function in this process.
3. Define the terms *membrane potential, threshold potential,* and *action potential.*
4. Explain the significance of cardiac tissue with a fast-response action potential vs. a slow-response action potential.
5. Define the terms *polarization, depolarization,* and *repolarization.*
6. Explain the cardiac action potential and correlate it with the waveforms produced on the ECG.
7. Define the absolute, relative refractory, and supernormal periods and their location in the cardiac cycle.
8. Describe the primary characteristics of cardiac cells.
9. Describe the normal sequence of electrical conduction through the heart.
10. Explain why the sinoatrial (SA) node is the dominant pacemaker in the normal heart.
11. Describe the location and function of the following structures: SA node, atrioventricular (AV) junction, bundle branches, and Purkinje fibers.
12. State the intrinsic rates of the SA node, AV junction, and Purkinje fibers.
13. Explain the primary mechanisms responsible for producing cardiac dysrhythmias.
14. Explain the terms *escape beat* and *escape rhythm.*
15. Explain the purpose and limitations of ECG monitoring.
16. List the leads that view the heart in the frontal plane and the horizontal plane.
17. Define the terms *augmented, bipolar, chest, limb, precordial, unipolar,* and *V leads.*
18. Describe the significance of Einthoven's triangle.
19. Describe correct electrode positioning and the area of the heart viewed by each lead of a standard 12-lead ECG.
20. Describe correct electrode positioning and the area of the heart viewed by leads MCL_1 and MCL_6.

21. Identify the numeric values assigned to the small and large boxes on ECG paper.
22. Define and describe the significance of each of the following as they relate to cardiac electrical activity: P wave, PR segment, PR interval, QRS complex, ST segment, T wave, QT interval, U wave.
23. Define the term *artifact* and explain methods that may be used to minimize its occurrence.
24. Describe four methods for calculating heart rate on an ECG rhythm strip.
25. Describe the steps in ECG rhythm strip analysis.

TYPES OF CARDIAC CELLS

Cardiac muscle cells (Table 2-1) have been studied and identified based on their anatomic characteristics. In general, cardiac cells have either a mechanical (contractile) or an electrical (pacemaker) function.

Myocardial cells (working or mechanical cells) contain contractile filaments. When these cells are electrically stimulated, these filaments slide together and the myocardial cell contracts. These myocardial cells form the muscular layer of the atrial walls and the thicker muscular layer of the ventricular walls (the myocardium). These cells do not normally spontaneously generate electrical impulses, depending on pacemaker cells for this function.

> **Myocardial cells:** Working cells of the myocardium that contain contractile filaments and form the muscular layer of the atrial walls and the thicker muscular layer of the ventricular walls

Pacemaker cells are specialized cells of the electrical conduction system responsible for the spontaneous generation and conduction of electrical impulses. Pacemaker cells are found in nodes, bundles, bundle branches, and branching networks (fascicles) in the heart.

> **Pacemaker cells:** Specialized cells of the heart's electrical conduction system capable of spontaneously generating and conducting electrical impulses

CARDIAC ACTION POTENTIAL

All living cells maintain a difference in the concentrations of ions across their cell membranes. Electrical impulses are the result of brief but rapid flow of ions (charged particles) back and forth across the cell membrane. The exchange of electrolytes in myocardial cells creates electrical activity, which appears on the ECG as waveforms. The major electrolytes that affect cardiac function are sodium (Na^+), potassium (K^+), and calcium (Ca^{++}).

> For electrical current to be generated, a difference between electrical charges must exist.

Differences in concentrations of these ions across the cell (ionic gradient) determine the cell's electrical charge. Normally, there is a slight excess of positive ions on the outside of the membrane and a slight excess of negative ions on the inside of the membrane. This results in a difference in electrical charge across the membrane called the **membrane potential. Threshold** is the membrane potential at which the cell

> **Membrane potential:** Difference in electrical charge across the cell membrane.

> **Threshold:** Membrane potential at which cell membrane will depolarize and generate an action potential.

TABLE 2-1 CARDIAC CELL TYPES			
Kinds of cardiac cells	Where found	Primary function	Primary property
Myocardial cells	Myocardium	Contraction and relaxation	Contractility
Pacemaker cells	Electrical conduction system	Generation and conduction of electrical impulses	Automaticity Conductivity

Modified from Huszar RJ: *Basic dysrhythmias: interpretation and management,* ed 2, St Louis, 1994, Mosby.

membrane will depolarize and generate an action potential. The **action potential** is a five-phase cycle that reflects the difference in the concentration of these ions across the cell membrane at any given time.

Cell membranes contain membrane channels. These channels are pores through which specific ions or other small, water-soluble molecules can cross the cell membrane from outside to inside (Figure 2-1). Permeability refers to the ability of a membrane channel to conduct ions once it is open.

A series of events causes the electrical charge inside the cell to change from its resting state (negative) to its depolarized (stimulated) state (positive) and back to its resting state (negative). The cardiac action potential is an illustration of these events in a single cardiac cell during polarization, depolarization, and repolarization. The stimulus that alters the gradient across the cell membrane may be electrical, mechanical, or chemical.

Types of Action Potentials

There are two types of action potentials in the heart: fast and slow. This classification is based on the rate of voltage change during depolarization of cardiac cells.

Fast-Response Action Potentials
Fast-response action potentials occur in the cells of the atria, ventricles, and Purkinje fibers. The fast-response action potential occurs because of the presence of many voltage-sensitive Na^+ channels that allow a rapid influx of Na^+ when these channels are open and prevent influx when they are closed. Myocardial fibers with a fast-response action potential can conduct impulses at relatively rapid rates.

Slow-Response Action Potentials
The SA and AV nodes do not possess fast Na^+ channels but have slow Ca^{++} and slow Na^+ channels. Slow-response action potentials normally occur in the SA and AV nodes but can occur abnormally anywhere in the heart, usually secondary to ischemia, injury, or an electrolyte imbalance.[1] The speed (velocity) of conduction is slower, and conduction is more likely to be blocked in cardiac tissues that have slow-response action potentials.

FIGURE 2-1 Cell membranes contain membrane channels. These channels are pores through which specific ions or other small, water-soluble molecules can cross the cell membrane from outside to inside.

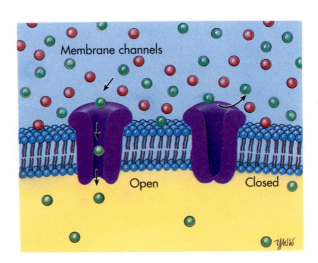

POLARIZATION, DEPOLARIZATION, AND REPOLARIZATION

Polarization

Polarization (also called the *resting membrane potential*) is the resting state during which no electrical activity occurs in the heart. When a cardiac muscle cell is polarized, the inside of the cell is more negative than the outside as a result of the numbers and types of ions found inside the cell. The primary intracellular ions include K^+ and several negatively charged ions (anions). During the resting state, K^+ ions leak out of the cell, leaving the negatively charged ions inside the cell. The result is a negative charge inside the cell (Figure 2-2).

Before the heart can mechanically contract and pump blood, cardiac muscle cell depolarization must take place. The terms *depolarization* and *repolarization* are used to describe

Polarized state: Period following repolarization of a myocardial cell (also called the *resting state*) when the outside of the cell is positive and the interior of the cell is negative.

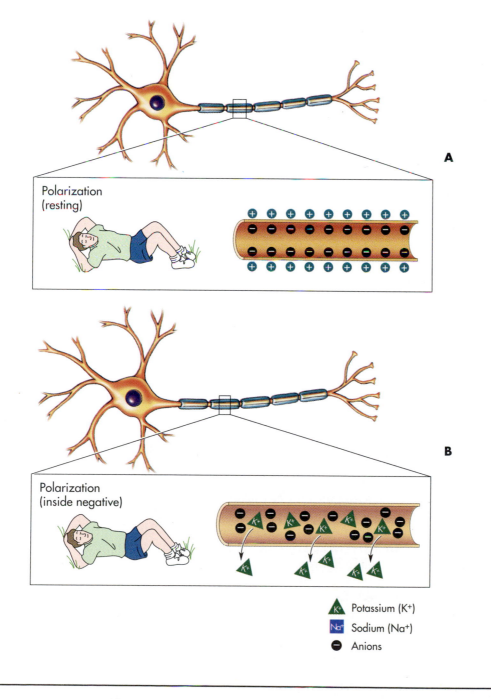

Polarization
(resting)

Polarization
(inside negative)

A

B

K⁺ Potassium (K^+)

Na⁺ Sodium (Na^+)

⊖ Anions

FIGURE **2-2**
Polarization.
A, Resting. **B,** Inside negative.

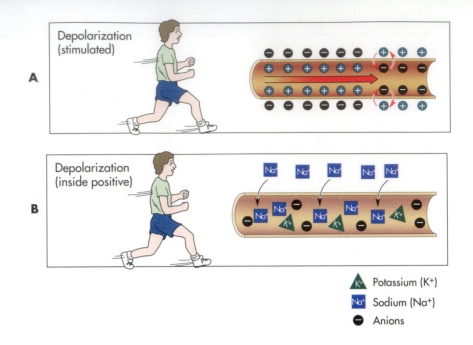

FIGURE **2-3**
Depolarization.
A, Stimulated.
B, Inside positive.

Potassium (K⁺)

Sodium (Na⁺)

Anions

the changes that occur in the heart when an impulse forms and spreads throughout the myocardium. Waveforms on the ECG correlate with depolarization and repolarization.

Depolarization

Depolarization: Movement of ions across a cell membrane causing the inside of the cell to become more positive.

When the cardiac muscle cell is stimulated, the cell is said to **depolarize** (Figure 2-3). The inside of the cell becomes more positive because of the entry of Na^+ ions into the cell through Na^+ membrane channels. Thus depolarization occurs because of the inward diffusion of Na^+.

Depolarization proceeds from the innermost layer of the heart (endocardium) to the outermost layer (epicardium). On the ECG, the P wave represents atrial depolarization and the QRS complex represents ventricular depolarization.

Depolarization is **not** the same as contraction. Depolarization is an electrical event expected to result in contraction (a mechanical event). It is possible to view electrical activity on the cardiac monitor, yet evaluation of the patient reveals no palpable pulse. This clinical situation is termed *pulseless electrical activity (PEA)*.

Repolarization

Repolarization: Movement of ions across a cell membrane causing the inside of the cell to be restored to its negative charge.

After the cell depolarizes, the diffusion of Na^+ into the cell stops. K^+ is allowed to diffuse out of the cell, leaving the anions (negatively charged ions) inside the cell. Thus **repolarization** occurs because of the outward diffusion of K^+. The membrane potential of the cell returns to its negative resting level (Figure 2-4). This causes the contractile proteins to separate (relax). The cell can then be stimulated again if another electrical impulse arrives at the cell membrane.

A cell cannot conduct another impulse until repolarization occurs.

Repolarization proceeds from the epicardium to the endocardium. On the ECG, the ST segment represents early ventricular repolarization, and the T wave represents ventricular repolarization.

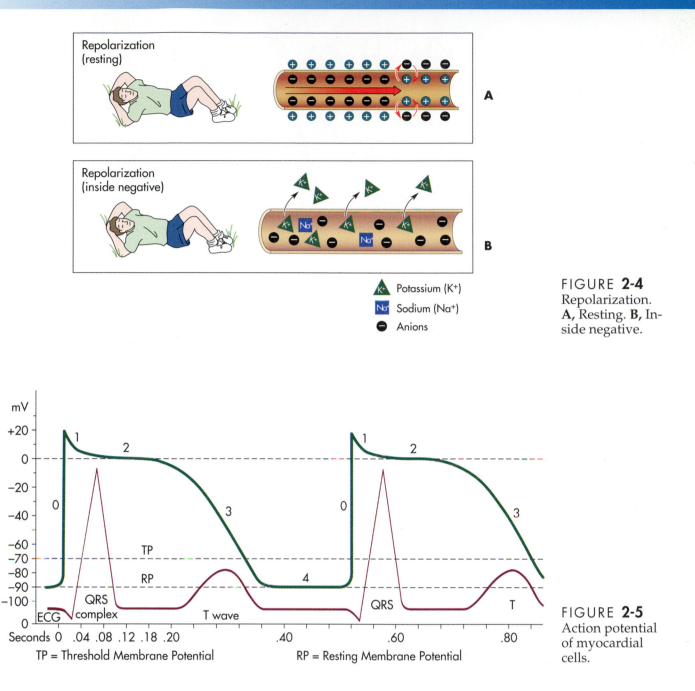

FIGURE **2-4**
Repolarization.
A, Resting. **B,** Inside negative.

K+ Potassium (K⁺)

Na⁺ Sodium (Na⁺)

⊖ Anions

FIGURE **2-5**
Action potential of myocardial cells.

Phases of the Cardiac Action Potential

The action potential of a cardiac cell consists of five phases labeled 0 to 4. These phases reflect the rapid sequence of voltage changes that occur across the cell membrane during the electrical cardiac cycle (Figure 2-5). Phases 1, 2, and 3 have been referred to as *electrical systole,* and phase 4 has been referred to as *electrical diastole.*

Phase 0 of the cardiac action potential (Figure 2-6) represents depolarization and is called the *rapid depolarization phase* (also known as the *upstroke, spike,* or *overshoot*). Phase 0 begins when the cell receives an impulse. Na^+ moves rapidly into the cell through the fast Na^+ channels, K^+ leaves the cell, and Ca^{++} moves slowly into the cell through slow Ca^{++} channels. The cell depolarizes and cardiac contraction begins.

Class I antidysrhythmic medications inhibit the fast Na^+ channels during depolarization. Phase 0 = depolarization.

FIGURE **2-6**
Phase 0 of cardiac action potential represents depolarization. Na+ moves rapidly into the cell through the fast Na+ channels, K+ leaves the cell, and Ca++ moves slowly into the cell through slow Ca++ channels.

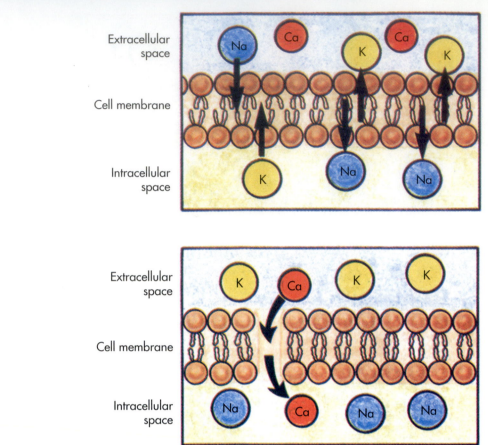

FIGURE **2-7**
Phase 2 (plateau phase) of the cardiac action potential is caused by slow inward movement of Ca++ and slow outward movement of K+ from the cell.

On the ECG the rapid depolarization phase of the cardiac action potential is represented by the QRS complex. Phase 0 (depolarization) is immediately followed by repolarization, which is divided into three phases.

Phase 1—Early Repolarization
Phase 1 of the cardiac action potential is an early, brief period of limited repolarization. During this period the fast Na^+ channels partially close, slowing the flow of Na^+ into the cell. At the same time, there is a transient outward movement of K^+ from the cell through K^+ channels. The result is a decrease in the number of positive electrical charges within the cell, producing a small negative deflection in the action potential (see Figure 2-5).

Phase 2—Repolarization (Plateau Phase)
Ca^{++} plays an important role in the process of contraction.

Phase 2 is the plateau phase of the action potential (Figure 2-7). The plateau occurs because of the slow, inward movement of Ca^{++} through slow Ca^{++} channels and the continued outward movement of K^+ through K^+ channels. The plateau phase allows cardiac muscle to sustain an increased period of contraction.

Phase 2 is responsible for the ST segment on the ECG and is part of the absolute refractory period. The ST segment reflects the early part of repolarization of the right and left ventricles.

Phase 3—Rapid Repolarization
Repolarization is complete by the end of phase 3.

Phase 3 begins with the downslope of the action potential and is the phase of late and rapid repolarization (see Figure 2-5). The cell rapidly completes repolarization as K^+ flows quickly out of the cell and the slow channels close, stopping the influx of Ca^{++}

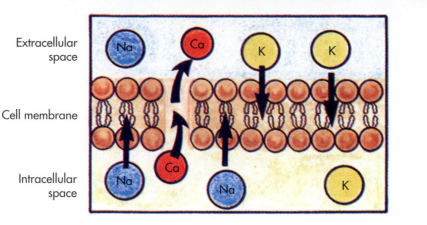

FIGURE **2-8**
Phase 4, there is an excess of Na+ inside the cell and an excess of K+ outside the cell. The Na+- K+ pump is activated to actively transport Na+ out of the cell and move K+ back into the cell.

and Na$^+$. The rapid efflux of K$^+$ from the cell causes it to become progressively more electrically negative. The cell gradually becomes more sensitive to external stimuli until its original sensitivity is restored (relative refractory period). Phase 3 of the action potential corresponds with the T wave (ventricular repolarization) on the ECG.

Phase 4—Resting Membrane Potential

Phase 4 is the resting membrane potential (return to resting state) (Figure 2-8). During phase 4 there is an excess of Na$^+$ inside the cell and an excess of K$^+$ outside the cell. The Na$^+$-K$^+$ pump is activated to actively transport Na$^+$ out of the cell and move K$^+$ back into the cell. The heart is "polarized" during this phase (ready for discharge). The cell will remain in this state until the cell membrane is reactivated by another stimulus.

Phase 4 of the cardiac action potential represents the fully polarized state of the resting cardiac cell.

REFRACTORY PERIODS

Refractoriness is a term used to describe the extent to which a cell is able to respond to a stimulus. In the heart the refractory period is longer than the contraction itself.

Refractoriness: Extent to which a cell is able to respond to a stimulus.

Absolute Refractory Period

The **absolute refractory period** (also known as the *effective refractory period*) corresponds with the onset of the QRS complex to the peak of the T wave and includes phases 0, 1, 2, and part of phase 3 of the cardiac action potential (Figure 2-9).

During this period the myocardial cell will not respond to further stimulation (the myocardial working cells cannot contract and the cells of the electrical conduction system cannot conduct an electrical impulse)—no matter how strong the stimulus. Because of this mechanism, tetanic (sustained) contractions cannot be induced in cardiac muscle.

Absolute refractory period: Corresponds with the onset of the QRS complex to approximately the peak of the T wave; during this period, cardiac cells cannot be stimulated to conduct an electrical impulse, no matter how strong the stimulus.

Relative Refractory Period

The **relative refractory period** (also known as the *vulnerable period*) corresponds with the downslope of the T wave. During this period, some cardiac cells have repolarized to their threshold potential and can be stimulated to respond (depolarize) to a stronger than normal stimulus (Figure 2-10).

Relative refractory period: Corresponds with downslope of T wave; cardiac cells can be stimulated to depolarize if stimulus is strong enough.

Supernormal Period

After the relative refractory period is a **supernormal period** during which a weaker than normal stimulus can cause depolarization of cardiac cells. This period extends from the

Supernormal period: Corresponds with end of T wave; cardiac cells can be depolarized by a weaker than normal stimulus.

FIGURE 2-9
Absolute and relative refractory periods correlated with the action potential of a cardiac muscle cell and an ECG tracing.

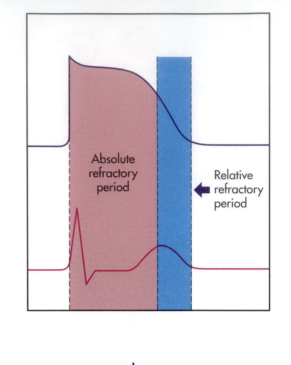

FIGURE 2-10
1, Absolute refractory period.
2, Relative refractory period.
3, Supernormal period.

🫀 The terms *arrhythmia* and *dysrhythmia* are used interchangeably by healthcare professionals to refer to an abnormal heart rhythm.

terminal portion of phase 3 of the action potential to the beginning of phase 4. On the ECG this corresponds with the end of the T wave. It is possible for cardiac dysrhythmias to develop during this period (see Figure 2-10).

PROPERTIES OF CARDIAC CELLS

Cardiac cells have four primary characteristics.

Automaticity: Ability of cardiac pacemaker cells to spontaneously initiate an electrical impulse without being stimulated from another source (such as a nerve).

Automaticity is the ability of cardiac pacemaker cells to spontaneously initiate an electrical impulse without being stimulated from another source (such as a nerve). The SA node, AV junction, and Purkinje fibers normally possess this characteristic. Normal concentrations of K^+, Na^+, and Ca^{++} are important in maintaining automaticity. Increased serum concentrations of these electrolytes decrease automaticity. Decreased serum concentrations of K^+ and Ca^{++} increase automaticity.

Excitability: Ability of cardiac muscle cells to respond to an outside stimulus.

Cardiac muscle is electrically irritable because of an ionic imbalance across the membranes of cells. **Excitability** (or **irritability**) is a characteristic shared by all cardiac cells and refers to the ability of cardiac muscle cells to respond to an external stimulus, such as that from a chemical, mechanical, or electrical source.

Conductivity: Ability of a cardiac cell to receive an electrical stimulus and conduct that impulse to an adjacent cardiac cell.

Conductivity refers to the ability of a cardiac cell to receive an electrical stimulus and conduct that impulse to an adjacent cardiac cell. All cardiac cells possess this characteristic. The intercalated disks present in the membranes of cardiac cells are responsible for the property of conductivity and allow an impulse in any part of the myocardium to spread throughout the heart. The speed of conduction can be altered by factors such as sympathetic and parasympathetic stimulation and medications.

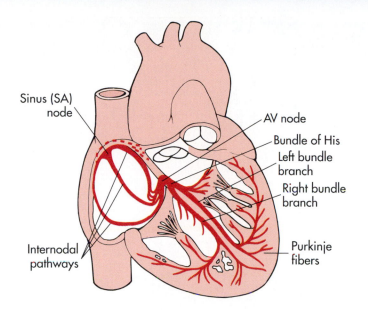

FIGURE **2-11**
Conduction
system.

Contractility refers to the ability of cardiac cells to shorten, causing cardiac muscle contraction in response to an electrical stimulus. Contractility can be enhanced with certain medications, such as digitalis, dopamine, and epinephrine.

Contractility: Ability of cardiac cells to shorten, causing cardiac muscle contraction in response to an electrical stimulus.

CONDUCTION SYSTEM

The specialized electrical (pacemaker) cells in the heart are arranged in a system of pathways called the *conduction system.* In the normal heart the cells of the conduction system are interconnected. The conduction system ensures that the chambers of the heart contract in a coordinated fashion. Normally, the pacemaker site with the fastest firing rate controls the heart.

Pacemaker cells may also be referred to as *conducting cells.*

Sinoatrial Node

The normal heartbeat is the result of an electrical impulse that originates in the sinoatrial (sinus or SA) node. The SA node is about 8-mm long and 2-mm thick and is located in the upper posterior portion of the right atrium at the junction of the superior vena cava and the right atrium (Figure 2-11).

The SA node contains two primary types of cells: (1) small round cells that have few myofibrils and organelles and (2) slender, elongated cells that are intermediate in appearance between the round and the ordinary atrial myocardial cells.[2] It is thought that the round cells are the pacemaker cells, and the transitional cells conduct impulses within the node and to its margins.

Normally, the cells of the SA node spontaneously reach threshold and depolarize more rapidly than other cardiac cells, dominating other areas that may be depolarizing at a slightly slower rate (overdrive suppression). Thus the SA node is normally the primary pacemaker of the heart. The SA node initiates electrical impulses at a rhythmic rate of 60 to 100 beats/min.

The SA node receives its blood supply from the SA node artery that runs lengthwise through the center of the node. The SA node artery originates from the right coronary artery in most individuals.

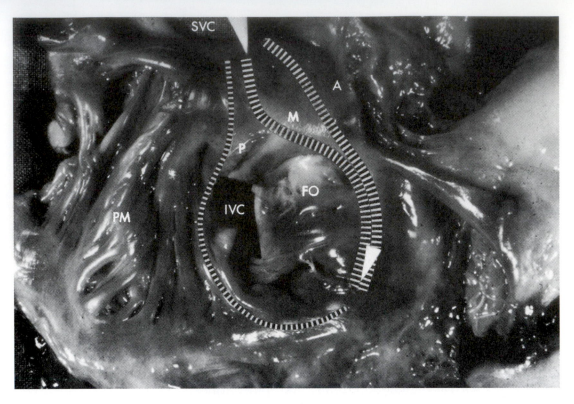

FIGURE 2-12
Right atrium has been opened. The *large white arrow* indicates the location of the SA node. The *small white arrow* shows the location of the AV node. *PM,* papillary muscle; *SVC,* superior vena cava; *IVC,* inferior vena cava; *FO,* fossa ovalis; *A,* anterior internodal pathway; *M,* middle internodal pathway; *P,* posterior internodal pathway.

Intrinsic rate: Rate at which a pacemaker of the heart normally generates impulses.

Other areas of the heart can take over control by discharging impulses more rapidly than the SA node or by passively taking over, either because the SA node has failed or because it is generating impulses too slowly. Pacemaker cells have an **intrinsic rate** that becomes slower and slower from the SA node down to the end of the His-Purkinje system.

The fibers of the SA node connect directly with the fibers of the atria. As the impulse leaves the SA node, it is spread from cell to cell in wavelike form across the atrial muscle, depolarizing the right atrium, the interatrial septum, and then the left atrium, resulting in almost simultaneous contraction of the right and left atria. Because a fibrous skeleton separates the atrial myocardium from the ventricular myocardium, the electrical stimulus affects only the atria.

The anterior internodal pathway (tract) is called *Bachmann's bundle,* the middle *Wenckebach's bundle,* and the posterior *Thorel's pathway.* Bachmann's bundle conducts impulses to the left atrium.[3,4]

It normally takes about 50 ms for an impulse to travel from the SA node, through the atrial muscle, and down to the AV node. Conduction through the AV node begins before atrial depolarization is completed. The impulse is spread to the AV node by means of three internodal pathways that have been identified as the anterior, middle, and posterior internodal pathways (Figure 2-12). These pathways consist of a mixture of ordinary myocardial cells and specialized conducting fibers.

Atrioventricular Junction

AV junction: AV node and the bundle of His.

The internodal pathways merge gradually with the cells of the AV node. Depolarization and repolarization are slow in the AV node, making this area vulnerable to blocks in conduction (AV blocks). The **AV junction** is the AV node and the nonbranching portion of the bundle of His (Figure 2-13). This area consists of specialized conduction tissue that provides the electrical links between the atrium and ventricle.[3] When the AV junction is bypassed by an abnormal pathway, the abnormal route is called an **accessory pathway.**

Accessory pathway: An extra muscle bundle consisting of working myocardial tissue that forms a connection between the atria and ventricles outside the normal conduction system.

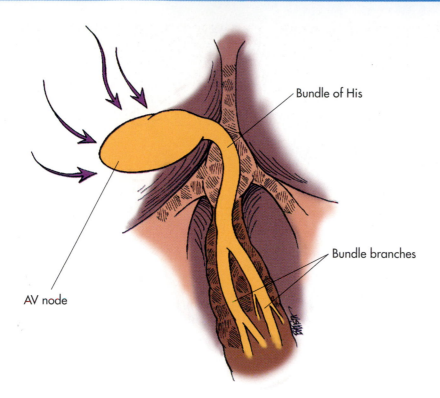

Bundle of His

Bundle branches

AV node

FIGURE **2-13**
AV junction con-
sists of the AV
node and the non-
branching portion
of the bundle of
His.

AV Node

The **AV node** is a group of cells located in the posterior septal wall of the right atrium immediately behind the tricuspid valve and near the opening of the coronary sinus. In the adult, the AV node is approximately 22 mm long, 10 mm wide, and 3 mm thick. In most individuals the AV node is supplied by the right coronary artery. In the remainder, the left circumflex artery provides the blood supply.

As the impulse from the atria enters the AV node, there is a delay in conduction of the impulse to the ventricles. This delay occurs in part because the fibers in the AV junction are smaller than those of atrial muscle and have few gap junctions. The delay in conduction allows time for the atria to empty their contents into the ventricles before the next ventricular contraction begins.

The AV node has been divided into three functional regions according to their action potentials and responses to electrical and chemical stimulation: (1) the atrionodal (AN) or upper junctional region (also called the *transitional zone*); (2) the nodal (N) region, the midportion of the AV node; and (3) the nodal-His (NH) or lower junctional region where the fibers of the AV node merge gradually with the bundle of His (Figure 2-14).

The upper and lower junctional areas possess cells that demonstrate automaticity and depolarize rapidly. Cells in the middle area lack automaticity, depolarize slowly, conduct slowly, and are difficult to stimulate electrically.[5] The primary delay in the passage of the electrical impulse from the atria to the ventricles occurs in the AN and N areas of the AV node (Figure 2-15).

Bundle of His

After passing through the AV node, the electrical impulse enters the **bundle of His** (also referred to as the *common bundle* or the *atrioventricular bundle*). The bundle of His is nor-

AV node: Specialized cells located in the lower portion of the right atrium; delays the electrical impulse to allow the atria to contract and complete filling of the ventricles.

When atrial rates are very fast (e.g., atrial fibrillation), the AV node helps regulate the number of impulses reaching the ventricles to protect them from dangerously fast rates.

Bundle of His: Cardiac muscle fibers located in the upper portion of the interventricular septum; connects the AV node with the two bundle branches.

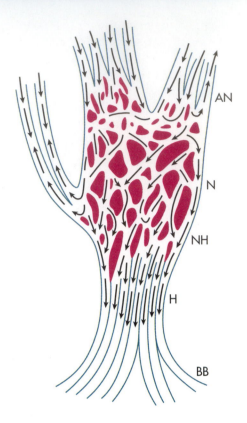

FIGURE 2-14
AV junction. *AN*, atrionodal; *N*, nodal; *NH*, nodal-His; *H*, bundle of His; *BB*, bundle branches.

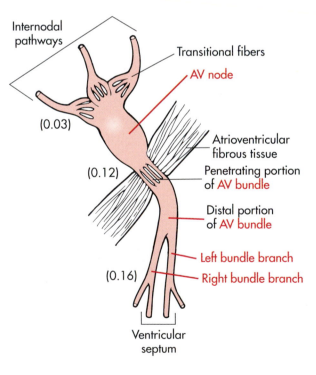

FIGURE 2-15
AV node, bundle of His (AV bundle), and bundle branches. The numbers represent the time from the origin of an impulse in the SA node.

Internodal pathways

Transitional fibers

AV node

(0.03)

Atrioventricular fibrous tissue

Penetrating portion of AV bundle

(0.12)

Distal portion of AV bundle

Left bundle branch

Right bundle branch

(0.16)

Ventricular septum

mally the only electrical connection between the atria and the ventricles. It is located in the upper portion of the interventricular septum and connects the AV node with the two bundle branches. The term **His-Purkinje system** or *His-Purkinje network* refers to the bundle of His, bundle branches, and Purkinje fibers.

The bundle of His receives a dual blood supply from branches of the left anterior and posterior descending coronary arteries, making this portion of the conduction system less vulnerable to ischemic damage.[1] The posterior descending artery is the right coronary artery in 90% of individuals.[6]

The bundle of His has pacemaker cells capable of discharging at a rate of 40 to 60 beats/min. The bundle of His conducts the electrical impulse to the right and left bundle branches.

Right and Left Bundle Branches

The right bundle branch innervates the right ventricle. The left bundle branch spreads the electrical impulse to the interventricular septum and left ventricle, which is thicker and more muscular than the right ventricle. The left bundle branch divides into three divisions (fascicles) called the *anterior fascicle, posterior fascicle,* and the *septal fascicle.*[1] The anterior fascicle spreads the electrical impulse to the anterior (superior) portions of the left ventricle. The posterior fascicle relays the impulse to the posterior (inferior) portions of the left ventricle, and the septal fascicle relays the impulse to the midseptum (Figure 2-16).

His-Purkinje system: Bundle of His, bundle branches, and Purkinje fibers.

Fascicle: Small bundle of nerve fibers.

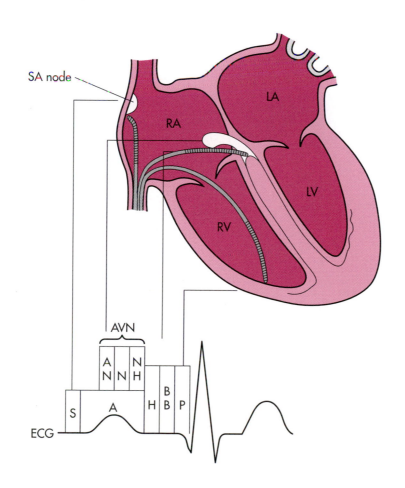

FIGURE **2-16** Sequence of activation through the conduction system. *S,* SA node conduction; *A,* atrial conduction; *AN,* atrionodal conduction; *N,* nodal conduction; *NH,* nodal–His conduction; *AVN,* AV nodal conduction; *H,* His bundle conduction; *BB,* bundle branch conduction; *P,* Purkinje fiber conduction; *RA,* right atrium; *LA,* left atrium, *RV,* right ventricle; *LV,* left ventricle.

Purkinje Fibers

The right and left bundle branches divide into smaller and smaller branches and then into a special network of fibers called the **Purkinje fibers.** These fibers spread from the interventricular septum into the papillary muscles and then continue downward to the apex of the heart, making up an elaborate web that penetrates about one third of the way into the ventricular muscle mass. The fibers then become continuous with the muscle cells of the right and left ventricles.

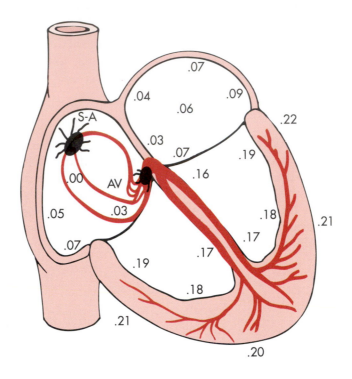

FIGURE 2-17 Transmission of the cardiac impulse through the heart, showing the time of appearance (in fractions of a second) of the impulse in different parts of the heart.

TABLE 2-2 SUMMARY OF THE CONDUCTION SYSTEM		
Structure	**Location**	**Function**
Sinoatrial node	Right atrial wall just inferior to opening of superior vena cava	Primary pacemaker; initiates impulse that is normally conducted throughout the left and right atria; intrinsic rate of 60 to 100 beats/min
Atrioventricular node	Posterior septal wall of the right atrium immediately behind the tricuspid valve and near the opening of the coronary sinus	Receives impulse from SA node and delays relay of the impulse to the bundle of His, allowing time for the atria to empty their contents into the ventricles before the onset of ventricular contraction
Bundle of His	Superior portion of interventricular septum	Receives impulse from AV node and relays it to right and left bundle branches; intrinsic pacemaker ability of 40 to 60 beats/min
Right and left bundle branches	Interventricular septum	Receives impulse from bundle of His and relays it to Purkinje fibers in ventricular myocardium
Purkinje fibers	Ventricular myocardium	Receives impulse from bundle branches and relays it to ventricular myocardium; intrinsic pacemaker ability of 20 to 40 beats/min

Conduction through the His-Purkinje system precedes ventricular contraction. The electrical impulse spreads rapidly through the right and left bundle branches and the Purkinje fibers to reach the ventricular muscle. The Purkinje fibers are very large and transmit impulses at a speed about 6 times faster than that in the usual cardiac muscle and 150 times faster than that in some portions of the AV fibers.[7]

The electrical impulse spreads from the endocardium to the myocardium, finally reaching the epicardial surface. The ventricular walls are stimulated to contract in a twisting motion that wrings blood out of the ventricular chambers and forces it into arteries. The Purkinje fibers have an intrinsic pacemaker ability of 20 to 40 beats/min (Figure 2-17).

A summary of the conduction system can be found in Table 2-2.

CAUSES OF DYSRHYTHMIAS

Enhanced Automaticity

Enhanced automaticity is an abnormal condition in which cardiac cells not normally associated with the property of automaticity begin to depolarize spontaneously or when escape pacemaker sites increase their firing rate beyond that which is considered normal. Enhanced automaticity may occur as the result of catecholamine administration (epinephrine), administration of atropine sulfate, digitalis toxicity, acidosis, alkalosis, hypoxia, myocardial ischemia or infarction, hypokalemia, or hypocalcemia.

Examples of rhythms associated with enhanced automaticity include atrial flutter; atrial fibrillation; supraventricular tachycardia; premature atrial, junctional, or ventricular complexes; ventricular tachycardia or ventricular fibrillation; junctional tachycardia; accelerated idioventricular rhythm, and accelerated junctional rhythm.

Reentry

Reentry is the propagation of an impulse through tissue already activated by that same impulse.[1] An electrical impulse is delayed or blocked (or both) in one or more divisions of the electrical conduction system while the impulse is conducted normally through the rest of the conduction system. This results in the delayed electrical impulse entering cardiac cells that have just been depolarized by the normally conducted impulse (Figure 2-18).

If the area the delayed impulse stimulates is relatively refractory, the impulse can cause depolarization of those cells, producing a single premature beat or repetitive electrical impulses, resulting in short periods of tachydysrhythmias. Common causes of reentry

Reentry: Propagation of an impulse through tissue already activated by that same impulse.

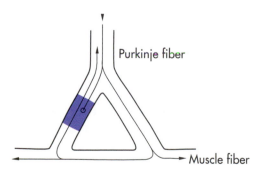

FIGURE **2-18**
Reentry.

produced by slowing or blocking conduction of electrical impulses include hyperkalemia, myocardial ischemia, and some antidysrhythmic drugs.

Examples of rhythms associated with reentry are paroxysmal supraventricular tachycardia (PSVT); ventricular tachycardia; and premature atrial, junctional, or ventricular complexes.

Escape Beats or Rhythms

Escape: Term used when the sinus node slows down or fails to initiate depolarization and a lower pacemaker site spontaneously produces electrical impulses, assuming responsibility for pacing the heart.

Escape is the term used when the SA node slows down or fails to initiate depolarization, and a lower site spontaneously produces electrical impulses, assuming responsibility for pacing the heart. Escape beats or rhythms are *protective* mechanisms to maintain cardiac output and originate in the AV junction or the ventricles.

Examples of escape beats or rhythms include junctional escape beats, junctional rhythm, idioventricular rhythm (also known as a *ventricular escape rhythm*), and ventricular escape beats.

Conduction Disturbances

Conduction disturbances may occur because of trauma, drug toxicity, electrolyte disturbances, myocardial ischemia, or infarction. Conduction may be too rapid or too slow. Examples of rhythms associated with disturbances in conductivity include AV blocks.

ELECTROCARDIOGRAM

The first ECG was introduced by Willem Einthoven, a Dutch physiologist, in the early 1900s.

The electrocardiogram (ECG) records the electrical activity of a large mass of atrial and ventricular cells as specific waveforms and complexes. Think of the ECG as a voltmeter that records the electrical voltages (potentials) generated by depolarization of heart muscle. The electrical activity within the heart can be observed by means of electrodes connected by cables to an ECG machine.

ECG monitoring may be used to monitor a patient's heart rate; evaluate the effects of disease or injury on heart function; evaluate pacemaker function; evaluate the response to medications (e.g., antidysrhythmics); and/or obtain a baseline recording before, during, and after a medical procedure.

The ECG *can* provide information about the orientation of the heart in the chest, conduction disturbances, electrical effects of medications and electrolytes, the mass of cardiac muscle, and the presence of ischemic damage. The ECG does *not* provide information about the mechanical (contractile) condition of the myocardium. The effectiveness of the heart's mechanical activity is evaluated by assessment of the patient's pulse and blood pressure.

Electrodes

To minimize artifact (distortion), be sure the conductive jelly in the center of the electrode is not dry and avoid placing the electrodes directly over bony prominences.

Three types of electrodes used for surface (skin) electrocardiography are the metal disk, metal suction cup, and the disposable disk. Metal disk and suction cup electrodes are used for obtaining a 12-lead ECG. The disposable disk electrode consists of an adhesive ring with a conductive substance in the center. This type of electrode is commonly used for monitoring. The conductive media of the electrode conducts skin surface voltage changes through color-coded wires to a cardiac monitor.

Electrodes are applied at specific locations on the patient's chest wall and extremities in combinations of two, three, four, or five to view the heart's electrical activity from different angles and planes. One end of a monitoring cable is attached to the electrode and the other end to an ECG machine (Figure 2-19).

Do not rely on the color coding of ECG cables. Colors are not standard and often vary.

Leads

A **lead** is a record of electrical activity between two electrodes. Each lead records the *average* current flow at a specific time in a portion of the heart.

Leads allow viewing the heart's electrical activity in two different planes: frontal (coronal) and horizontal (transverse). Frontal plane leads view the heart from the front of the body. Directions in the frontal plane are superior, inferior, right, and left. Horizontal plane leads view the heart as if the body were sliced in half horizontally. Directions in the horizontal plane are anterior, posterior, right, and left. A 12-lead ECG provides views of the heart in both the frontal and horizontal planes and views the surfaces of the left ventricle from 12 different angles.

There are three types of leads: standard limb leads, augmented leads, and precordial (chest) leads. Each lead has a negative (−) and positive (+) electrode (pole). Moving the lead selector on the ECG machine allows any of the electrodes to be made positive or negative.

Think of the positive electrode as an eye. The position of the positive electrode on the body determines the portion of the heart "seen" by each lead. Each lead senses the magnitude and direction of the electrical forces caused by the spread of waves of depolarization and repolarization throughout the heart (Figure 2-20).

If the wave of depolarization (electrical impulse) moves toward the *positive* electrode, the waveform recorded on ECG graph paper will be upright (positive deflection). If the wave of depolarization moves toward the *negative* electrode, the waveform recorded will be inverted (downward or negative deflection). A *biphasic* (partly positive, partly

The term equiphasic may be used instead of biphasic to describe a waveform that has no net positive or negative deflection.

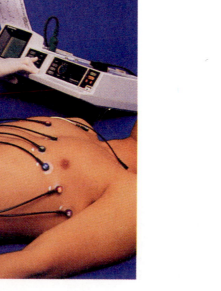

FIGURE **2-19**
Electrodes are applied at specific locations on the patient's chest wall and extremities to view the heart's electrical activity from different angles and planes.

FIGURE **2-20**
Each lead has a negative (−) and positive (+) electrode. The position of the positive electrode on the body determines the portion of the heart "seen" by each lead.

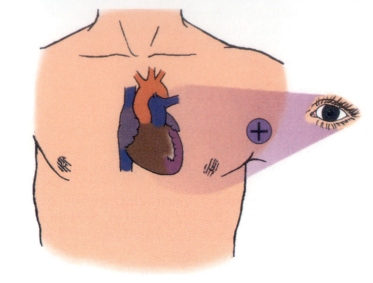

FIGURE **2-21**
A, If wave of depolarization moves toward positive electrode, waveform recorded on ECG graph paper will be upright. **B,** If wave of depolarization moves toward negative electrode, waveform produced will be inverted. **C,** Biphasic (partly positive, partly negative) waveform is recorded when wave of depolarization moves perpendicularly to positive electrode.

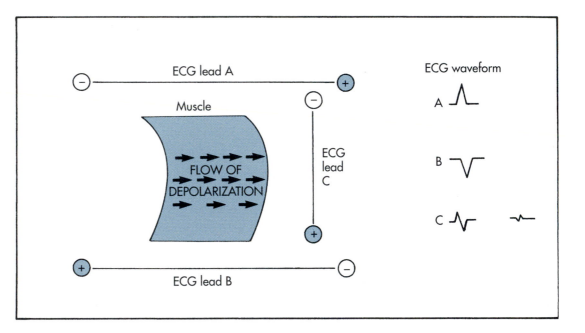

negative) waveform or a straight line is recorded when the wave of depolarization moves perpendicularly to the positive electrode (Figure 2-21).

Each waveform produced is related to a specific electrical event in the heart. When electrical activity is not detected, a straight line is recorded called the **baseline** or **isoelectric line.**

Baseline: Straight line recorded on ECG graph paper when no electrical activity is detected.

Frontal Plane Leads
Six leads view the heart in the frontal plane as if the body were flat: three bipolar leads and three unipolar leads. A **bipolar lead** consists of two electrodes of opposite polarity (positive and negative). Each lead records the difference in electrical potential between

Bipolar lead: ECG lead consisting of a positive and negative electrode.

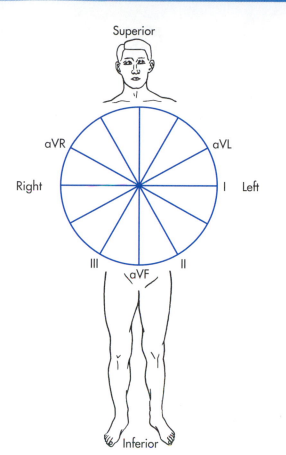

Superior

aVR   aVL

Right   I   Left

III   II
aVF

Inferior

FIGURE **2-22**
Frontal plane
leads.

two selected electrodes. Leads I, II, and III are called *standard limb leads* or *bipolar leads* (Figure 2-22).

A lead that consists of a single positive electrode and a reference point is called a **unipolar lead.** These leads are also called *unipolar limb leads* or *augmented limb leads*. The reference point (with zero electrical potential) lies in the center of the heart's electrical field (left of the interventricular septum and below the AV junction).

Unipolar lead: Lead that consists of a single positive electrode and a reference point.

Leads aVR, aVL, and aVF are augmented limb leads. The "a" in aVR, aVL, and aVF refers to *augmented*. The "V" refers to *voltage*. The "R" refers to *right arm*, the "L" to *left arm*, and the "F" to *left foot (leg)*. The electrical potential produced by the augmented leads is normally relatively small. The ECG machine augments (magnifies) the amplitude of the electrical potentials detected at each extremity by approximately 50% over those recorded at the bipolar leads. The augmented leads record the difference in electrical potential at one location relative to zero potential rather than relative to the electrical potential of another extremity, as in the bipolar leads.

Horizontal Plane Leads

Six precordial (chest or V) leads view the heart in the horizontal plane allowing a view of the front and left side of the heart. The precordial leads are identified as V_1, V_2, V_3, V_4, V_5, and V_6. Each electrode placed in a "V" position is a positive electrode. The negative electrode is a zero reference point (central terminal) that combines information from the limb leads. This negative electrode is found at the electrical center of the heart (Figure 2-23). Thus the precordial leads are also unipolar leads.

The precordial leads record differences in electrical potential via electrodes positioned on the chest wall.

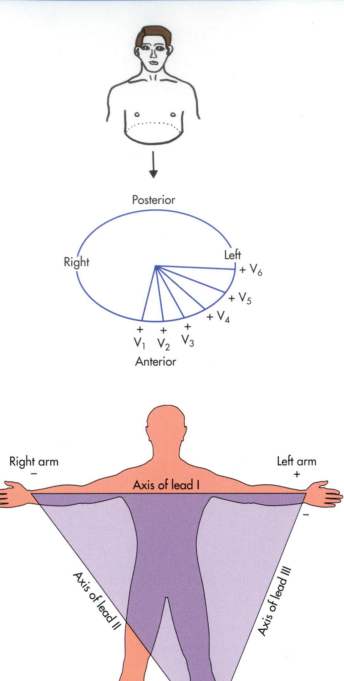

FIGURE **2-23**
Horizontal plane
leads.

FIGURE **2-24**
Einthoven's
triangle.

Standard Limb Leads

Leads I, II, and III make up the standard limb leads. If an electrode is placed on the right arm, left arm, and left leg, three leads are formed. An imaginary line joining the positive and negative electrodes of a lead is called the **axis** of the lead. The axes of these three limb leads form an equilateral triangle with the heart at the center (Einthoven's triangle) (Figure 2-24). Although placement of the left leg electrode may appear to make the trian-

Axis: Imaginary line joining the positive and negative electrodes of a lead.

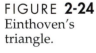

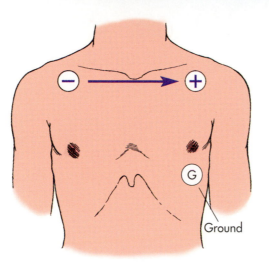

FIGURE **2-25**
Lead I.

gle out of balance, it is nevertheless an equilateral triangle because all electrodes are about equidistant from the electrical field of the heart.[6]

Einthoven's triangle is a means of illustrating that the two arms and the left leg form apices of a triangle surrounding the heart. The two apices at the upper part of the triangle represent the points at which the two arms connect electrically with the fluids around the heart. The lower apex is the point at which the left leg connects with the fluids.[7]

Einthoven expressed the relationship between leads I, II, and III as follows: the sum of any complex in leads I and III equals that of lead II. Thus leads I + III = II. Stated another way, the voltage of a waveform in lead I plus the voltage of the same waveform in lead III equals the voltage of the same waveform in lead II. For example, when viewing leads I, II, and III, if the R wave in lead II does not appear to be the sum of the voltage of the R waves in leads I and III, the leads may have been incorrectly applied.

Lead I + lead III = lead II.

In the bipolar leads, the right arm electrode is always the electrically negative pole and the left leg electrode is always the electrically positive pole. Over the years, electrode placement for leads I, II, and III has been altered and moved to the patient's chest to allow for patient movement and to minimize muscle artifact. However, proper electrode positioning for these leads includes placement on the patient's extremities. Where the electrodes are placed on the extremity does not matter as long as bony prominences are avoided.

Lead I
Lead I records the difference in electrical potential between the left arm (+) and right arm (−) electrodes. The positive electrode is placed just below the left clavicle (or on the left arm), and the negative electrode is placed just below the right clavicle (or on the right arm). The third electrode is a ground that minimizes electrical activity from other sources (Figure 2-25).

Lead I views the lateral surface of the left ventricle. The QRS in lead I is normally predominantly positive because the direction of depolarization is toward the positive electrode.

Lead II
Lead II records the difference in electrical potential between the left leg (+) and right arm (−) electrodes. The positive electrode is placed below the left pectoral muscle (or on

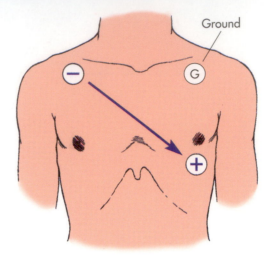

FIGURE **2-26**
Lead II.

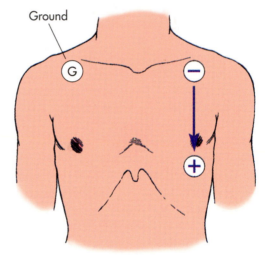

FIGURE **2-27**
Lead III.

the left leg), and the negative electrode is placed just below the right clavicle (or on the right arm) (Figure 2-26).

Lead II views the inferior surface of the left ventricle. The QRS in lead II is normally positive because the direction of depolarization is predominantly toward the positive electrode. This lead is commonly used for cardiac monitoring because positioning of the positive and negative electrodes in this lead most closely resembles the pathway of current flow in normal atrial and ventricular depolarization.

Lead III
Lead III records the difference in electrical potential between the left leg (+) and left arm (−) electrodes. In lead III the positive electrode is placed below the left pectoral muscle (or on the left leg), and the negative electrode is placed just below the left clavicle (or on the left arm) (Figure 2-27).

Lead III views the inferior surface of the left ventricle. P waves seen in this lead may normally be positive, negative, or biphasic and are usually of lower amplitude than in lead II (Figure 2-28). The QRS in lead III is normally predominantly positive although the R wave is not as tall as in lead II.

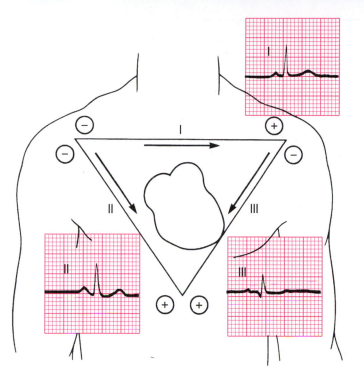

FIGURE **2-28**
Comparison of
the waveforms
recorded in the
standard limb
leads.

Modified Chest Leads

The modified chest leads (MCL) are bipolar precordial (chest) leads that are variations of the unipolar precordial leads. Each modified chest lead consists of a positive and negative electrode applied to a specific location on the thorax. Accurate placement of the positive electrode is important.

The modified chest leads are useful in detecting bundle branch blocks, differentiating right and left premature beats, and differentiating supraventricular tachycardia (SVT) from ventricular tachycardia (VT).

Lead MCL$_1$
Lead MCL$_1$ is a variation of the precordial lead V$_1$ and views the ventricular septum. The negative electrode is placed below the left clavicle toward the left shoulder, and the positive electrode is placed to the right of the sternum in the fourth intercostal space (Figure 2-29, *A*). In this lead the positive electrode is in a position to the right of the left ventricle. Because the primary wave of depolarization is directed toward the left ventricle, the QRS complex recorded in this lead will normally appear negative (Figure 2-29, *B*).

Lead MCL$_6$
Lead MCL$_6$ is a variation of the precordial lead V$_6$ and views the low lateral wall of the left ventricle. The negative electrode is placed below the left clavicle toward the left shoulder and the positive electrode is placed at the fifth intercostal space, left midaxillary line (Figure 2-29, *C*).

A summary of the standard limb leads can be found in Table 2-3.

Augmented Limb Leads

Leads aVR, aVL, and aVF make up the augmented limb leads. Each letter of an augmented lead refers to a specific term: "a" = augmented, "V" = voltage, "R" = right arm,

Leads II, MCL$_1$, and MCL$_6$ are the most commonly used for continuous ECG monitoring.

46   ECGs Made Easy

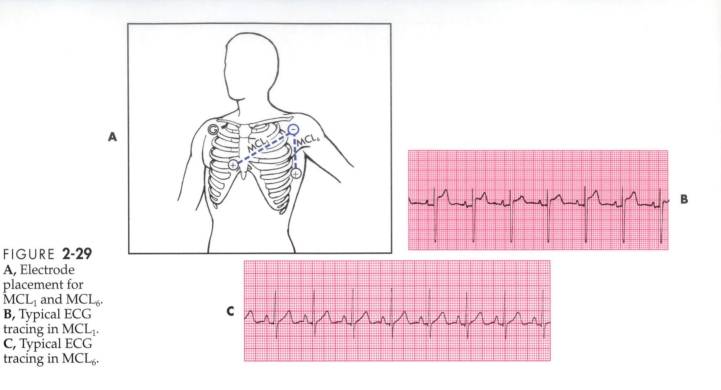

FIGURE **2-29**
A, Electrode placement for MCL_1 and MCL_6.
B, Typical ECG tracing in MCL_1.
C, Typical ECG tracing in MCL_6.

TABLE **2-3**	SUMMARY OF STANDARD LIMB LEADS		
Lead	**Positive electrode**	**Negative electrode**	**Heart surface viewed**
Lead I	Left arm	Right arm	Lateral
Lead II	Left leg	Right arm	Inferior
Lead III	Left leg	Left arm	Inferior

"L" = left arm, and "F" = foot (usually the left leg). The augmented limb leads are unipolar consisting of only one electrode (a positive electrode) on the body surface (Figure 2-30).

Lead aVR
Lead aVR views the heart from the right shoulder (the positive electrode) and views the base of the heart (primarily the atria and the great vessels). This lead does not view any wall of the heart. P waves and QRS complexes are normally negative in this lead because the direction of depolarization is away from the positive electrode.

Lead aVL
Lead aVL views the heart from the left shoulder (the positive electrode) and is oriented to the lateral wall of the left ventricle. The QRS in lead aVL is neither primarily positive nor negative because the direction of depolarization is essentially perpendicular to the positive and negative electrodes.

Lead aVF
Lead aVF views the heart from the left foot (leg) (positive electrode) and views the inferior surface of the left ventricle. The QRS in lead aVF is positive because the direction of depolarization is primarily toward the positive electrode.

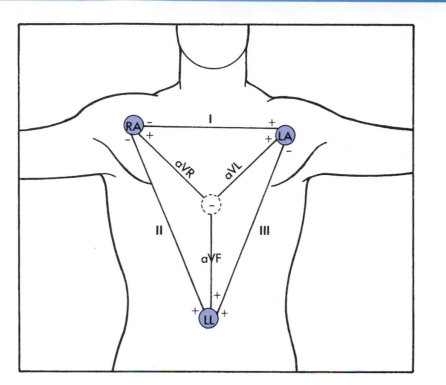

FIGURE **2-30**
View of the standard limb leads and augmented leads.

TABLE **2-4** SUMMARY OF AUGMENTED LEADS		
Lead	**Positive electrode**	**Heart surface viewed**
Lead aVR	Right arm	None
Lead aVL	Left arm	Lateral
Lead aVF	Left leg	Inferior

A summary of augmented leads can be found in Table 2-4.

Precordial (Chest) Leads

The six precordial leads are unipolar leads that view the heart in the horizontal plane. The precordial leads are identified as V_1, V_2, V_3, V_4, V_5, and V_6. Each electrode placed in a V position is a positive electrode. Leads V_1 and V_2 lie over the right ventricle. Leads V_3 and V_4 lie over the interventricular septum. Leads V_5 and V_6 lie over the left ventricle.

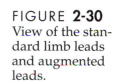 Because their location varies, do not use the nipples as landmarks for precordial electrode placement.

The wave of ventricular depolarization normally moves from right to left. In the right precordial leads (V_1 and V_2), the QRS deflection is predominantly negative (moving away from the positive precordial electrode). As the precordial electrode is placed further left, the wave of depolarization is moving toward the positive electrode. Thus the QRS deflection recorded as the electrode is moved to the left becomes progressively more positive.

Lead V_1
Lead V_1 is recorded with the positive electrode in the fourth intercostal space, just to the right of the sternum (Figure 2-31). The P waves in this lead may be positive, negative, or biphasic. The QRS in this lead is normally negative.

Leads MCL_1 and V_1 are similar but not identical. In V_1, the negative electrode is calculated by the ECG machine at the center of the heart. In MCL_1, the negative electrode is located just below the left clavicle.

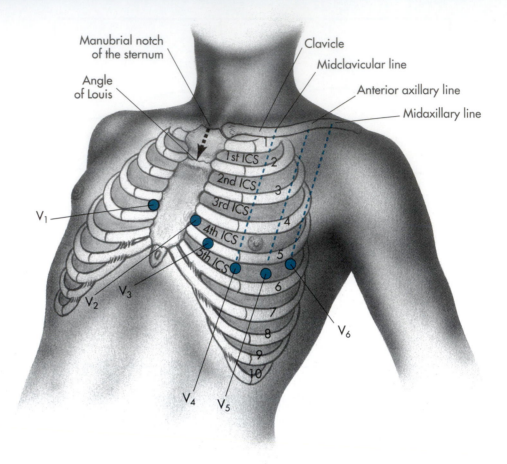

FIGURE 2-31
Anatomic place-
ment of the pre-
cordial leads.

Lead V₂

Lead V_2 is recorded with the positive electrode in the fourth intercostal space, just to the left of the sternum. P waves in this lead may be positive, negative, or biphasic. The QRS is typically biphasic.

Lead V₃

Lead V_3 is recorded with the positive electrode on a line midway between V_2 and V_4. P waves in this lead should be upright. The QRS may be biphasic.

Lead V₄

Lead V_4 is recorded with the positive electrode in the left midclavicular line in the fifth intercostal space. P waves in this lead should be upright. The QRS may be biphasic.

If a *right* ventricular MI is suspected, lead V_4 may be moved to the same anatomic location but on the *right* side of the chest. The lead is then called V_4R and is viewed for ECG changes consistent with acute MI.

Lead V₅

In the female patient, the electrode for leads V_5 and V_6 should be placed **under** the breast.

Lead V_5 is recorded with the positive electrode in the left anterior axillary line at the same level as V_4. P waves and QRS complexes should be upright in this lead.

Lead V₆

Lead V_6 is recorded with the positive electrode in the left midaxillary line at the same level as V_4. P waves and QRS complexes should be upright in this lead.

A summary of precordial leads can be found in Table 2-5.

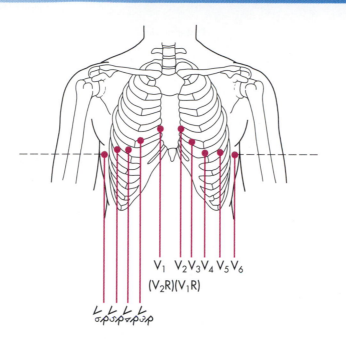

V_1 $V_2V_3V_4$ V_5V_6
$(V_2R)(V_1R)$

FIGURE **2-32**
Anatomic place-
ment of the left
and right precor-
dial leads.

TABLE 2-5	SUMMARY OF PRECORDIAL LEADS	
Lead	**Positive electrode position**	**Heart surface viewed**
Lead V_1	Right side of sternum, fourth intercostal space	Septum
Lead V_2	Left side of sternum, fourth intercostal space	Septum
Lead V_3	Midway between V_2 and V_4	Anterior
Lead V_4	Left midclavicular line, fifth intercostal space	Anterior
Lead V_5	Left anterior axillary line at same level as V_4	Lateral
Lead V_6	Left midaxillary line at same level as V_4	Lateral

Right Precordial Leads

Other precordial leads that are not part of a standard 12-lead ECG may be used to view specific surfaces of the heart. When a right ventricular myocardial infarction is suspected, right precordial leads are used. Placement of right precordial leads is identical to placement of the standard precordial leads except it is done on the right side of the chest (Figure 2-32). If time does not permit obtaining all of the right precordial leads, the lead of choice is V_4R. The right precordial leads and their placement are:

Lead V_1R = Lead V_2
Lead V_2R = Lead V_1
Lead V_3R = Midway between V_2R and V_4R
Lead V_4R = Right midclavicular line, fifth intercostal space
Lead V_5R = Right anterior axillary line at same level as V_4R
Lead V_6R = Right midaxillary line at same level as V_4R

Posterior Precordial Leads

On a standard 12-lead ECG, no leads directly face the posterior surface of the heart. Additional precordial leads may be used for this purpose. These leads are placed further left and toward the back. All of the leads are placed on the same horizontal line as V_4 to V_6. Lead V_7 is placed at the posterior axillary line. Lead V_8 is placed at the angle of the scapula (posterior scapular line) and lead V_9 is placed over the left border of spine (Figure 2-33).

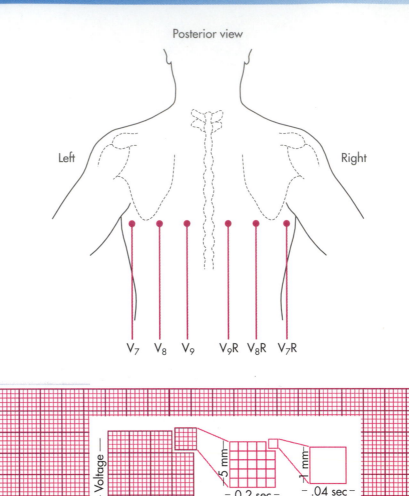

FIGURE 2-33
Posterior precordial lead placement.

FIGURE 2-34
The horizontal axis represents time. The vertical axis represents amplitude or voltage.

ECG Paper

ECG paper is graph paper made up of small and large boxes measured in millimeters. The smallest boxes are 1-mm wide and 1-mm high. The horizontal axis of the paper corresponds with *time.* Time is stated in seconds (Figure 2-34). ECG paper normally records at a constant speed of 25 mm/sec. Thus each horizontal unit (1-mm box) represents 0.04 sec (25 mm/sec × 0.04 sec = 1 mm). The lines between every five small boxes on the paper are heavier and indicate one large box. Because each large box is the width of five small boxes, a large box represents 0.20 sec. Five large boxes, each consisting of five small boxes, represent 1 sec. Fifteen large boxes equal an interval of 3 sec. Thirty large boxes represent 6 sec.

The vertical axis of the graph paper represents *voltage* or *amplitude* of the ECG waveforms or deflections. Voltage may appear as a positive or negative value because voltage is a force with direction as well as amplitude.[8] The size or amplitude of a waveform is measured in millivolts (mV) or millimeters (mm).

The ECG machine's sensitivity must be calibrated so that a 1-mV electrical signal will produce a deflection measuring exactly 10-mm tall (Figure 2-35). When properly cali-

ECG paper records at a speed of 25 mm/sec. Horizontally then, 1 mm (1 small box) = 0.04 sec, and 5 mm (1 large box) = 0.20 sec.

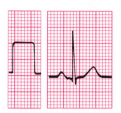

FIGURE **2-35**
When the ECG
machine is prop-
erly calibrated, a
1-mV electrical
signal will pro-
duce a deflection
measuring exactly
10-mm tall.

TABLE **2-6**	TERMINOLOGY AND DEFINITIONS
Waveform	Movement away from the baseline in either a positive or negative direction
Segment	A line between waveforms; named by the waveform that precedes or follows it
Interval	A waveform and a segment
Complex	Several waveforms

brated, a small box is 1-mm high (0.1 mV), and a large box (equal to five small boxes) is 5-mm high (0.5 mV). Clinically, the height of a waveform is usually stated in millimeters not millivolts.

WAVEFORMS

A **waveform** or deflection is movement away from the baseline in either a positive (up-ward) or negative (downward) direction (Table 2-6). A waveform that is partly positive and partly negative is *biphasic*. A waveform or deflection that rests on the baseline is *isoelectric*.

P Wave

Electrical impulses originating in the SA node produce various waves on the ECG as they spread throughout the heart. The first wave in the cardiac cycle is the *P wave* (Fig-ure 2-36). The first half of the P wave is recorded when the electrical impulse that origi-nated in the SA node stimulates the right atrium and reaches the AV node. The down-slope of the P wave reflects stimulation of the left atrium. Thus the P wave represents atrial depolarization and the spread of the electrical impulse throughout the right and left atria. The atria contract a fraction of a second after the P wave begins. A waveform representing atrial repolarization is usually not seen on the ECG because it is small and buried in the QRS complex.

The beginning of the P wave is recognized as the first abrupt or gradual deviation from the baseline; its end is the point at which the waveform returns to the baseline (Figure 2-37).

Normal Characteristics of the P Wave
- Smooth and rounded
- No more than 2.5 mm in height
- No more than 0.11 sec in duration (width)
- Positive in leads I, II, aVF, and V_2 through V_6
- May be positive, negative, or biphasic in leads III, aVL, and V_1

Activation of the SA node occurs before the on-set of the P wave and is not observed on the ECG.

The AV node is stim-ulated at approximately the peak of the P wave.

A P wave normally precedes each QRS complex.

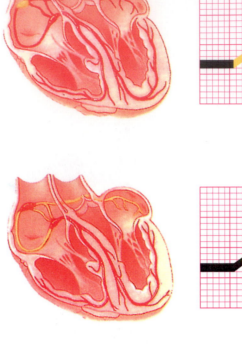

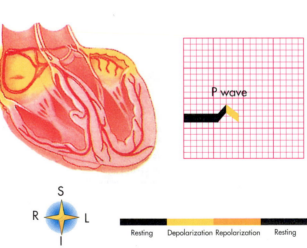

FIGURE 2-36

First wave in the cardiac cycle is the P wave. First half of the P wave reflects stimulation of the right atrium. Down-slope of the P wave reflects stimulation of the left atrium.

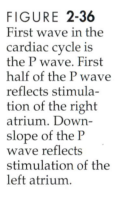

FIGURE 2-37

The normal P wave is usually no more than 2.5 mm in height and 0.11 sec in duration.

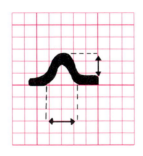

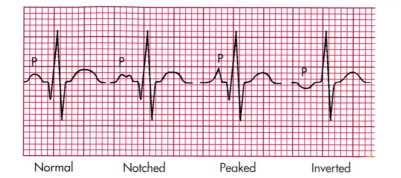

Normal   Notched   Peaked   Inverted

FIGURE **2-38**
Abnormal P
waves may be
notched, tall
and pointed
(peaked), or in-
verted (negative).

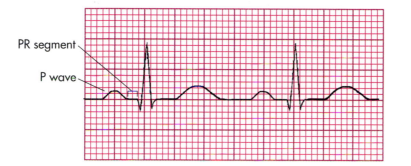

PR segment

P wave

FIGURE **2-39**
PR segment.

Abnormal P Waves

Tall and pointed (peaked) or wide and notched P waves may be seen in conditions such as chronic obstructive pulmonary disease (COPD), congestive heart failure (CHF), or in valvular disease and may be indicative of atrial enlargement (Figure 2-38).

Ectopic P waves may be either positive or negative in lead II. If the ectopic pacemaker is in the atria, the P wave will be upright; if the ectopic pacemaker is in the AV junction, the P wave will be negative (inverted) in lead II.

In right atrial enlarge-
ment, the initial part of the
P wave is abnormally tall.
In left atrial enlargement,
the latter part of the P
wave is prominent.

PR Segment

A segment is a line between waveforms and is named by the waveform that precedes or follows it. The *PR segment* is part of the PR interval and is the horizontal line between the end of the P wave and the beginning of the QRS complex (Figure 2-39). The PR segment is normally isoelectric. The His-Purkinje system is activated during the PR segment. The duration of the PR segment depends on duration of the P wave and impulse conduction through the AV junction.[9]

The PR segment is
used as a baseline from
which to evaluate ST
segment elevation or
depression.

PR Interval

An interval is a waveform and a segment. The P wave plus the PR segment equals the *PR interval* (PRI) (Figure 2-40). The PR interval reflects depolarization of the right and left atria (P wave) and the spread of the impulse through the AV node, bundle of His, right and left bundle branches, and the Purkinje fibers (PR segment) (Figure 2-41). It does not include the duration of conduction from the SA node to the right atrium. The PR interval is measured from the point where the P wave leaves the baseline to the beginning of the QRS complex.

P wave + PR segment
= PR interval (PRI).

The term *PQ interval*
is preferred by some be-
cause it is the period actually measured unless a Q
wave is absent.

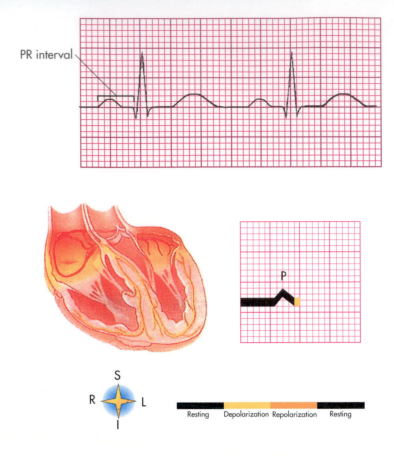

FIGURE 2-40
PR interval.

FIGURE 2-41
PR interval represents the interval between the onset of atrial depolarization and ventricular depolarization.

⟡ Measuring how quickly or slowly an electrical impulse spreads through the heart provides important information about the condition of the heart's conduction system and the muscle itself.

Normal Characteristics of the PR Interval

- A normal PR interval indicates the electrical impulse was conducted normally through the atria, AV node, bundle of His, bundle branches, and Purkinje fibers
- Normally measures 0.12 to 0.20 sec in adults; may be shorter in children and longer in older persons
- Normally shortens as heart rate increases

Abnormal PR Intervals

A long PR interval (greater than 0.20 sec) indicates the impulse was delayed as it passed through the atria or AV node. Prolonged PR intervals may be seen in first-degree AV block, hypothyroidism, and digitalis toxicity, among other conditions. The P wave associated with a prolonged PR interval may be normal or abnormal.

A PR interval of *less* than 0.12 sec may be seen when the impulse originates in an ectopic pacemaker in the atria close to the AV node or in the AV junction. A shortened PR interval may also occur if the electrical impulse progresses from the atria to the ventricles through an abnormal conduction pathway that bypasses the AV node and depolarizes the ventricles earlier than usual. Wolff-Parkinson-White and Lown-Ganong-Levine syndromes are examples of conditions in which this may be seen.

QRS Complex

⟡ Atrial repolarization usually takes place during this time, but the QRS complex overshadows it on the ECG.

A **complex** consists of several waveforms. The *QRS complex* consists of the Q wave, R wave, and S wave and represents the spread of the electrical impulse through the ventricles (ventricular depolarization. Depolarization triggers contraction of ventricular tissue. Thus, shortly after the QRS complex begins, the ventricles contract (Figure 2-42). The QRS complex is significantly larger than the P wave because depolarization of the

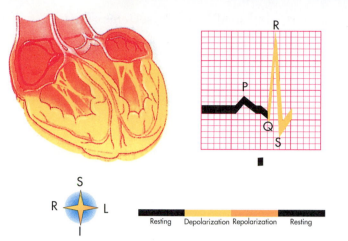

Resting   Depolarization Repolarization   Resting

FIGURE **2-42**
QRS complex
represents
ventricular
depolarization.

ventricles involves a considerably greater muscle mass than depolarization of the atria. A QRS complex normally follows each P wave. One or even two of the three waveforms that make up the QRS complex may not always be present.

Q Wave
The QRS complex begins as a downward deflection, the *Q wave.* A Q wave is **always** a negative waveform. The Q wave represents depolarization of the interventricular septum, which is activated from left to right. In lead II, the direction of the current flow is almost perpendicular to it, and more current is moving away from the positive electrode than is moving toward it. (In lead MCL_1, depolarization of the interventricular septum will appear as a small, upright R wave. In this lead, this is the first deflection of a normal QRS complex).

It is important to differentiate normal (physiologic) Q waves from pathologic Q waves. With the exception of leads III and aVR, a normal Q wave in the limb leads is less than 0.04 sec in duration and less than 25% of the amplitude of the R wave in that lead. With the exception of leads III and aVR, an abnormal (pathologic) Q wave is more than 0.04 sec in duration and more than 25% of the amplitude of the following R wave in that lead.

Myocardial infarction is one possible cause of pathologic Q waves.

R and S Waves
The QRS complex continues as a large, upright, triangular waveform known as the *R wave.* The *S wave* is the negative waveform following the R wave. The R and S waves represent simultaneous depolarization of the right and left ventricles. Because of its greater muscle mass, the QRS complex generally represents the electrical activity occurring in the left ventricle.

An R wave is **always** positive and an S wave is **always** negative.

Variations of the QRS Complex
Although the term *QRS complex* is used, not every QRS complex contains a Q wave, R wave, and S wave. To review, when the first deflection of the QRS complex is negative (below the baseline), the waveform is called a *Q wave.* The *R wave* is the first positive deflection (above the baseline) in the QRS complex. A negative deflection following the R wave is called an *S wave.*

If the QRS complex consists entirely of a positive waveform, it is called an *R wave.* If the complex consists entirely of a negative waveform, it is called a *QS wave.* If there are two positive deflections in the same complex, the second is called *R prime* and is written *R'.* If there are two negative deflections following an R wave, the second is called *S prime* and is written *S'.* Capital (upper case) letters are used to designate waveforms of relatively large amplitude, and small (lower case) letters are used to label relatively small waveforms (Figure 2-43).

Measuring the Duration of the QRS Complex

The width of a QRS complex is most accurately determined when it is viewed and measured in more than one lead. The measurement should be taken from the QRS complex with the longest duration and clearest onset and end. The beginning of the QRS complex is measured from the point where the first wave of the complex begins to deviate from the baseline. The point at which the last wave of the complex begins to level out at, above, or below the baseline marks the end of the QRS complex.

The QRS complex may appear predominantly positive, negative, or biphasic, depending on the lead. It is predominantly positive in leads that view the heart from the left (I, aVL, V_5, V_6) and in leads that look at the heart's inferior surface (II, III, aVF). In leads that view the heart from the right side, the QRS complex is predominantly negative (aVR, V_1, V_2). The QRS is normally biphasic in leads V_3, V_4, and sometimes III.[10]

Normal Characteristics of the QRS Complex

About half of all adults have a QRS duration of 0.08 sec. A 0.11 sec duration may sometimes be observed in healthy individuals. Men tend to have slightly longer QRS durations than women.[9]

- Normal duration of the QRS complex in an adult varies between 0.06 and 0.10 sec
- With the exception of leads III and aVR, a normal Q wave is less than 0.04 sec in duration and less than 25% of the amplitude of the R wave in that lead
- QRS complex is predominantly positive in leads I, aVL, V_5, V_6 and in II, III, aVF, predominantly negative in leads aVR, V_1, V_2, and normally biphasic in leads V_3, V_4, and sometimes III

Abnormal QRS Complexes

If the spread of the impulse through the ventricles is slowed, the duration of the QRS is prolonged as seen in conditions such as ventricular hypertrophy or conduction defects (e.g., bundle branch block).

- Duration of an abnormal QRS complex is greater than 0.10 sec
- Duration of a QRS caused by an electrical impulse originating in an ectopic pacemaker in the Purkinje network or ventricular myocardium is usually greater than 0.12 sec and often 0.16 sec or greater
- If the electrical impulse originates in a bundle branch, the duration of the QRS may be only slightly greater than 0.10 sec
- Enlargement of the right ventricle produces an abnormally prominent R wave; left ventricular enlargement produces an abnormally prominent S wave

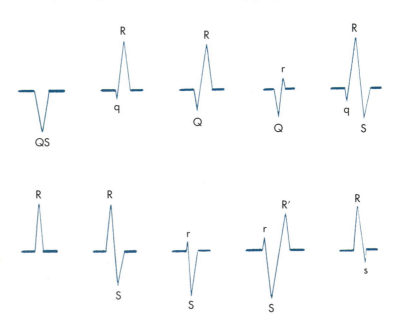

FIGURE **2-43**
QRS complex may appear in various forms.

ST Segment

The portion of the ECG tracing between the QRS complex and the T wave is the ST segment (Figure 2-44). The term *ST segment* is used regardless of whether the final wave of the QRS complex is an R or an S wave. The point where the QRS complex and the ST segment meet is called the *junction* or *J point* (Figure 2-45).

The ST segment represents the early part of repolarization of the right and left ventricles. The normal ST segment begins at the isoelectric line, extends from the end of the S wave, and curves gradually upward to the beginning of the T wave.

Various conditions may cause displacement of the ST segment from the isoelectric line in either a positive or negative direction. ST segment depression (deviation of the segment below the baseline) may reflect myocardial ischemia or hypokalemia. ST segment elevation (deviation of the segment above the baseline) may represent a normal variant, myocardial injury, pericarditis, or ventricular aneurysm.

Pericarditis causes ST-segment elevation in all or virtually all leads.

The PR segment is used as the baseline from which to evaluate the degree of displacement of the ST segment from the isoelectric line. To determine the degree of displacement, measure at a point 0.04 sec (one small box) after the J point. The ST segment is considered *elevated* if the segment is deviated above the baseline and is considered *depressed* if the segment is deviated below it (Figure 2-46). ST segment elevation or depression is considered "significant" if the displacement is more than 1 mm (one box) and is seen in two or more leads facing the same anatomic area of the heart.

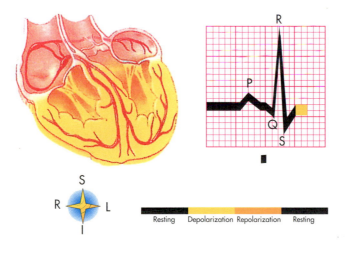

Resting   Depolarization Repolarization   Resting

FIGURE 2-44
ST segment represents the early part of repolarization of the right and left ventricles.

J point

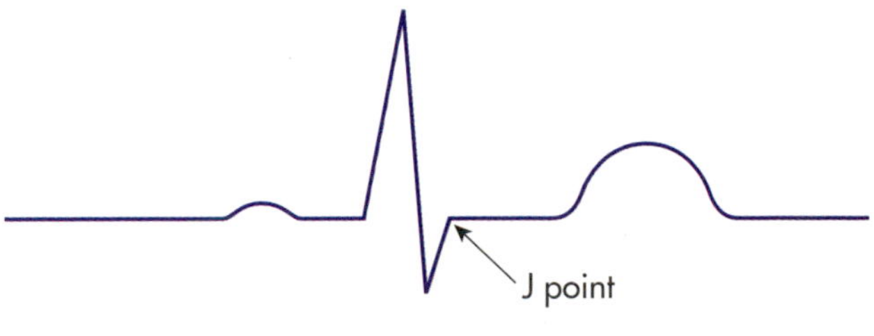

FIGURE 2-45
The point where the QRS complex and the ST segment meet is called the *junction* or *J point*.

Normal Characteristics of the ST Segment

- Begins with the end of the QRS complex and ends with the onset of the T wave
- In the limb leads, the normal ST segment is isoelectric (flat) but may normally be slightly elevated or depressed (usually by less than 1 mm)
- In the left precordial leads, ST segment elevation is not normally more than 1 to 2 mm

Abnormal ST Segments

- ST segment depression of more than 1 mm is suggestive of myocardial ischemia; ST segment elevation of more than 1 mm in the limb leads or 2 mm in the precordial leads is suggestive of myocardial injury
- A horizontal ST segment (forming a sharp angle with the T wave) is suggestive of ischemia
- Digitalis causes a depression (scoop) of the ST segment sometimes referred to as a "dig dip" (Figure 2-47)

ST segment elevation is most common and marked in leads V_2 and V_3 where the amplitude may reach 3 mm.[9]

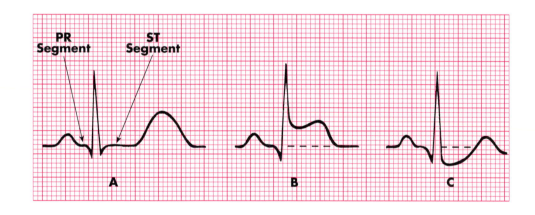

FIGURE 2-46
ST segment.
A, The PR segment is used as the baseline from which to determine the presence of ST segment elevation or depression. **B,** ST segment elevation. **C,** ST segment depression.

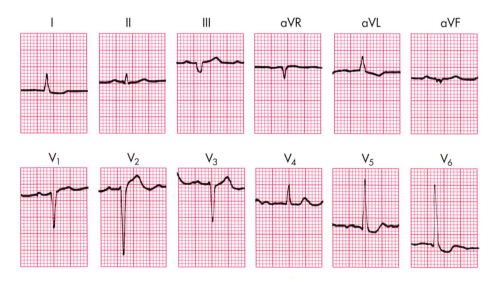

FIGURE 2-47
Digitalis may produce a characteristic "scooping" of the ST segment, shown here in leads V_5 and V_6.

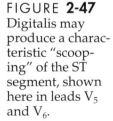

T Wave

Ventricular repolarization is represented on the ECG by the *T wave* (Figure 2-48). The absolute refractory period is still present during the beginning of the T wave. At the peak of the T wave, the relative refractory period has begun. It is during the relative refractory period that a stronger than normal stimulus may produce ventricular dysrhythmias.

The normal T wave is slightly asymmetric: the peak of the waveform is closer to its end than to the beginning, and the first half has a more gradual slope than the second half. The beginning of the T wave is identified as the point where the slope of the ST segment appears to become abruptly or gradually steeper. The T wave ends when it returns to the baseline. It may be difficult to clearly determine the onset and end of the T wave (Figure 2-49).

The T wave is normally oriented in the same direction as the preceding QRS complex. This is because epicardial cells repolarize earlier than endocardial cells. This causes the wave of repolarization to spread in the direction opposite depolarization. The result is a T wave deflected in the same direction as the QRS complex.[11]

Normal Characteristics of the T Wave

- Slightly asymmetric
- T wave is not normally more than 5 mm in height in any limb lead or 10 mm in any precordial lead; T waves are not normally less than 0.5 mm in height in leads I and II
- T waves are normally positive in leads I, II, V_2 to V_6; negative in lead aVR, positive in leads aVL and aVF but may be negative if the QRS complex is less than 6 mm in height; and may be positive or negative in leads III and V_1

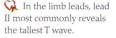 In the limb leads, lead II most commonly reveals the tallest T wave.

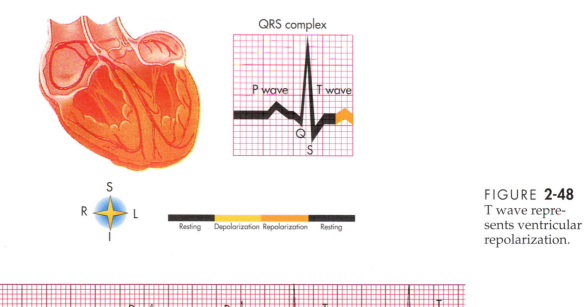

FIGURE **2-48**
T wave represents ventricular repolarization.

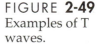

FIGURE **2-49**
Examples of T waves.

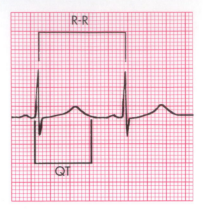

FIGURE **2-50**
Measuring the QT
interval. Abnor-
mal QT interval
prolongation in a
patient taking
quinidine.

Abnormal T Waves

- T wave following an abnormal QRS complex is usually opposite in direction of the QRS
- Negative T waves suggest myocardial ischemia
- Tall, pointed (peaked) T waves are commonly seen in hyperkalemia
- Significant cerebral disease (e.g., subarachnoid hemorrhage) may be associated with deeply inverted T waves, often called *cerebral T waves*

QT Interval

The QT interval represents total ventricular activity—the time from ventricular depolarization (activation) to repolarization (recovery). The term *QT interval* is used regardless of whether the QRS complex begins with a Q or R wave.

The QT interval is measured from the beginning of the QRS complex to the end of the T wave. In the absence of a Q wave, the QT interval is measured from the beginning of the R wave to the end of the T wave.

The duration of the QT interval varies according to age, gender, and particularly heart rate. As the heart rate increases, the QT interval decreases. As the heart rate decreases, the QT interval increases. Because of the variability of the QT interval with heart rate, it can be measured more accurately if it is corrected for the patient's heart rate. This is represented by QTc and is determined by dividing the QT interval by the square root of the R-R interval.

$$QT_c = \frac{QT}{\sqrt{R\text{-}R}}$$

To more rapidly, but less accurately, determine the QT interval, measure the interval between two consecutive R waves (R-R interval) and divide the number by two. Measure the QT interval. If the measured QT interval is less than half the R-R interval, it is probably normal (Figure 2-50). A QT interval that is approximately half the R-R interval is considered borderline. A QT interval that is more than half the R-R interval is considered prolonged.

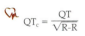 Digitalis and hyper-
calcemia shorten the QT
interval.

A prolonged QT interval indicates a lengthened relative refractory period (vulnerable period), which puts the ventricles at risk for life-threatening dysrhythmias, such as torsades de pointes (TdP). A prolonged QT interval may be congenital or acquired.

U Wave

A *U wave* is a small waveform that, when seen, follows the T wave (Figure 2-51). The mechanism of the U wave is not definitely known. One theory suggests that it represents repolarization of the Purkinje fibers. U waves are most easily seen when the heart

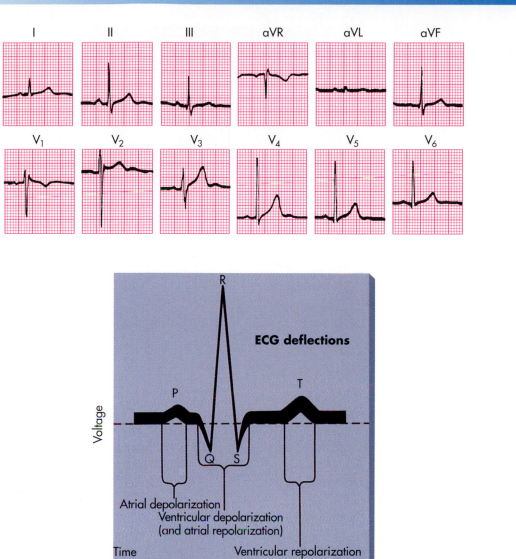

I   II   III   aVR   aVL   aVF

V_1 V_2 V_3 V_4 V_5 V_6

FIGURE **2-51**
Normal U waves
(best viewed in
leads V_2 through
V_4) in a 22-year-
old male.

ECG deflections

R

P   T

Q   S

Voltage

Atrial depolarization
Ventricular depolarization
(and atrial repolarization)
Time   Ventricular repolarization

FIGURE **2-52**
ECG waveforms:
P, QRS, and T.

rate is slow and are difficult to identify when the rate exceeds 90 beats/min. When seen, U waves are normally tallest in leads V_2 and V_3.

The amplitude of the normal U wave is usually proportional to the T wave in the same lead, ranging between 5% and 25% of the T wave's amplitude. Although the average height of a U wave is 0.33 mm, it may reach a height of 2 mm.[9] In general, a U wave taller than 1.5 mm in any lead is considered abnormal and may be the result of electrolyte imbalance (e.g., hypokalemia, hypomagnesemia, hypercalcemia), medications (e.g., quinidine, procainamide, disopyramide, amiodarone, digitalis, phenothiazines), hyperthyroidism, central nervous system disease, and long QT syndrome, among other causes. Negative U waves are strongly suggestive of organic heart disease and may be seen in patients with ischemic heart disease.

One group of researchers found that U wave inversion at rest or exercise-induced is a marker of severe stenosis of the left anterior descending artery.

Characteristics of the U Wave
- Rounded and symmetric
- Usually less than 2 mm in height and smaller than that of the preceding T wave
- In general, a U wave more than 1.5 mm in height in any lead is considered abnormal

Figure 2-52 displays the ECG waveforms, and Figure 2-53 displays the principal ECG intervals discussed in this chapter.

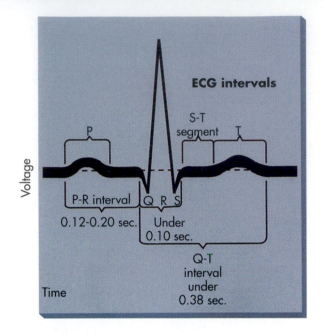

FIGURE **2-53**
ECG segments
and intervals: PR
interval, QRS du-
ration, ST seg-
ment, QT interval.

ARTIFACT

Artifact: Distortion of an
ECG tracing by electrical
activity that is noncardiac
in origin.

Accurate ECG rhythm recognition requires a tracing in which the waveforms and intervals are free of distortion. Distortion of an ECG tracing by electrical activity that is noncardiac in origin is called **artifact.** Because artifact can mimic various cardiac dysrhythmias, including ventricular fibrillation, it is essential to evaluate the patient before
initiating any medical intervention.

Artifact may be caused by loose electrodes, broken ECG cables or broken wires,
muscle tremor, patient movement, external chest compressions, and 60-cycle interference. Proper preparation of the patient's skin and evaluation of the monitoring
equipment (electrodes, wires) before use can minimize the problems associated with
artifact.

Loose Electrodes

An irregular baseline may be identified by bizarre, irregular deflections of the baseline
on the ECG paper. This may be the result of a broken lead wire, poor electrical contact,
or a loose electrode (Figure 2-54). Before applying electrodes, cleanse the patient's skin
by rubbing briskly with an alcohol swab to remove surface skin oils.

Patient Movement/Muscle Activity

A wandering baseline may occur because of normal respiratory movement (particularly
when electrodes have been applied directly over the ribs) or because of poor electrode
contact with the patient's skin. Seizures, shivering, tense muscles, or Parkinson's disease
may cause muscle tremor artifact (Figure 2-55). Consider clipping the ECG cable to the
patient's clothing to minimize excessive movement.

60-Cycle (AC) Interference

A phenomenon known as 60-cycle interference may be caused by improperly grounded
electrical equipment or other electrical interference (Figure 2-56). If 60-cycle interference

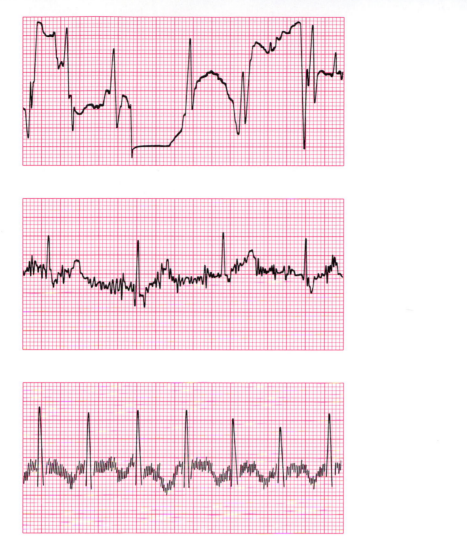

FIGURE **2-54**
Loose electrode.

FIGURE **2-55**
Artifact caused by muscle tremors.

FIGURE **2-56**
60-cycle interference.

is observed, check for crossing of cable wires with other electrical wires (e.g., bed control) or frayed and broken wires. Verify that all electrical equipment is properly grounded and that the cable electrode connections are clean.

RATE MEASUREMENT

There are several methods used for calculating heart rate (Figure 2-57).

Method 1: Six-Second Method

Most ECG paper in use today is printed with 1-sec or 3-sec markers on the top or bottom of the paper. To determine the ventricular rate, count the number of *complete* QRS complexes within a period of 6 seconds and multiply that number by 10 to find the number of complexes in 1 minute. This method may be used for regular and irregular rhythms and is the simplest, quickest, and most commonly used method of rate measurement.

5 large boxes = 1 second.

15 large boxes = 3 seconds.

30 large boxes = 6 seconds.

Method 2: Large Boxes

To determine the ventricular rate, count the number of large boxes between two consecutive R waves (R-R interval) and divide into 300. To determine the atrial rate, count the

FIGURE **2-57**
Calculating heart rate. *Method 1:* Number of R-R intervals in 6 seconds × 10 (e.g., 8 × 10 = 80/min). *Method 2:* Number of large boxes between QRS complexes divided into 300 (e.g., 300 divided by 4 = 75/min). *Method 3:* Number of small boxes between QRS complexes divided into 1500 (e.g., 1500 divided by 18 = 84/min).

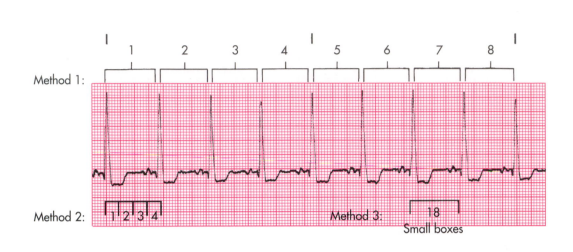

TABLE **2-7**	HEART RATE DETERMINATION BASED ON THE NUMBER OF LARGE BOXES		
Number of large boxes	Heart rate (beats/min)	Number of large boxes	Heart rate (beats/min)
1	300	6	50
2	150	7	43
3	100	8	38
4	75	9	33
5	60	10	30

♥ Large box method is best used if rhythm is regular; however, it may be used if rhythm is irregular and a rate range (slowest and fastest rate) is given.

♥ Small box method is time-consuming but accurate. If the rhythm is irregular, a rate range should be given.

number of large boxes between two consecutive P waves (P-P interval) and divide into 300 (Table 2-7).

Method 3: Small Boxes

Each 1-mm box on the graph paper represents 0.04 sec. There are 1500 boxes in 1 minute (60 secs/min divided by 0.04 sec/box = 1500 boxes/min). To calculate the ventricular rate, count the number of small boxes between two consecutive R waves and divide into 1500. To determine the atrial rate, count the number of small boxes between two consecutive P waves and divide into 1500.

Method 4: Sequence Method

To determine ventricular rate, select an R wave that falls on a dark vertical line. Number the next 6 consecutive dark vertical lines as follows: 300, 150, 100, 75, 60, and 50 (Figure 2-58). Note where the next R wave falls in relation to the 6 dark vertical lines already marked. This is the heart rate.

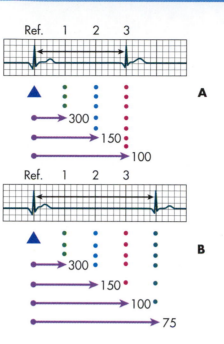

RHYTHM/REGULARITY

The term *rhythm* is used to indicate the site of origin of an electrical impulse (e.g., sinus rhythm, junctional rhythm) and to describe the regularity or irregularity of waveforms.

The waveforms on an ECG strip are evaluated for regularity by measuring the distance between the P waves and QRS complexes. If the rhythm is regular, the R-R intervals (or P-P intervals, if assessing atrial rhythm) are the same. Generally, a variation of plus or minus 10% is acceptable. For example, if there are 10 small boxes in an R-R interval, an R wave could be "off" by 1 small box and still be considered regular.

For accuracy, the R-R or P-P intervals should be evaluated across an entire 6-second rhythm strip.

Ventricular Rhythm

To evaluate the regularity of the ventricular rhythm, measure the distance between two consecutive R-R intervals. Place one point of a pair of calipers (or make a mark on a piece of paper) on the beginning of an R wave. Place the other point of the calipers (or make a second mark on the paper) on the beginning of the R wave of the next QRS complex. Without adjusting the calipers, evaluate each succeeding R-R interval. (If paper is used, lift the paper and move it across the rhythm strip). Compare the distance measured with the other R-R intervals. If the ventricular rhythm is regular, the R-R intervals will measure the same.

Rhythm/regularity may also be determined by counting the small boxes between intervals and comparing the intervals with each other.

Atrial Rhythm

To determine if the atrial rhythm is regular or irregular, follow the same procedure previously described for evaluation of ventricular rhythm but measure the distance between two consecutive P-P intervals (instead of R-R intervals) and compare that distance with the other P-P intervals. The P-P intervals will measure the same if the atrial rhythm is regular.

Terminology

Various terms may be used to describe an irregular rhythm. If the variation between the shortest and longest R-R intervals (or P-P intervals) is less than four small boxes (0.16 sec), the rhythm is termed *essentially regular*. For example, the underlying rhythm may be regular but the pattern may be periodically interrupted by ectopic beats that arise from a part of the heart other than the SA node.

If the shortest and longest R-R intervals vary by more than 0.16 sec, the rhythm is considered *irregular*. A *regularly irregular* rhythm is one in which the R-R intervals are not the same, the shortest and longest R-R intervals vary by more than 0.16 sec, and there is a repeating pattern of irregularity. An *irregularly irregular* rhythm is one in which the R-R intervals are not the same, there is no repeating pattern of irregularity, and the shortest and longest R-R intervals vary by more than 0.16 sec.

ANALYZING A RHYTHM STRIP

A methodic approach should be used when analyzing a rhythm strip to ensure accurate interpretation. Begin analyzing the rhythm strip from left to right.

Assess the Rate

To determine the ventricular rate, measure the distance between two consecutive R waves (R-R interval). To determine the atrial rate, measure the distance between two consecutive P waves (P-P interval). *Tachycardia* exists if the rate is more than 100 beats/min. *Bradycardia* exists if the rate is less than 60 beats/min.

Assess Rhythm/Regularity

To determine if the ventricular rhythm is regular or irregular, measure the distance between two consecutive R-R intervals and compare that distance with the other R-R intervals. If the ventricular rhythm is regular, the R-R intervals will measure the same.

To determine if the atrial rhythm is regular or irregular, measure the distance between two consecutive P-P intervals and compare that distance with the other P-P intervals. If the atrial rhythm is regular, the P-P intervals will measure the same.

Identify and Examine P Waves

To locate P waves, look to the left of each QRS complex. Normally, one P wave precedes each QRS complex, they occur regularly, and appear similar in size, shape, and position. If no P wave is present, the rhythm originated in the AV junction or the ventricles.

If one P wave is present before each QRS and the QRS is *narrow:*

- Is the P wave positive? If so, the rhythm probably originated from the SA node.
- Is the P wave negative or absent? If so, and the QRS complexes occur regularly, the rhythm probably originated from the AV junction.

Assess Intervals (Evaluate Conduction)

PR Interval

Measure the PR interval. The PR interval is measured from the point where the P wave leaves the baseline to the beginning of the QRS complex. The normal PR interval is 0.12 to 0.20 sec. If the PR intervals are the same, they are said to be constant. If the PR inter-

---

An irregular rhythm may be normal, fast, or slow.

A regularly irregular rhythm may be the result of grouped beating.

An irregularly irregular rhythm may also be called a *grossly* or *totally irregular* rhythm.

It is essential to develop a systematic approach to rhythm analysis and consistently apply it when interpreting a rhythm strip.

Generally, a variation of plus or minus 10% is acceptable, and the rhythm is still considered regular.

Some dysrhythmias, such as atrial fibrillation, junctional rhythms, and ventricular rhythms, may not have a P wave before the QRS complex.

Dysrhythmias such as AV blocks are associated with abnormal PR intervals.

vals are different, is there a pattern? In some dysrhythmias, the duration of the PR interval will increase until a P wave appears with no QRS after it. This is referred to as "lengthening" of the PR interval. PR intervals that vary in duration and have no pattern are said to be "variable."

QRS Duration

Identify the QRS complexes and measure their duration. The beginning of the QRS is measured from the point where the first wave of the complex begins to deviate from the baseline. The point at which the last wave of the complex begins to level out at, above, or below the baseline marks the end of the QRS complex. QRS is considered narrow (normal) if it measures 0.10 sec or less and wide if it measures more than 0.10 sec.

A QRS complex of 0.10 sec or less (narrow) is presumed to be supraventricular in origin.

QT Interval

Measure the QT interval in the leads that show the largest amplitude T waves. The QT interval is measured from the beginning of the QRS complex to the end of the T wave. In the absence of a Q wave, the QT interval is measured from the beginning of the R wave to the end of the T wave. If the measured QT interval is less than half the R-R interval, it is probably normal. This method of QT interval measurement works well as a general guideline until the ventricular rate exceeds 100 beats/min.

A prolonged QT interval indicates a lengthened relative refractory period (vulnerable period), which can put the ventricles at risk for life-threatening dysrhythmias such as TdP.

Evaluate the Overall Appearance of the Rhythm

ST Segment

The ST segment is usually isoelectric in the limb leads. ST segment elevation or depression is determined by measuring at a point 0.04 sec (one small box) after the end of the QRS complex. The PR segment is used as the baseline from which to evaluate the degree of displacement of the ST segment from the isoelectric line (elevation or depression).

The ST segment is considered *elevated* if the segment is deviated above the baseline of the PR segment and is considered *depressed* if the segment deviates below it. ST segment elevation or depression is considered "significant" if the displacement is more than 1 mm (one box) and is seen in two or more leads facing the same anatomic area of the heart.

T Wave

Evaluate the T waves. Are the T waves upright and of normal height? The T wave following an abnormal QRS complex is usually opposite in direction of the QRS. Negative T waves suggest myocardial ischemia. Tall, pointed (peaked) T waves are commonly seen in hyperkalemia.

A summary of normal waveform configuration can be found in Table 2-8.

Interpret the Rhythm and Evaluate Its Clinical Significance

Interpret the rhythm, specifying the site of the origin (pacemaker site) of the rhythm (sinus), the mechanism (bradycardia), and the ventricular rate. For example, "sinus bradycardia at 38/min." Evaluate the patient's clinical presentation to determine how he or she is tolerating the rate and rhythm.

TABLE 2-8   Summary of Normal Waveform Configuration

Lead type	Heart surface viewed	Lead	P wave	Q wave	R wave	S wave	ST segment	T wave
Limb	Lateral	Lead I	Positive	Small	Largest waveform	Small (<R) or none	May vary from +1 to −0.5 mm	Positive
Limb	Inferior	Lead II	Positive	Small or none	Large	Small (<R) or none	May vary from +1 to −0.5 mm	Positive
Limb	Inferior	Lead III	Positive, negative, or biphasic	Small or none; if large, must also be present in aVF to be diagnostic	None to large	None to large	May vary from +1 to −0.5 mm	Positive, negative, or biphasic
Limb	None	aVR	Negative	Small, none, or large	Small or none	Large (may be QS)	May vary from +1 to −0.5 mm	Negative
Limb	Lateral	aVL	Positive, negative, or biphasic	Small, none, or large; if large, must also be present in lead I, V_5, or V_6 to be diagnostic	Small, none, or large	None to large	May vary from +1 to −0.5 mm	Positive, negative, or biphasic
Limb	Inferior	aVF	Positive	Small or none	Small, none, or large	None to large	May vary from +1 to −0.5 mm	Positive, negative, or biphasic
Precordial	Septum	V_1	Positive, negative, or biphasic	None; possible QS	<S wave or none (QS)	Large (may be QS)	May vary from 0 to +3 mm	Positive, negative, or biphasic
Precordial	Septum	V_2	Positive	None; possible QS	<S wave or none (QS); progressively larger; small R' may be present	Large (may be QS)	May vary from 0 to +3 mm	Positive
Precordial	Anterior	V_3	Positive	Small or none	R < S, R > S, or R = S; progressively larger	Large; S > R, S < R, or S = R	May vary from 0 to +3 mm	Positive
Precordial	Anterior	V_4	Positive	Small or none	Progressively larger waveform; R > S	Progressively smaller; S < R	Usually isoelectric; may vary from +1 to −0.5 mm	Positive
Precordial	Lateral	V_5	Positive	Small	Progressively larger waveform; <26 mm	Progressively smaller; <S wave in V_4	Usually isoelectric; may vary from +1 to −0.5 mm	Positive
Precordial	Lateral	V_6	Positive	Small	Largest waveform; <26 mm	Smallest; <S wave in V_5	Usually isoelectric; may vary from +1 to −0.5 mm	Positive

Modified from Goldman MJ: *Principles of electrocardiography*, ed 10, California, 1979, Lange Medical Publications.

REFERENCES

1. Marriott HJL, Conover MB: *Advanced concepts in arrhythmias,* ed 3, St Louis, 1998, Mosby.
2. Berne RM, Levy MN: *Cardiovascular physiology,* ed 7, St Louis, 1997, Mosby.
3. Braunwauld E, Scheinman M, editors: *Arrhythmias: electrophysiologic principles,* Vol IX, Singapore, 1996, Current Medicine/Mosby.
4. Padrid PJ, Kowey PR, editors: *Cardiac arrhythmia: mechanisms, diagnosis, and management,* Baltimore, 1995, Williams & Wilkins.
5. Clochesy JM, Breau C, Cardin S, Whittaker AA, Rudy EB: *Critical care nursing,* ed 2, Philadelphia, 1996, WB Saunders.
6. Conover MB: *Understanding electrocardiography,* ed 7, St Louis, 1996, Mosby.
7. Guyton AC, Hall JE: *Textbook of medical physiology,* ed 9, Philadelphia, 1996, WB Saunders.
8. Taylor G: *150 practice ECGs: interpretation and board review,* Cambridge, 1997, Blackwell Science.
9. Chou T, Knilans TK: *Electrocardiography in clinical practice: adult and pediatric,* Philadelphia, 1996, WB Saunders.
10. Lipman BC, Cascio T: *ECG assessment and interpretation,* Philadelphia, 1994, FA Davis.
11. Wagner GS: *Marriott's practical electrocardiography,* ed 9, Baltimore, 1994, Williams & Wilkins.

BIBLIOGRAPHY

Anderson KN, Anderson LE, Glanze WD, editors: *Mosby's medical, nursing, and allied health dictionary,* ed 4, St Louis, 1994, Mosby.

Berne RM, Levy MN: *Cardiovascular physiology,* ed 7, St Louis, 1997, Mosby.

Braunwauld E, Scheinman M, editors: *Arrhythmias: electrophysiologic principles,* Vol IX, Singapore, 1996, Current Medicine/Mosby.

Chou T, Knilans TK: *Electrocardiography in clinical practice: adult and pediatric,* Philadelphia, 1996, WB Saunders.

Clochesy JM, Breau C, Cardin S, Whittaker AA, Rudy EB: *Critical care nursing,* ed 2, Philadelphia, 1996, WB Saunders.

Conover MB: *Understanding electrocardiography,* ed 7, St Louis, 1996, Mosby.

Crawford MH, editor: *Current diagnosis and treatment in cardiology,* Norwalk, 1995, Appleton & Lange.

Ganong WF: *Review of medical physiology,* ed 17, Norwalk, 1995, Appleton & Lange.

Goldberger AL: *Clinical electrocardiography: a simplified approach,* ed 6, St Louis, 1999, Mosby.

Guyton AC, Hall JE: *Textbook of medical physiology,* ed 9, Philadelphia, 1996, WB Saunders.

Johnson R, Swartz MH: *A simplified approach to electrocardiography,* Philadelphia, 1986, WB Saunders.

Kinney MR, editor: *Andreoli's comprehensive cardiac care,* ed 8, St Louis, 1996, Mosby.

Lipman BC, Cascio T: *ECG assessment and interpretation,* Philadelphia, 1994, FA Davis.

Lounsbury P, Frye SJ: *Cardiac rhythm disorders: a nursing process approach,* ed 2, St Louis, 1992, Mosby.

Marriott HJL, Conover MB: *Advanced concepts in arrhythmias,* ed 3, St Louis, 1998, Mosby.

Padrid PJ, Kowey PR, editors: *Cardiac arrhythmia: mechanisms, diagnosis, and management,* Baltimore, 1995, Williams & Wilkins.

Thelan LA, Davie JK, Urden LD, Lough ME: *Critical care nursing: diagnosis and management,* ed 2, St Louis, 1994, Mosby.

Thibodeau GA, Patton KT: *Anatomy and physiology,* ed 2, St. Louis, 1993, Mosby.

Wagner GS: *Marriott's practical electrocardiography,* ed 9, Baltimore, 1994, Williams & Wilkins.

MATCHING

___ 1. QT interval
___ 2. Intrinsic rate of AV junction
___ 3. Excitability
___ 4. Refractoriness
___ 5. Repolarization
___ 6. Intrinsic rate of ventricles
___ 7. Myocardial cells
___ 8. Absolute refractory period
___ 9. Depolarization
___ 10. Pacemaker cells
___ 11. Intrinsic rate of SA node
___ 12. Inferior
___ 13. Bipolar limb leads
___ 14. Relative refractory period
___ 15. Lateral
___ 16. Time
___ 17. Unipolar limb leads
___ 18. Amplitude/voltage

A. 60 to 100 beats/min
B. Corresponds with the downslope of the T wave
C. Movement of ions across a cell membrane causing the inside of the cell to become more positive
D. Surface of the left ventricle viewed by leads II, III, and aVF
E. Working cells of the myocardium that contain contractile filaments
F. Measured on the vertical axis of ECG paper
G. 40 to 60 beats/min
H. Extent to which a cell is able to respond to a stimulus
I. Specialized cells of the heart's electrical conduction system capable of spontaneously generating and conducting electrical impulses
J. Ability of cardiac muscle cells to respond to an external stimulus
K. Corresponds with the onset of the QRS complex to the peak of the T wave
L. I, II, III
M. Measured on the horizontal axis of ECG paper
N. aVR, aVL, aVF
O. Represents total ventricular activity—the time from ventricular depolarization to repolarization
P. Surface of the left ventricle viewed by leads I, aVL, V_5, and V_6
Q. Movement of ions across a cell membrane in which the inside of the cell is restored to its negative charge
R. 20 to 40 beats/min

IDENTIFICATION AND MEASUREMENTS—PRACTICE RHYTHM STRIPS

For each of the following rhythm strips determine the atrial and ventricular rates; label the P wave, QRS complex and T wave; and measure the PR interval, QRS duration, and QT interval. *Not all waveforms will be present in each of the following rhythm strips.*

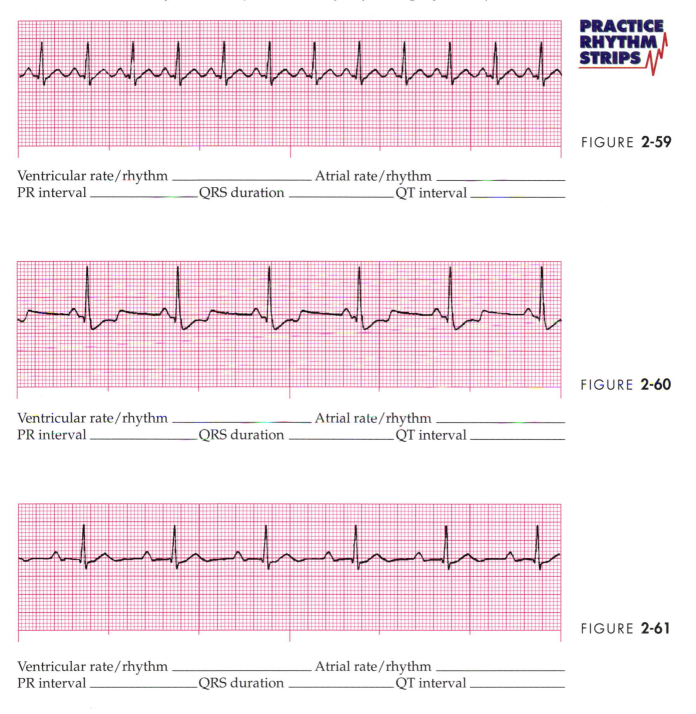

PRACTICE RHYTHM STRIPS

FIGURE **2-59**

Ventricular rate/rhythm _____ Atrial rate/rhythm _____
PR interval _____ QRS duration _____ QT interval _____

FIGURE **2-60**

Ventricular rate/rhythm _____ Atrial rate/rhythm _____
PR interval _____ QRS duration _____ QT interval _____

FIGURE **2-61**

Ventricular rate/rhythm _____ Atrial rate/rhythm _____
PR interval _____ QRS duration _____ QT interval _____

PRACTICE RHYTHM STRIPS

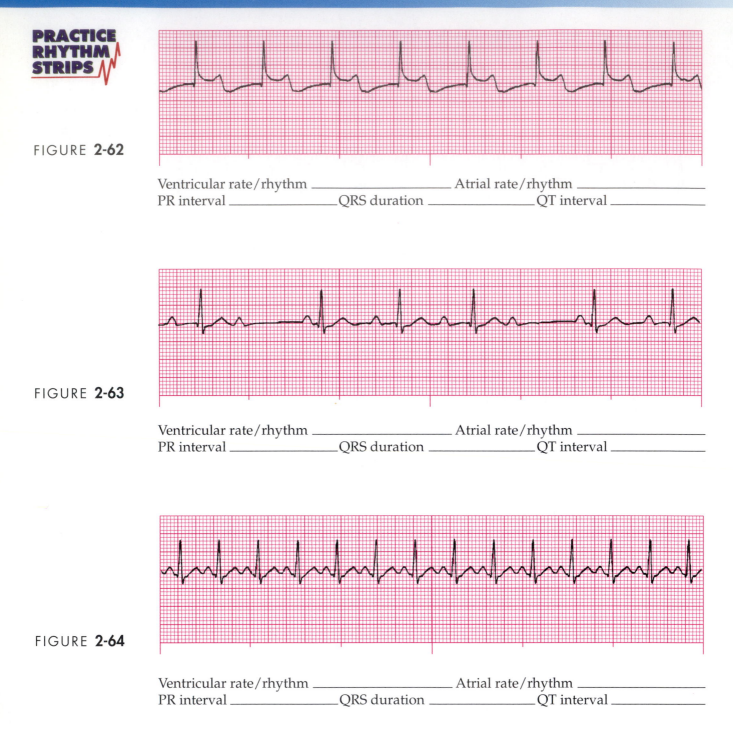

FIGURE **2-62**

Ventricular rate/rhythm _____ Atrial rate/rhythm _____
PR interval _____ QRS duration _____ QT interval _____

FIGURE **2-63**

Ventricular rate/rhythm _____ Atrial rate/rhythm _____
PR interval _____ QRS duration _____ QT interval _____

FIGURE **2-64**

Ventricular rate/rhythm _____ Atrial rate/rhythm _____
PR interval _____ QRS duration _____ QT interval _____

CHAPTER 3

Sinus Mechanisms

OBJECTIVES

On completion of this chapter, you will be able to:

1. Describe the ECG characteristics of a sinus rhythm.
2. Describe the ECG characteristics, possible causes, signs and symptoms, and emergency management of each of the following dysrhythmias that originate in the sinoatrial node:
   a. Sinus bradycardia
   b. Sinus tachycardia
   c. Sinus arrhythmia
   d. Sinoatrial block
   e. Sinus arrest

OVERVIEW

The normal heartbeat is the result of an electrical impulse that originates in the sinoatrial (SA) node. Normally, pacemaker cells within the SA node spontaneously depolarize more rapidly than other cardiac cells, thus dominating other areas that may be depolarizing at a slightly slower rate. The impulse is then transmitted to transitional cells at the periphery of the SA node and subsequently to the myocardial cells of the surrounding atrium. A rhythm originating from the SA node will have one positive (upright) P wave before each QRS complex.

Dysrhythmia: Any disturbance or abnormality in a normal rhythmic pattern; any cardiac rhythm other than a sinus rhythm.

A **dysrhythmia** (also called an *arrhythmia*) is a manifestation of abnormal electrical activity. The transmission of an electrical impulse from the SA node may be affected by medications, diseases, or conditions that delay the emergence of the impulse from the SA node or prevent it altogether.[1] Variations in rhythms originating from the SA node include differences in rate (i.e., fast/slow) and/or pattern and rhythm (regularity).

SINUS RHYTHM

Sinus rhythm is sometimes referred to as *regular sinus rhythm (RSR)* or *normal sinus rhythm (NSR)*.

The SA node normally initiates electrical impulses at a rate of 60 to 100 beats/min. This rate is faster than any other part of the conduction system. As a result, the SA node is normally the primary pacemaker of the heart. **Sinus rhythm** is the name given to the rhythm reflecting normal electrical activity—that is, the rhythm originates in the SA node and follows the normal pathway of conduction through the atria, AV junction, bundle branches, and ventricles, resulting in atrial and ventricular depolarization.

ECG Criteria

A sinus rhythm (Figure 3-1) is characterized by a regular atrial and ventricular rhythm occurring at a rate of 60 to 100 beats/min. One positive P wave (in lead II) precedes each QRS complex. The P waves are uniform in appearance. The PR interval measures 0.12 to 0.20 sec and is constant from beat to beat. The duration of the QRS complex measures 0.10 sec or less. The QRS may appear widened when a delay in conduction occurs within the ventricles (Table 3-1).

TABLE 3-1	CHARACTERISTICS OF SINUS RHYTHM
Rate	60-100 beats/min
Rhythm	Regular
P waves	Uniform in appearance, positive (upright) in lead II, one precedes each QRS complex
PR interval	0.12-0.20 sec and constant from beat to beat
QRS duration	0.10 sec or less

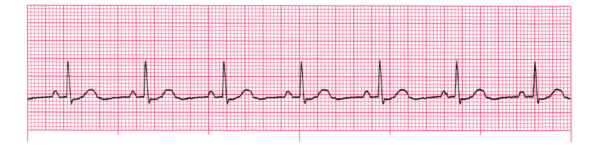

FIGURE **3-1**
Sinus rhythm at 70 beats/min.

SINUS BRADYCARDIA

If the SA node discharges fewer than 60 beats/min, the rhythm is termed **sinus brady-cardia**—the rhythm originates in the SA node and follows the normal pathway of conduction through the atria, AV junction, bundle branches, and ventricles, resulting in atrial and ventricular depolarization.

Bradycardia: A heart rate slower than 60 beats/min; *brady* = slow.

ECG Criteria

Sinus bradycardia (Figure 3-2) is characterized by a regular atrial and ventricular rhythm occurring at a rate less than 60 beats/min. One positive P wave precedes each QRS complex in lead II. The P waves are uniform in appearance. The PR interval measures 0.12 to 0.20 sec and is constant from beat to beat. The duration of the QRS complex usually measures 0.10 sec or less (Table 3-2).

Causes and Clinical Significance

Sinus bradycardia may be normal in physically conditioned adults and during sleep. However, sinus bradycardia is the most common dysrhythmia associated with acute myocardial infarction,[2] and is often seen in patients with inferior and posterior infarction. Other causes of sinus bradycardia include disease of the SA node, increased vagal (parasympathetic) tone (vomiting, increased intracranial pressure, vagal maneuvers, carotid sinus pressure), hypoxia, hypothermia, anorexia nervosa, hypothyroidism, hyperkalemia, uremia, glaucoma, sleep apnea syndrome, and administration of medications such as calcium channel blockers (verapamil, diltiazem), digitalis, and beta-blockers (propranolol).

Remember that cardiac output = stroke volume × heart rate. Therefore a decrease in either stroke volume *or* heart rate may result in a decrease in cardiac output. Decreasing cardiac output will eventually produce myocardial ischemia and further hemodynamic compromise. Clinical signs and symptoms of hemodynamic compromise include hypotension, chest pain, shortness of breath, changes in mental status, left ventricular failure, a fall in urine output, and cold, clammy skin.

TABLE 3-2	CHARACTERISTICS OF SINUS BRADYCARDIA
Rate	Less than 60 beats/min
Rhythm	Regular
P waves	Uniform in appearance, positive (upright) in lead II, one precedes each QRS complex
PR interval	0.12-0.20 sec and constant from beat to beat
QRS duration	0.10 sec or less

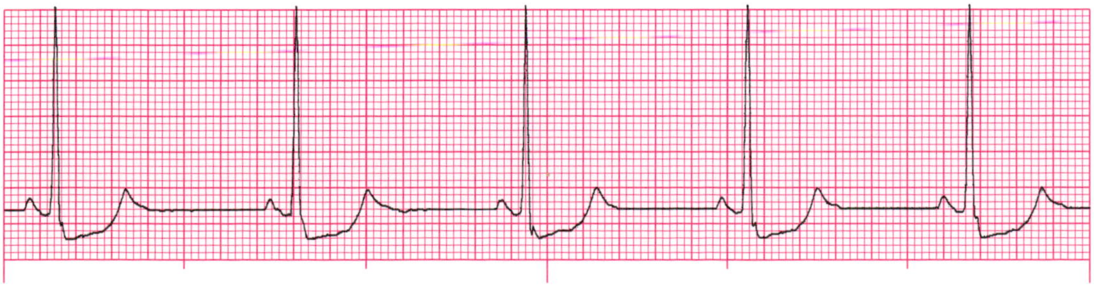

FIGURE **3-2**
Sinus bradycardia at 48 beats/min; ST depression.

Intervention

No intervention is necessary if the patient is asymptomatic. If the patient is symptomatic because of the bradycardia, interventions may include oxygen, IV access, and administration of atropine and/or transcutaneous pacing.

SINUS TACHYCARDIA

Tachycardia: A heart rate greater than 100 beats/min; *tachy* = fast.

If the SA node discharges at a rate greater than 100 beats/min, the rhythm is termed **sinus tachycardia**—the rhythm originates in the SA node and follows the normal pathway of conduction through the atria, AV junction, bundle branches, and ventricles, resulting in atrial and ventricular depolarization.

ECG Criteria

Sinus tachycardia (Figure 3-3) is characterized by a regular atrial and ventricular rhythm occurring at a rate greater than 100 beats/min. In adults, the rate associated with sinus tachycardia is typically between 101 and 180 beats/min.

One positive P wave precedes each QRS complex in lead II. The P waves are uniform in appearance. The PR interval measures 0.12 to 0.20 sec and is constant from beat to beat. The duration of the QRS complex usually measures 0.10 sec or less. At very fast rates, it may be difficult to distinguish between a P wave and T wave. Sinus tachycardia begins and ends gradually (Table 3-3).

Causes and Clinical Significance

Sinus tachycardia occurs as a normal response to the body's demand for increased oxygen because of fever, pain and anxiety, hypoxia, congestive heart failure, acute myocardial infarction, infection, sympathetic stimulation, shock, hypovolemia, dehydration, exercise, and fright. Sinus tachycardia may also occur as the result of administration of

TABLE 3-3	CHARACTERISTICS OF SINUS TACHYCARDIA
Rate	101-180 beats/min
Rhythm	Regular
P waves	Uniform in appearance, positive (upright) in lead II, one precedes each QRS complex; at very fast rates it may be difficult to distinguish a P wave from a T wave
PR interval	0.12-0.20 sec and constant from beat to beat
QRS duration	0.10 sec or less

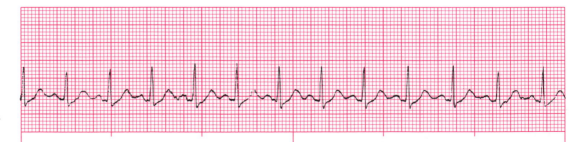

FIGURE **3-3**
Sinus tachycardia at 129 beats/min.

medications such as epinephrine, atropine, dopamine, and dobutamine, or substances such as caffeine-containing beverages, nicotine, and cocaine.

Sinus tachycardia is seen in about one third of patients with acute myocardial infarction,[3] especially those with an anterior infarction.[4] In the setting of acute MI, sinus tachycardia is a warning signal for heart failure, hypovolemia, and increased risk for serious dysrhythmias.

Intervention

Interventions are directed at correcting the underlying cause—i.e., fluid replacement, relief of pain, removal of offending medications or substances, reducing fever, and/or anxiety. Sinus tachycardia in a patient with an acute MI may be treated with beta-blockers. Beta-blockers are administered to slow the heart rate and decrease myocardial oxygen demand, provided there are no signs of heart failure or other contraindications to beta-blocker therapy.

SINUS ARRHYTHMIA

Sinus arrhythmia occurs when the SA node discharges irregularly. Sinus arrhythmia that is associated with the phases of respiration and changes in intrathoracic pressure is commonly referred to as *respiratory sinus arrhythmia.* Sinus arrhythmia that is not related to the respiratory cycle is called *nonrespiratory sinus arrhythmia.*

The term *arrhythmia* refers to an abnormal heart rhythm.

ECG Criteria

Sinus arrhythmia (Figure 3-4) originates in the SA node and follows the normal pathway of conduction through the atria, AV junction, bundle branches, and ventricles, resulting in atrial and ventricular depolarization. The rhythm is characterized

TABLE 3-4	CHARACTERISTICS OF SINUS ARRHYTHMIA
Rate	Usually 60-100 beats/min, but may be slower or faster
Rhythm	Irregular, phasic with respiration; heart rate increases gradually during inspiration (R-R intervals shorten) and decreases with expiration (R-R intervals lengthen)
P waves	Uniform in appearance, positive (upright) in lead II, one precedes each QRS complex
PR interval	0.12-0.20 sec and constant from beat to beat
QRS duration	0.10 sec or less

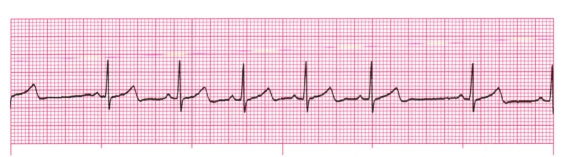

FIGURE **3-4**
Sinus arrhythmia at 54 to 88 beats/min.

by an irregular atrial and ventricular rhythm, usually occurring at a rate of 60 to 100 beats/min. If sinus arrhythmia is associated with a bradycardic rate, it is called *sinus brady-arrhythmia.* If the rhythm is associated with a tachycardic rate, it is known as *sinus tachy-arrhythmia.*

Respiratory sinus arrhythmia is characterized by a heart rate that increases grad-ually during inspiration (R-R intervals shorten) and decreases with expiration (R-R intervals lengthen). One positive P wave precedes each QRS complex in lead II. The P waves are uniform in appearance, and the P-P intervals typically vary by more than 0.16 sec. The PR interval measures 0.12 to 0.20 sec and is constant from beat to beat. The duration of the QRS complex usually measures 0.10 sec or less (Table 3-4).

Causes and Clinical Significance

Respiratory sinus arrhythmia is a normal phenomenon that occurs with changes in in-trathoracic pressure. The heart rate increases with inspiration (R-R intervals shorten) and decreases with expiration (R-R intervals lengthen). Sinus arrhythmia is most commonly observed in infants and children but may be seen in any age group.

Nonrespiratory sinus arrhythmia is more likely in older individuals and in those with heart disease. It is common after acute inferior wall MI and may be seen with increased intracranial pressure. Nonrespiratory sinus arrhythmia may be the result of effects of medications, such as digitalis and morphine, or carotid sinus pressure.[3]

Intervention

If a patient's pulse is irregular, it should be counted for 1 full minute.

Sinus arrhythmia does not usually require intervention unless it is accompanied by a bradycardia that causes hemodynamic compromise. If hemodynamic compromise is present, IV atropine may be indicated.

SINOATRIAL (SA) BLOCK

SA block is also called *sinus exit block.*

In sinoatrial (SA) block, an impulse is initiated by the pacemaker cells within the SA node but is blocked as it exits the SA node. This is thought to occur because of failure of the transitional cells in the SA node to conduct the impulse from the pacemaker cells to the surrounding atrium. Thus SA block is a disorder of conductivity.

The rhythmicity of the SA node is unaffected by SA block, thus impulses are generated regularly. However, because an impulse is blocked as it exits the SA node, the atria are not acti-vated. This appears on the ECG as a single missed beat (a P wave, QRS complex, and T wave are missing). The pause caused by the missed beat is the same as (or an exact multi-ple of) the distance between two P-P intervals of the underlying rhythm.

ECG Criteria

SA block (Figure 3-5) is characterized by an irregular rhythm caused by pause(s) result-ing from the block. If several impulses are blocked as they exit the SA node, the overall rate may be bradycardic. A positive P wave (in lead II) precedes each QRS complex, and the P waves are uniform in appearance. The P-P interval is an exact multiple of the dis-tance between two P-P intervals of the underlying rhythm. This occurs because im-pulses are generated regularly but periodically fail to exit the SA node.

When present, the PR interval measures 0.12 to 0.20 sec and is constant from beat to beat. The duration of the QRS complex usually measures 0.10 sec or less unless an intra-

TABLE 3-5	CHARACTERISTICS OF SINOATRIAL (SA) BLOCK
Rate	Usually normal but varies because of the pause
Rhythm	Irregular because of the pause(s) caused by the SA block—each pause is the same as (or an exact multiple of) the distance between two other P-P intervals
P waves	Uniform in appearance, positive (upright) in lead II; when present, one precedes each QRS complex
PR interval	0.12-0.20 sec and constant from beat to beat
QRS duration	0.10 sec or less

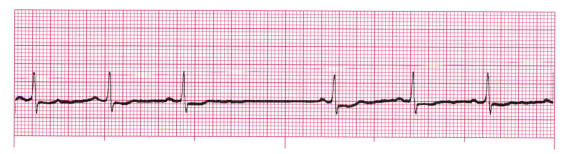

FIGURE **3-5**
Sinoatrial (SA) block.

ventricular conduction delay exists. Because this dysrhythmia occurs as the result of a specific event and the remainder of the rhythm is regular, its regularity (rhythm) may be described as irregular or regular except for the event (Table 3-5).

Causes and Clinical Significance

SA block is relatively uncommon but may occur as a result of acute MI; digitalis, quinidine, procainamide, or salicylate administration; coronary artery disease; myocarditis; congestive heart failure; carotid sinus sensitivity; or increased vagal tone.

If episodes of SA block are frequent and/or accompanied by a slow heart rate, the patient may show signs and symptoms of hemodynamic compromise. Clinical signs and symptoms of hemodynamic compromise include hypotension, chest pain, shortness of breath, changes in mental status, left ventricular failure, a fall in urine output, and cold, clammy skin.

Intervention

If the episodes of SA block are transient and there are no significant signs or symptoms, the patient is observed. If signs of hemodynamic compromise are present and are the result of medication toxicity, the offending agents should be withheld. If the episodes of SA block are frequent, IV atropine, temporary pacing, or insertion of a permanent pacemaker may be warranted.

SINUS ARREST

Sinus arrest is a disorder of the property of automaticity. In sinus arrest, the pacemaker cells of the SA node fail to initiate an electrical impulse (depolarize) for one or more beats. When the SA node fails to initiate an impulse, an escape pacemaker site (the AV junction or ventricles) should assume responsibility for pacing the heart. If they do not, absent PQRST complexes are observed on the ECG.

Sinus arrest is also called *sinus pause* or *SA arrest.*

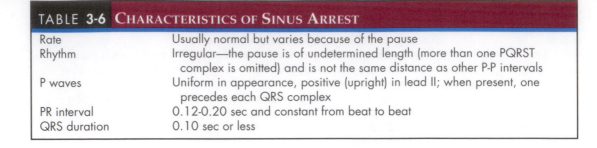

TABLE **3-6**	CHARACTERISTICS OF SINUS ARREST
Rate	Usually normal but varies because of the pause
Rhythm	Irregular—the pause is of undetermined length (more than one PQRST complex is omitted) and is not the same distance as other P-P intervals
P waves	Uniform in appearance, positive (upright) in lead II; when present, one precedes each QRS complex
PR interval	0.12-0.20 sec and constant from beat to beat
QRS duration	0.10 sec or less

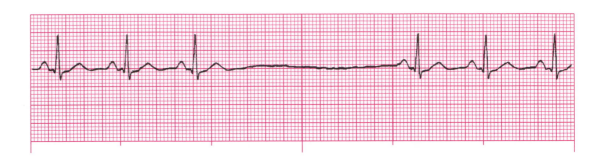

FIGURE **3-6**
Sinus arrest.

ECG Criteria

Sinus arrest (Figure 3-6) is characterized by an irregular rhythm caused by the pause(s) resulting from the sinus arrest. When present, a positive P wave (in lead II) precedes each QRS complex, and the P waves are uniform in appearance. Because the SA node periodically fails to generate impulses, the P-P intervals are not exact multiples of other P-P intervals. When present, the PR interval measures 0.12 to 0.20 sec and is constant from beat to beat. The duration of the QRS complex usually measures 0.10 sec or less unless an intraventricular conduction delay exists (Table 3-6).

Because the rhythmicity of this dysrhythmia occurs as the result of a specific event and the remainder of the rhythm is regular, the regularity (rhythm) may be described as irregular or as regular except for the event. Identification of this dysrhythmia should include the underlying rhythm and the duration of the sinus arrest. For example, "sinus bradycardia at 48 beats/min with a 3.8 sec period of sinus arrest."

Causes and Clinical Significance

Causes of sinus arrest include hypoxia, myocardial ischemia or infarction, hyperkalemia, digitalis toxicity, reactions to medications such as beta-blockers and calcium channel blockers, carotid sinus sensitivity, or increased vagal tone. Signs of hemodynamic compromise such as weakness, lightheadedness, dizziness, or syncope may be associated with this dysrhythmia.

Intervention

If the episodes of sinus arrest are transient and there are no significant signs or symptoms, the patient is observed. If hemodynamic compromise is present, IV atropine may be indicated. If the episodes of sinus arrest are frequent and/or prolonged (more than 3 seconds), temporary pacing or insertion of a permanent pacemaker may be warranted.

A summary of the characteristics of sinus mechanisms can be found in Table 3-7.

TABLE 3-7   SINUS MECHANISMS: SUMMARY OF CHARACTERISTICS

	Sinus rhythm	Sinus bradycardia	Sinus tachycardia	Sinus arrhythmia	SA block	Sinus arrest
Rate	60-100	<60	101-180	Usually 60-100	Varies	Varies
Rhythm	Regular	Regular	Regular	Irregular, typically phasic with respiration	Regular except for the event; pause is the same as (or an exact multiple of) the distance between two P-P intervals of underlying rhythm	Regular except for the event; pause of undetermined length, not a multiple of other P-P intervals
P waves (lead II)	Positive, one precedes each QRS	Positive, one precedes each QRS	Positive, one precedes each QRS	Positive, one precedes each QRS	When present, positive, one precedes each QRS	When present, positive, one precedes each QRS
PR interval	0.12-0.20 sec	0.12-0.20 sec	0.12-0.20 sec	0.12-0.20 sec	When present, 0.12-0.20 sec	When present, 0.12-0.20 sec
QRS	0.10 sec or less	0.10 sec or less	0.10 sec or less	0.10 sec or less	0.10 sec or less	0.10 sec or less
Clinical significance		May be asymptomatic; if decreased cardiac output occurs because of the slow rate, fatigue, syncope, lightheadedness, and/or hypotension may result	Normal response to increased demand for oxygen resulting from fever, pain, anxiety, hypoxia, CHF, fright, stress, etc; may be asymptomatic	Does not usually require intervention unless accompanied by a bradycardia that causes hemodynamic compromise	Usually asymptomatic; may be associated with signs/symptoms of decreased cardiac output, including altered mental status, dizziness, near-syncope, syncope, hypotension	May be associated with signs/symptoms of decreased cardiac output, including altered mental status, dizziness, near-syncope, syncope, hypotension

REFERENCES

1. Phillips RE, Feeney MK: *The cardiac rhythms: a systematic approach to interpretation,* ed 3, Philadelphia, 1990, WB Saunders.
2. Weil MH, Tang W, editors: *CPR: resuscitation of the arrested heart,* Philadelphia, 1999, WB Saunders.
3. Chou T, Knilans TK, *Electrocardiography in clinical practice: adult and pediatric,* Philadelphia, 1996, WB Saunders.
4. Murphy JG, *Mayo clinical cardiology review,* ed 2, Philadelphia, 2000, Lippincott, Williams & Wilkins.

BIBLIOGRAPHY

Anderson KN, Anderson LE, Glanze WD, editors: *Mosby's medical, nursing, and allied health dictionary,* ed 4, St Louis, 1994, Mosby.

Berne RM, Levy MN: *Cardiovascular physiology,* ed 7, St Louis, 1997, Mosby.

Chou T, Knilans TK: *Electrocardiography in clinical practice: adult and pediatric,* Philadelphia, 1996, WB Saunders.

Crawford MV, Spence MI: *Common sense approach to coronary care,* ed 6, St Louis, 1995, Mosby.

Ganong WF: *Review of medical physiology,* ed 17, Norwalk, Conn, 1995, Appleton & Lange.

Goldberger AL: *Clinical electrocardiography: a simplified approach,* ed 6, St Louis, 1999, Mosby.

Huszar RJ: *Basic dysrhythmias: interpretation and management,* ed 2, St Louis, 1994, Mosby.

Marriott HJL, Conover MB: *Advanced concepts in arrhythmias,* ed 3, St Louis, 1998, Mosby.

Murphy JG: *Mayo clinical cardiology review,* ed 2, Philadelphia, 2000, Lippincott, Williams & Wilkins.

Padrid PJ, Kowey PR, editors: *Cardiac arrhythmia: mechanisms, diagnosis, and management,* Baltimore, 1995, Williams & Wilkins.

Phillips RE, Feeney MK: *The cardiac rhythms: a systematic approach to interpretation,* ed 3, Philadelphia, 1990, WB Saunders.

Ryan TJ, Anderson JL, Antman EM, et al: ACC/AHA guidelines for the management of patients with acute myocardial infarction: a report of the American College of Cardiology/American Heart Association Task Force on Practice Guidelines (Committee on Management of Acute Myocardial Infarction), *J Am Coll Cardiol,* 28:1328-1428, 1996.

Thelan LA, Davie JK, Urden LD, Lough ME: *Critical care nursing: diagnosis and management,* ed 2, St Louis, 1994, Mosby.

Wagner GS: *Marriott's practical electrocardiography,* ed 9, Baltimore, 1994, Williams & Wilkins.

Woods SL, Sivarajan Froelicher ES, Motzer SA: *Cardiac nursing,* ed 4, Philadelphia, 2000, Lippincott, Williams & Wilkins.

MATCHING

_____ 1. Common dysrhythmia associated with respiratory rate
_____ 2. Appearance of P waves that originate from the SA node
_____ 3. Rate associated with a sinus bradycardia
_____ 4. If the SA node fails to generate an impulse, the next (escape) pacemaker that should generate an impulse
_____ 5. Dysrhythmia with a pause that is the same as (or an exact multiple of) the distance between two other P-P intervals
_____ 6. Normal rate for a sinus rhythm
_____ 7. Pacemaker with an intrinsic rate of 20 to 40 beats/min
_____ 8. Dysrhythmia that originates from the SA node and has a ventricular rate of 101 to 180 beats/min
_____ 9. Dysrhythmia with a pause of undetermined length that is not the same distance as other P-P intervals
_____ 10. Normal QRS duration in an adult

A. Sinus arrest
B. 60 to 100 beats/min
C. Sinus tachycardia
D. Ventricles
E. Less than 0.10 sec
F. Less than 60 beats/min
G. AV junction
H. Sinus arrhythmia
I. Sinoatrial (SA) block
J. Positive (upright) in lead II, one precedes each QRS

IDENTIFICATION AND MEASUREMENTS—PRACTICE RHYTHM STRIPS

For each of the following rhythm strips, determine the atrial and ventricular rates, measure the PR interval, QRS duration, and QT interval, and then identify the rhythm. All strips lead II unless otherwise noted.

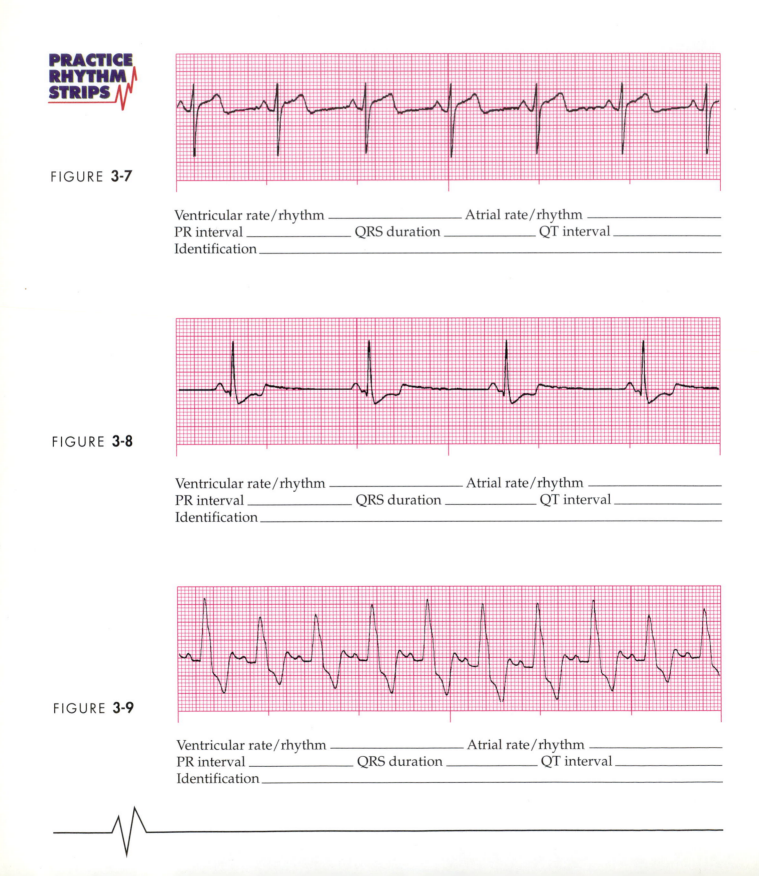

PRACTICE RHYTHM STRIPS

FIGURE **3-7**

Ventricular rate/rhythm _____ Atrial rate/rhythm _____
PR interval _____ QRS duration _____ QT interval _____
Identification _____

FIGURE **3-8**

Ventricular rate/rhythm _____ Atrial rate/rhythm _____
PR interval _____ QRS duration _____ QT interval _____
Identification _____

FIGURE **3-9**

Ventricular rate/rhythm _____ Atrial rate/rhythm _____
PR interval _____ QRS duration _____ QT interval _____
Identification _____

The rhythm strip below is from a 76-year-old female experiencing a syncopal episode. BP 80 by palpation, respirations 20. History of similar episodes recently. Home medications include propranolol.

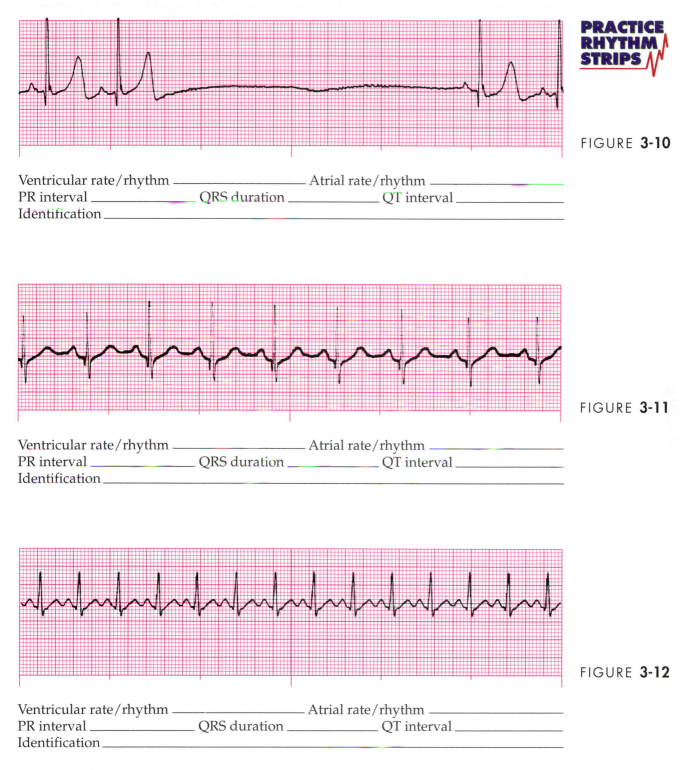

PRACTICE RHYTHM STRIPS

FIGURE **3-10**

Ventricular rate/rhythm _____ Atrial rate/rhythm _____
PR interval _____ QRS duration _____ QT interval _____
Identification _____

FIGURE **3-11**

Ventricular rate/rhythm _____ Atrial rate/rhythm _____
PR interval _____ QRS duration _____ QT interval _____
Identification _____

FIGURE **3-12**

Ventricular rate/rhythm _____ Atrial rate/rhythm _____
PR interval _____ QRS duration _____ QT interval _____
Identification _____

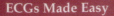

PRACTICE RHYTHM STRIPS

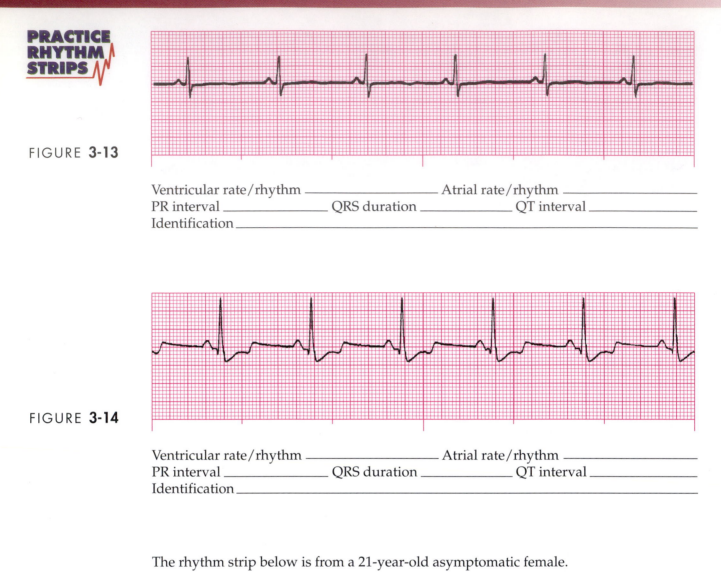

FIGURE **3-13**

Ventricular rate/rhythm _____ Atrial rate/rhythm _____
PR interval _____ QRS duration _____ QT interval _____
Identification _____

FIGURE **3-14**

Ventricular rate/rhythm _____ Atrial rate/rhythm _____
PR interval _____ QRS duration _____ QT interval _____
Identification _____

The rhythm strip below is from a 21-year-old asymptomatic female.

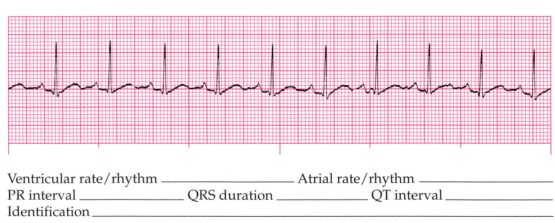

FIGURE **3-15**

Ventricular rate/rhythm _____ Atrial rate/rhythm _____
PR interval _____ QRS duration _____ QT interval _____
Identification _____

The rhythm strip below is from a 73-year-old male complaining of chest pain. History of hypertension and lung disease. Medications include aspirin, albuterol, and Lotensin.

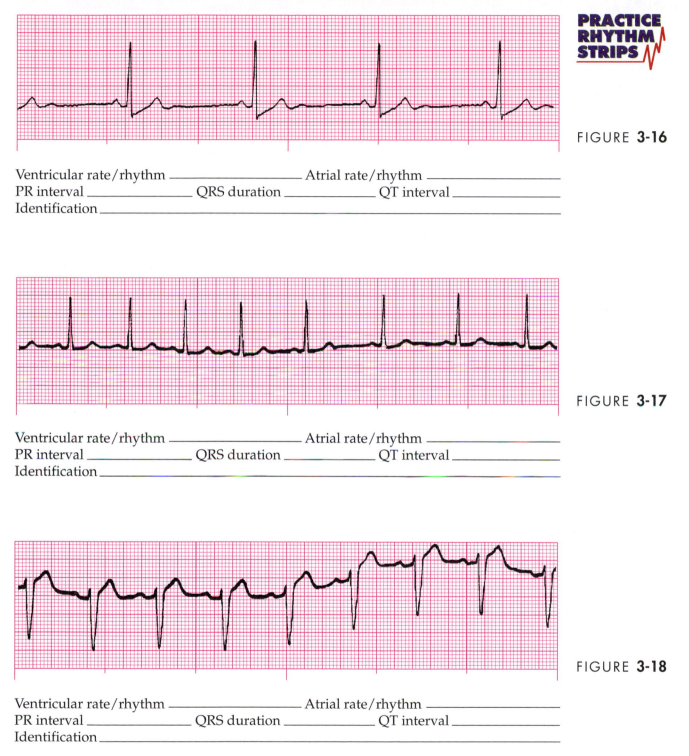

PRACTICE RHYTHM STRIPS

FIGURE **3-16**

Ventricular rate/rhythm _____ Atrial rate/rhythm _____
PR interval _____ QRS duration _____ QT interval _____
Identification _____

FIGURE **3-17**

Ventricular rate/rhythm _____ Atrial rate/rhythm _____
PR interval _____ QRS duration _____ QT interval _____
Identification _____

FIGURE **3-18**

Ventricular rate/rhythm _____ Atrial rate/rhythm _____
PR interval _____ QRS duration _____ QT interval _____
Identification _____

PRACTICE RHYTHM STRIPS

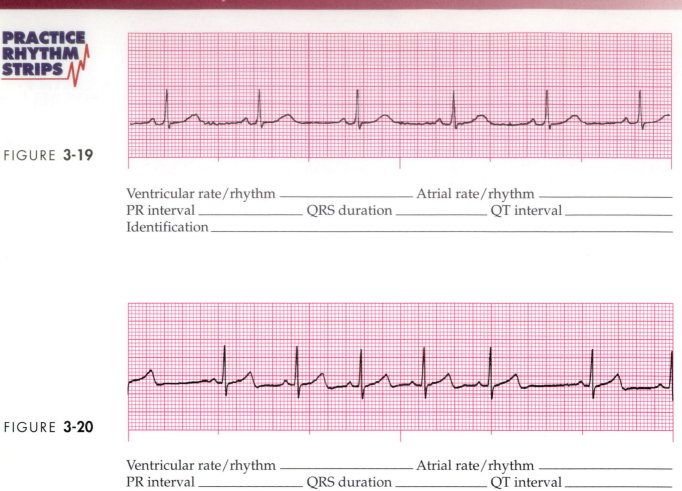

FIGURE **3-19**

Ventricular rate/rhythm ———————————— Atrial rate/rhythm ————————————
PR interval ———————— QRS duration ———————— QT interval ————————
Identification ————————————————————————————————————

FIGURE **3-20**

Ventricular rate/rhythm ———————————— Atrial rate/rhythm ————————————
PR interval ———————— QRS duration ———————— QT interval ————————
Identification ————————————————————————————————————

CHAPTER 4

Atrial Rhythms

OBJECTIVES

On completion of this chapter, you will be able to:

1. Describe the ECG characteristics, possible causes, signs and symptoms, and emergency management of each of the following dysrhythmias:
   a. Premature atrial complexes (PACs)
   b. Wandering atrial pacemaker (multiformed atrial rhythm)
   c. Multifocal atrial tachycardia (MAT)
   d. Supraventricular tachycardia (SVT)
   e. Atrioventricular nodal reentrant tachycardia (AVNRT)
   f. Atrioventricular reentrant tachycardia (AVRT)
   g. Wolff-Parkinson-White (WPW) syndrome
   h. Atrial flutter
   i. Atrial fibrillation (Afib)
2. Explain the concepts of altered automaticity, triggered activity, and reentry.
3. Explain the difference between a compensatory and noncompensatory pause.
4. Explain the terms *bigeminy, trigeminy, quadrigeminy,* and *"run"* when used to describe premature complexes.
5. Explain the terms *wandering atrial pacemaker* and *multifocal atrial tachycardia.*
6. Explain the term *paroxysmal supraventricular tachycardia (PSVT).*
7. List the three primary types of PSVT.
8. Compare and contrast supraventricular tachycardia and multifocal atrial tachycardia.
9. Explain the classification of AV nodal passive and AV nodal active supraventricular tachycardia.
10. List four examples of vagal maneuvers.
11. Discuss the indications and procedure for synchronized cardioversion.
12. Discuss preexcitation syndrome and name its three major forms.
13. Explain the terms *controlled* and *uncontrolled* when used to describe atrial fibrillation.
14. Explain why there is an increased risk of stroke associated with atrial fibrillation.

OVERVIEW

The atria are thin-walled, low-pressure chambers that receive blood from the systemic circulation and lungs. There is normally a continuous flow of blood from the superior and inferior vena cavae into the atria. Approximately 70% of this blood flows directly through the atria and into the ventricles before the atria contract. With atrial contraction, an additional 30% is added to filling of the ventricles. This additional contribution of blood because of atrial contraction is called **atrial kick.**

P waves reflect atrial depolarization. A rhythm originating from the SA node has one positive (upright) P wave before each QRS complex. A rhythm originating from the atria will have a positive P wave that is shaped differently than SA node–initiated P waves. This difference in P wave configuration occurs because the impulse originates in the atria and follows a different conduction pathway to the AV node.

Atrial Dysrhythmias: Mechanisms

The SA node, AV junction, and ventricular conduction system normally possess the property of automaticity—the ability to spontaneously depolarize. Atrial dysrhythmias reflect abnormal electrical impulse formation and conduction in the atria. They result from altered automaticity, triggered activity, or reentry. Altered automaticity and triggered activity are disorders in impulse *formation*. Reentry is a disorder in impulse *conduction*.

Altered Automaticity

Sinus tachycardia is an example of altered automaticity in normal pacemaker cells.

Altered automaticity occurs in normal pacemaker cells and in atrial, Purkinje, and ventricular fibers (myocardial working cells) that do not normally function as pacemaker sites. In altered automaticity, these cells depolarize and initiate impulses before a normal impulse.

Conditions that may predispose cardiac cells to altered automaticity include ischemia, drug toxicity, hypocalcemia, and an imbalance of electrolytes across the cardiac cell membrane. Atrial dysrhythmias associated with altered automaticity include premature atrial complexes, supraventricular tachycardia, atrial flutter, and atrial fibrillation.

Triggered Activity

Triggered activity results from abnormal electrical impulses that sometimes occur during repolarization (afterdepolarizations), when cells are normally quiet. Triggered activity requires a stimulus to initiate depolarization and occurs when escape pacemaker and myocardial working cells depolarize more than once after stimulation by a single impulse.

Causes of triggered activity include hypoxia, an increase in catecholamines, hypomagnesemia, myocardial ischemia and injury, and medications that prolong repolarization (e.g., quinidine). Triggered activity can result in atrial or ventricular beats that occur singly, in pairs, in "runs" (three or more beats), or as a sustained ectopic rhythm.

Reentry

Reentry (reactivation) is a condition in which an impulse returns to stimulate tissue that was previously depolarized. Reentry requires (1) a potential conduction circuit or circular conduction pathway, (2) a block within part of the circuit, and (3) delayed conduction within the remainder of the circuit[1] (Figure 4-1).

Normally, an impulse spreads through the heart only once after it is initiated by pacemaker cells. In reentry, however, an electrical impulse is delayed or blocked (or both) in

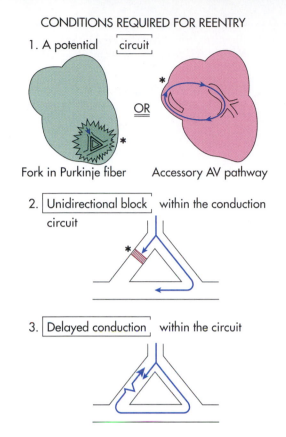

CONDITIONS REQUIRED FOR REENTRY

1. A potential | circuit |

OR

Fork in Purkinje fiber   Accessory AV pathway

2. | Unidirectional block | within the conduction circuit

3. | Delayed conduction | within the circuit

FIGURE 4-1
Reentry requires
(1) a potential
conduction circuit
or circular con-
duction pathway,
(2) a block within
part of the circuit,
and **(3)** delayed
conduction
within the re-
mainder of the
circuit.

one or more divisions of the conduction system while being conducted normally through the rest of the system. This results in the delayed electrical impulse entering cardiac cells that have just been depolarized by the normally conducted impulse.

If the delayed impulse stimulates a relatively refractory area, the impulse can cause depolarization of those cells, producing a single premature beat or repetitive electrical impulses, resulting in short periods of tachydysrhythmias. Common causes of reentry include hyperkalemia, myocardial ischemia, and some antidysrhythmic medications. Atrial dysrhythmias associated with reentry include premature atrial complexes (PACs) and paroxysmal supraventricular tachycardia (PSVT).

Most atrial dysrhythmias are not life-threatening, but some may be associated with extremely fast ventricular rates. Increases in heart rate shorten all phases of the cardiac cycle, but the most important is a decrease in the length of time spent in diastole. If diastole is shortened, there is less time for adequate ventricular filling. Thus an excessively rapid heart rate may compromise cardiac output.

Factors that influence heart rate include hormone levels (e.g., thyroxin, epinephrine, norepinephrine), medications, stress, anxiety, fear, and body temperature.

PREMATURE ATRIAL COMPLEXES (PACs)

ECG Criteria

Premature beats may be produced by the atria, AV junction, or the ventricles. Premature beats appear *early*, that is, they occur before the next expected beat.

Premature beats are identified by their site of origin (atrial, junctional, or ventricular). A **premature atrial complex (PAC)** occurs when an irritable site (focus) within the atria discharges before the next SA node impulse is due to discharge, thus interrupting the

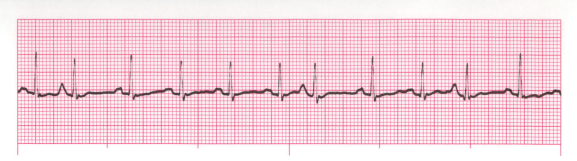

FIGURE 4-2
Sinus tachycardia with three PACs. From the left, beats 2, 7, and 10 are PACs.

FIGURE 4-3
PACs with and without abnormal conduction (aberrancy). First PAC *(arrow)* was conducted abnormally, producing a wide QRS complex. Second PAC *(arrow)* was conducted normally. Compare T waves preceding each PAC with those of underlying sinus bradycardia.

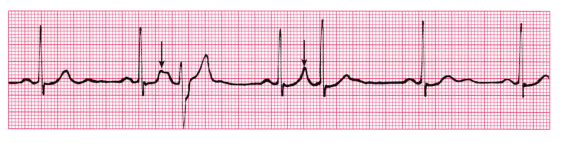

 The term *complex* is used instead of *contraction* to correctly identify an early beat because the ECG depicts electrical activity not mechanical function of the heart.

sinus rhythm. If the irritable site is close to the SA node, the atrial P wave will look very similar to the P waves initiated by the SA node. The P wave of a PAC may be biphasic (partly positive, partly negative), flattened, notched, or pointed.

When compared with the P-P intervals of the underlying rhythm, a PAC is premature—occurring before the next expected sinus P wave (Figure 4-2). Premature atrial complexes are identified by:

- Early (premature) P waves
- Positive (upright) P waves (in lead II) that differ in shape from sinus P waves
- Early P wave that may or may not be followed by a QRS complex

The PR interval of the PAC may be normal or prolonged, depending on the prematurity of the beat. QRS complexes associated with a PAC are typically identical or similar in shape and duration to those of the underlying rhythm because the impulse is conducted normally through the AV junction, bundle branches, and ventricles.

Aberrantly Conducted PACs
If a PAC occurs very early, the right bundle branch can be particularly slow to respond to the impulse *(refractory)*. The impulse travels down the left bundle branch without difficulty. Stimulation of the left bundle branch subsequently results in stimulation of the right bundle branch. Because of this delay in ventricular depolarization, the QRS will appear wide (greater than 0.10 sec). PACs associated with a wide QRS complex are called **aberrantly conducted PACs,** indicating conduction through the ventricles is abnormal (Figure 4-3).

Noncompensatory vs. Compensatory Pause
A **noncompensatory (incomplete) pause** often follows a PAC and represents the delay during which the SA node resets its rhythm for the next beat. A **compensatory (complete) pause** often follows premature ventricular complexes (PVCs) (Box 4-1).

Noncompensatory pause: A pause is termed *noncompensatory (or incomplete)* if the normal beat following the premature complex occurs before it was expected.

BOX 4-1 | DETERMINING NONCOMPENSATORY VS. COMPENSATORY PAUSES

To determine whether or not the pause following a premature complex is compensatory or noncompensatory, measure the distance between three normal beats. Then compare that measurement to the distance between three beats, one of which includes the premature complex.

A pause is termed **noncompensatory (or incomplete)** if the normal beat following the premature complex occurs before it was expected (i.e., the period between the complex before and after the premature beat is less than two normal R-R intervals).

A pause is termed **compensatory (or complete)** if the normal beat following the premature complex occurs when expected (i.e., the period between the complex before and after the premature beat is the same as two normal R-R intervals).

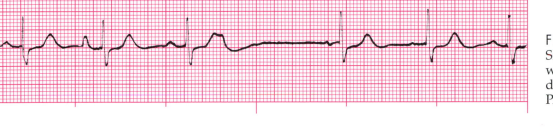

FIGURE **4-4**
Sinus rhythm with a nonconducted (blocked) PAC.

TABLE 4-1 | CHARACTERISTICS OF PREMATURE ATRIAL COMPLEXES (PACs)

Rate	Usually within normal range but depends on underlying rhythm
Rhythm	Regular with premature beats
P waves	Premature (occurring earlier than the next expected sinus P wave), positive (upright) in lead II, one precedes each QRS complex, often differ in shape from sinus P waves—may be flattened, notched, pointed, biphasic, or lost in the preceding T wave
PR interval	May be normal or prolonged, depending on the prematurity of the beat
QRS duration	Usually less than 0.10 sec but may be wide (aberrant) or absent, depending on the prematurity of the beat; the QRS of the PAC is similar in shape to those of the underlying rhythm unless the PAC is abnormally conducted

A PAC is not an entire rhythm—it is a single beat. Therefore it is important to identify the underlying rhythm and the ectopic beat(s), i.e., "sinus bradycardia at 46 beats/min with a PAC."

Nonconducted PACs

Sometimes, when the PAC occurs very prematurely and close to the T wave of the preceding beat, only a P wave may be seen with no QRS after it (appearing as a pause) (Figure 4-4). This type of PAC is termed a *nonconducted* or *blocked* PAC because the P wave occurred too early to be conducted. Nonconducted PACs occur because the AV junction is still refractory to stimulation and unable to conduct the impulse to the ventricles (thus no QRS complex).

Look for the early P wave in the T wave of the preceding beat. The T wave of the preceding beat may be of higher amplitude than other T waves or have an extra "hump," suggesting the presence of a hidden P wave (Table 4-1).

Compensatory pause: A pause is termed *compensatory (or complete)* if the normal beat following a premature complex occurs when expected.

When PACs occur in pairs, they are known as an *atrial couplet*.

PACs: Patterns
PACs may occur in patterns:

- *Pairs (coupled):* Two sequential PACs
- *"Runs" or "bursts":* Three or more sequential PACs; often called *paroxysmal* (meaning "sudden") *atrial tachycardia (PAT)* or *paroxysmal supraventricular tachycardia (PSVT)*
- *Atrial bigeminy (bigeminal PACs):* Every other beat is a PAC
- *Atrial trigeminy (trigeminal PACs):* Every third beat is a PAC
- *Atrial quadrigeminy (quadrigeminal PACs):* Every fourth beat is a PAC

Causes and Clinical Significance

PACs may be the result of enhanced automaticity or reentry.

PACs are very common. Their presence does not necessarily imply underlying cardiac disease. PACs may occur because of emotional stress, congestive heart failure, myocardial ischemia or injury, mental and physical fatigue, atrial enlargement, digitalis toxicity, hypokalemia, hypomagnesemia, hyperthyroidism, or excessive intake of caffeine, tobacco, or alcohol. PACs may be present in up to half of all patients with acute myocardial infarction.[2]

The patient may complain of a "skipped beat" or occasional "palpitations" (if PACs are frequent) or may be unaware of their occurrence. Because the rhythm is irregular, count the patient's pulse for a full minute.

Intervention

PACs usually do not require treatment if they are infrequent; however, frequent PACs may initiate episodes of atrial fibrillation, atrial flutter, or PSVT. Frequent PACs are treated by correcting the underlying cause: reducing stress, reducing consumption of caffeine-containing beverages, treating congestive heart failure, or correcting electrolyte imbalances. If needed, frequent PACs may be treated with beta-blockers, calcium channel blockers, and/or antianxiety medications.

WANDERING ATRIAL PACEMAKER

ECG Criteria

Multiformed atrial rhythm is an updated term for the rhythm formerly known as **wandering atrial pacemaker.** With this rhythm, the size, shape, and direction of the P waves vary, sometimes from beat to beat. The differences in P wave configuration reflect gradual shifting of the dominant pacemaker between the SA node, the atria, and/or the AV junction (Figure 4-5). At least three different P wave configurations, seen in the same lead, are required for a diagnosis of wandering atrial pacemaker.

Lead II (continuous)

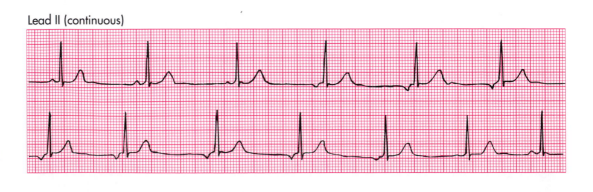

FIGURE 4-5
Wandering atrial pacemaker.

TABLE 4-2	CHARACTERISTICS OF WANDERING ATRIAL PACEMAKER (MULTIFORMED ATRIAL RHYTHM)
Rate	Usually 60-100 beats/min but may be slow; if the rate is greater than 100 beats/min, the rhythm is termed *multifocal* (or *chaotic*) *atrial tachycardia*
Rhythm	May be irregular as the pacemaker site shifts from the SA node to ectopic atrial locations and the AV junction
P waves	Size, shape, and direction may change from beat to beat; at least three different P wave configurations are required for a diagnosis of wandering atrial pacemaker or multifocal atrial tachycardia
PR interval	Variable
QRS duration	Usually less than 0.10 sec unless an intraventricular conduction delay exists

Wandering atrial pacemaker is associated with a normal or slow rate and irregular P-P, R-R, and PR intervals because of the different sites of impulse formation. The QRS duration is normally less than 0.10 sec because conduction through the ventricles is usually normal (Table 4-2).

Causes and Clinical Significance

Wandering atrial pacemaker may be observed in normal, healthy hearts (particularly in athletes) and during sleep. It may also occur with some types of organic heart disease and with digitalis toxicity. This dysrhythmia usually produces no signs and symptoms unless it is associated with a bradycardic rate.

Because the patient's pulse is irregular with MAT, count the patient's pulse for a full minute.

Interventions

If the rhythm occurs because of digitalis toxicity, the drug should be withheld.

MULTIFOCAL ATRIAL TACHYCARDIA

ECG Criteria

When the wandering atrial pacemaker is associated with a ventricular response of 100 beats/min or greater, the rhythm is termed **multifocal atrial tachycardia (MAT)** (Figure 4-6). MAT is also called *chaotic atrial tachycardia.* In MAT, multiple ectopic sites stimulate the atria. Multifocal atrial tachycardia may be confused with atrial fibrillation because both rhythms are irregular; however, P waves (although varying in size, shape, and direction) are clearly visible in MAT.

Causes and Clinical Significance

Multifocal atrial tachycardia is most commonly observed in elderly individuals and in persons with severe chronic obstructive pulmonary disease (COPD), acute myocardial

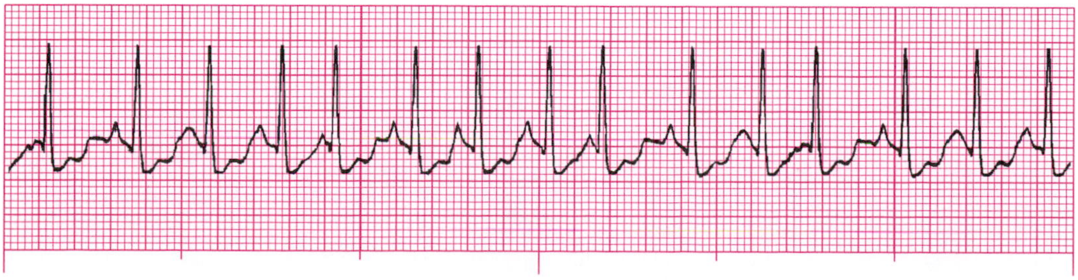

FIGURE **4-6**
Multifocal atrial tachycardia (MAT).

infarction, hypoxia, and theophylline toxicity. Also electrolyte imbalances, such as hypokalemia and hypomagnesemia, have been reported as the etiology of this dysrhythmia.[3]

Intervention

Treatment of MAT is directed at the underlying cause. If the patient is stable but symptomatic and has normal cardiac function, interventions may include medications such as calcium channel blockers, beta-blockers, or amiodarone. Carotid sinus pressure has no effect on MAT. Treatment of the stable but symptomatic patient with impaired cardiac function may include the use of amiodarone or diltiazem.

SUPRAVENTRICULAR TACHYCARDIA (SVT)

The term **supraventricular tachycardia (SVT)** may be used in two ways. First, it describes all tachydysrhythmias that originate above the bifurcation of the bundle of His. Thus SVTs can include sinus tachycardia, atrial tachycardia, atrial flutter, atrial fibrillation, and junctional tachycardia. Second, the term refers to a dysrhythmia with a rapid ventricular rate (tachycardia) and a narrow-QRS complex, but whose specific origin (atrial or junctional) is uncertain.

The term **paroxysmal** is used to describe the sudden onset or cessation of a dysrhythmia. Correct use of the term *paroxysmal* requires observing the onset or cessation of the dysrhythmia and identification of the underlying rhythm that preceded it. An SVT that starts or ends suddenly is called **paroxysmal supraventricular tachycardia (PSVT)** (Figure 4-7). In PSVT, the QRS is narrow unless there is an intraventricular conduction delay (bundle branch block).

SVT may occur because of altered automaticity, triggered activity, or reentry. The three primary types of PSVT are:

- Atrial tachycardia
- Atrioventricular nodal reentrant tachycardia (AVNRT)
- Atrioventricular reentrant tachycardia (AVRT)

Passive AV nodal SVTs include atrial tachycardia, atrial flutter, and atrial fibrillation.

"Supraventricular tachycardias can be classified into those that are AV nodal passive and those that are AV nodal active. AV nodal *passive* SVTs are those in which the AV node does not play a part in the maintenance of the tachycardia but serves only to conduct passively the supraventricular rhythm into the ventricles. AV nodal passive SVTs include atrial tachycardia, atrial flutter, and atrial fibrillation, all of which arise from

TABLE 4-3	CHARACTERISTICS OF SUPRAVENTRICULAR TACHYCARDIA (SVT)
Rate	150-250 beats/min
Rhythm	Regular
P waves	Atrial P waves may be observed that differ from sinus P waves
PR interval	If P waves are seen, the PRI will usually measure 0.12-0.20 sec
QRS duration	Less than 0.10 sec unless an intraventricular conduction delay exists

FIGURE **4-7**
Paroxysmal
supraventricular
tachycardia
(PSVT).

within the atria and do not need the AV node's participation to sustain the atrial arrhythmia. AV nodal *active* tachycardias require participation of the AV node in the maintenance of the tachycardia."[4] Regular, narrow-QRS tachycardias are most commonly caused by AVNRT and AVRT, both of which require the AV node as part of the reentry circuit that sustains the tachycardia (Table 4-3).

Atrial Tachycardia

ECG Criteria

Three or more sequential premature atrial complexes (PACs) occurring at a rate of more than 100/min is called **atrial tachycardia.** Atrial tachycardia that starts or ends suddenly is called **paroxysmal atrial tachycardia (PAT).** Paroxysmal atrial tachycardia may last for minutes, hours, or days.

Atrial tachycardia (Figure 4-8) is a series of rapid beats from an atrial ectopic focus, often precipitated by a PAC. This very rapid atrial rate overrides the SA node and becomes the pacemaker. Conduction of the atrial impulse to the ventricles is frequently 1:1 (i.e., every atrial impulse is conducted to the ventricles). Carotid sinus pressure, when used in an attempt to slow this type of paroxysmal atrial tachycardia, will either abruptly convert the dysrhythmia to a sinus rhythm or have no effect.

With very rapid atrial rates, the AV node begins to filter some of the impulses coming to it, thus protecting the ventricles from excessively rapid rates. When the AV node selectively filters conduction of some of these impulses, the dysrhythmia is called *paroxysmal atrial tachycardia (PAT) with block.* PAT with block is frequently associated with digitalis toxicity.

Atrial tachycardia is characterized by a regular atrial and ventricular rhythm occurring at a rate of 150 to 250 beats/min. One positive P wave precedes each QRS complex in lead II but the P waves differ in shape from sinus P waves. With rapid rates, it is difficult to distinguish P waves from T waves. The PR interval may be shorter or longer than normal and may be difficult to measure because P waves may be hidden in T waves. The QRS complex usually measures 0.10 sec or less unless an intraventricular conduction delay is present (Table 4-4).

A rhythm that lasts from three beats up to 30 seconds is called *nonsustained.* A *sustained* rhythm is one that lasts more than 30 seconds.

In healthy hearts, the AV node can rarely conduct 1:1 atrial impulses exceeding 180 beats/min.[5]

When the AV node blocks every other atrial impulse from traveling to the ventricles, the dysrhythmia is called *PAT with 2:1 block.*

When PAT with block exists, more than one P wave is present before each QRS.

TABLE 4-4 CHARACTERISTICS OF ATRIAL TACHYCARDIA	
Rate	150-250 beats/min
Rhythm	Regular
P waves	One positive P wave precedes each QRS complex in lead II but the P waves differ in shape from sinus P waves; with rapid rates, it is difficult to distinguish P waves from T waves
PR interval	May be shorter or longer than normal and may be difficult to measure because P waves may be hidden in T waves
QRS duration	0.10 sec or less unless an intraventricular conduction delay exists

FIGURE **4-8**
Atrial tachycardia.

AV Nodal Reentrant Tachycardia (AVNRT)

ECG Criteria

Although technically a dysrhythmia of junctional origin, AVNRT is discussed here because it was once thought to be a type of paroxysmal atrial tachycardia.

AVNRT is the most common type of PSVT. As its name implies, AV nodal reentrant tachycardia is caused by a reentrant focus in the area of the AV node. Two conduction pathways exist within the AV node that conduct impulses at different speeds and recover at different rates. The fast pathway conducts impulses rapidly but has a long refractory period (slow recovery time). The slow pathway conducts impulses slowly but has a short refractory period (fast recovery time)[6] (Figure 4-9). Under the right conditions, the fast and slow pathways can form an electrical circuit or loop. As one side of the loop is repolarizing, the other is depolarizing. Normally, conduction occurs down the fast pathway to activate the bundle of His and ventricles.

AVNRT is usually precipitated by a PAC that is propagated by the electrical circuit. This allows the impulse to spin around in a circle indefinitely, reentering the normal electrical pathway with each pass around the circuit. The result is a very rapid and regular rhythm that ranges from 150 to 250 beats/min (typically 170 to 250 beats/min).

Because AVNRT originates in the area of the AV node, the impulse spreads simultaneously to the atria and ventricles. This results in P waves that are often hidden in the QRS complex. If the ventricles are stimulated first and then the atria, a negative (inverted) P wave will appear after the QRS in leads II, III, and aVF. When the atria are depolarized after the ventricles, the P wave typically distorts the end of the QRS complex. P waves are not seen before the QRS complex; therefore, the PR interval is not measurable. The ventricular rhythm is usually very regular. The QRS is usually narrow (0.10 sec or less) because conduction through the ventricles is normal but may be wide if an intraventricular conduction delay exists (Table 4-5).

TABLE 4-5	CHARACTERISTICS OF AV NODAL REENTRANT TACHYCARDIA (AVNRT)
Rate	150-250 beats/min; typically 170-250 beats/min
Rhythm	Ventricular rhythm is usually very regular
P waves	P waves are often hidden in the QRS complex; if the ventricles are stimulated first and then the atria, a negative (inverted) P wave will appear after the QRS in leads II, III, and a VF; when the atria are depolarized after the ventricles, the P wave typically distorts the end of the QRS complex
PR interval	P waves are not seen before the QRS complex; therefore, the PR interval is not measurable
QRS duration	Less than 0.10 sec unless an intraventricular conduction delay exists

FIGURE 4-9 Schematic for typical AV nodal reentrant tachycardia (AVNRT). *AV*, AV node; *NSR*, normal sinus rhythm; *PAC*, premature atrial complex; *SVT*, supraventricular tachycardia.

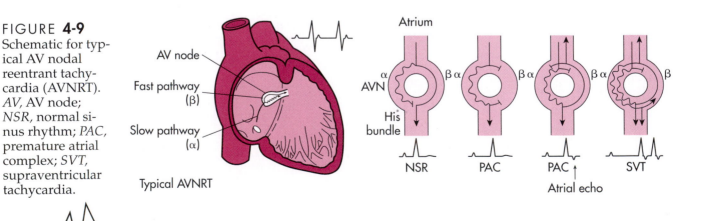

Causes and Clinical Significance

AVNRT is common in young, healthy individuals with no structural heart disease as well as in individuals with atherosclerotic or hypertensive heart disease. AVNRT is often precipitated by a premature complex. The primary symptom during AVNRT is palpitations. Rapid ventricular rates may be associated with lightheadedness, dyspnea, weakness, nervousness, chest pain or pressure, nausea, diaphoresis, dizziness, syncope, and possible signs of shock, depending on the duration and rate of the tachycardia and the presence of structural heart disease. Recurrent episodes vary in frequency, duration, and severity from several times a day to every 2 to 3 years.

Intervention

Intervention depends on the severity of the patient's signs and symptoms. Stable but symptomatic patients are treated with oxygen therapy, IV access, and vagal maneuvers such as coughing, gagging, holding one's breath, bearing down (Valsalva maneuver), or carotid sinus pressure (Box 4-2) (Figure 4-10). When vagal maneuvers are performed, baroreceptors in the carotid arteries are stimulated to slow AV conduction, resulting in slowing of the heart rate. If vagal maneuvers do not slow the rate or cause conversion of the tachycardia to a sinus rhythm, pharmacologic treatment may be necessary.

Premature complexes may be triggered by stress, caffeine, nicotine, alcohol, or medications that increase heart rate (beta-receptor agonists).

Although there is some overlap of the right and left vagus nerves, it is thought that the right vagus nerve has more fibers to the SA node and atrial muscle and the left vagus more fibers to the AV node and some ventricular muscle.

BOX 4-2 VAGAL MANEUVERS

Vagal maneuvers are methods used to stimulate baroreceptors located in the internal carotid arteries and the aortic arch. Stimulation of these receptors results in reflex stimulation of the vagus nerve and release of acetylcholine. Acetylcholine slows conduction through the AV node, resulting in slowing of the heart rate.

Examples of vagal maneuvers include:

- Coughing
- Bearing down
- Squatting
- Breath-holding
- Carotid sinus pressure (see Figure 4-10)
- Immersion of the face in ice water
- Stimulation of the gag reflex

Carotid pressure should be avoided in older patients. Simultaneous, bilateral carotid pressure should **never** be performed.

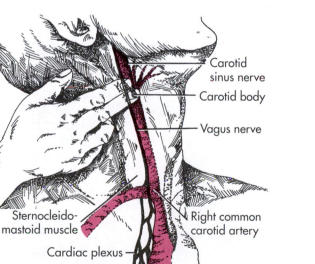

Carotid sinus nerve
Carotid body
Vagus nerve
Sternocleido-mastoid muscle
Right common carotid artery
Cardiac plexus

FIGURE 4-10 Carotid sinus pressure. The carotid sinus (carotid body) is located at the bifurcation of the carotid artery at the angle of the jaw.

Signs and symptoms of hemodynamic compromise include shock, chest pain, hypotension, shortness of breath, pulmonary congestion, congestive heart failure, acute MI, and/or decreased level of consciousness. The unstable patient should be treated with oxygen therapy, IV access, consideration of medication administration, possible sedation (if awake and time permits), followed by synchronized cardioversion (Box 4-3).

Recurrent AVNRT may require treatment with a long-acting calcium channel blocker (sustained-release verapamil, long-acting diltiazem) or long-acting beta-blockers. Class Ia (procainamide and quinidine) or Class Ic (propafenone and flecainide) antidysrhythmic medications may also be used.

BOX 4-3   ELECTRICAL THERAPY: SYNCHRONIZED CARDIOVERSION

DESCRIPTION AND PURPOSE

Synchronized cardioversion reduces the potential for delivery of energy during the vulnerable period of the T wave (relative refractory period). A synchronizing circuit allows the delivery of a countershock to be "programmed." The machine searches for the highest (R wave deflection) or deepest (QS deflection) part of the QRS complex and delivers the shock a few milliseconds after this portion of the complex.

INDICATIONS (UNSTABLE PATIENT)
- Supraventricular tachycardia
- Atrial fibrillation
- Atrial flutter
- Ventricular tachycardia with a pulse

PROCEDURE
1. Administer sedation if the patient is awake and time permits.
2. Apply conductive material to the defibrillator paddles (gel) or chest wall (disposable defibrillator pads). Remove nitroglycerin paste/patches from the patient's chest if present.
3. Turn on the defibrillator.
4. Select the appropriate energy level for the clinical situation/dysrhythmia.
5. Press the synchronizer switch/button.
6. Ensure machine sensing of the QRS complex.
7. Place the defibrillator paddles (or self-adhesive defib pads) on the patient's chest. If using manual defibrillator paddles, apply firm pressure (Figure 4-11).
8. Charge the paddles and recheck the ECG rhythm.
9. LOOK (360 degrees) to be sure the area is clear. Call "Clear!"
10. Depress both discharge buttons on the paddles simultaneously to deliver the shock.
11. Reassess the ECG rhythm and patient.

FIGURE 4-11
Paddle placement for synchronized cardioversion (and defibrillation). The sternum paddle is placed to the right of the upper sternum just below the clavicle. The apex paddle is placed in the left midaxillary line.

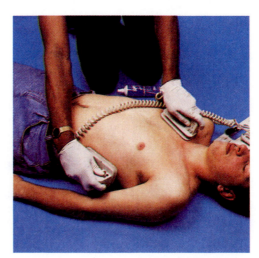

Patients who are resistant to drug therapy or who do not wish to remain on life-long medications for AVNRT are candidates for radiofrequency catheter ablation. Radiofrequency catheter ablation is rapidly becoming the treatment of choice in the management of patients with symptomatic recurrent episodes of AVNRT. Electrophysiologic studies are done to locate the abnormal pathways and reentry circuits. Once localized, a special ablation catheter is placed at the site of the abnormal pathway. Low-energy, high-frequency current is delivered through this catheter. With each burst of energy from the catheter, an area of tissue is destroyed (ablated). The energy is applied in various areas until the unwanted pathway is no longer functional and the circuit is broken. Catheter ablation is more than 95% successful in permanently interrupting the circuit and curing the dysrhythmia.[7]

AV Reentrant Tachycardia (AVRT)

The next most common type of PSVT is AV reentrant tachycardia (AVRT). **Preexcitation** is a term used to describe rhythms that originate from above the ventricles but in which the impulse travels via a pathway other than the AV node and bundle of His. Thus the supraventricular impulse excites the ventricles earlier than would be expected if the impulse traveled by way of the normal conduction system. Patients with preexcitation syndromes are prone to AVRT.

Preexcitation: A term used to describe rhythms that originate from above the ventricles but in which the impulse travels via a pathway other than the AV node and bundle of His— thus the supraventricular impulse excites the ventricles earlier than normal.

During fetal development, strands of myocardial tissue form connections between the atria and ventricles, outside the normal conduction system. These strands normally become nonfunctional shortly after birth; however, in patients with preexcitation syndrome, these connections persist as congenital malformations of working myocardial tissue. Because these connections bypass part or all of the normal conduction system, they are called **accessory pathways.** The term **bypass tract** is used when one end of an accessory pathway is attached to normal conductive tissue. This pathway may connect the right atrial and ventricular walls, the left atrial and ventricular walls, or connect the atrial and ventricular septa on either the right or the left side.

There are three major forms of preexcitation syndrome, each differentiated by its accessory pathway or bypass tract[1] (Figure 4-12).

1. In **Wolff-Parkinson-White (WPW) syndrome,** the accessory pathway is called the *Kent bundle.* This bundle connects the atria directly to the ventricles, completely bypassing the normal conduction system.
2. In **Lown-Ganong-Levine (LGL) syndrome,** the accessory pathway is called the *James bundle.* This bundle connects the atria directly to the lower portion of the AV node, thus partially bypassing the AV node. In LGL syndrome, one end of the James bundle is attached to normal conductive tissue. This congenital pathway may be called a *bypass tract.*

Delta waves are produced with accessory pathways that insert directly into ventricular muscle.

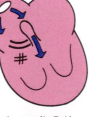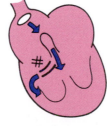

Kent (W-P-W) short P-R with Δ wave

James (L-G-L) short P-R without Δ wave

Mahaim normal P-R with Δ wave

FIGURE **4-12** Three major forms of preexcitation. Note location of the accessory pathways and corresponding ECG characteristics.

3. Another unnamed preexcitation syndrome involves the *Mahaim fibers*. These fibers do not bypass the AV node but originate below the AV node and insert into the ventricular wall, bypassing part or all of the ventricular conduction system.

Because WPW is the most common type of preexcitation syndrome, it will be the focus of our discussion regarding AVRT.

ECG Criteria

In WPW associated with a sinus rhythm, the P wave is of normal shape, and the PR interval is less than 0.12 sec because the normal delay in the AV node is bypassed. The QRS duration typically exceeds 0.12 sec because part of the ventricle receives the impulse early through the accessory pathway and begins to depolarize in a cell-to-cell fashion before the rest of the ventricle is activated by the normal conduction system.

This preexcitation of the ventricles results in distortion of the initial portion of the QRS complex, observed as an initial slurring and slowly rising onset of the QRS in some leads (delta wave) (Figure 4-13). The delta wave is the initial slurred deflection at the beginning of the QRS complex that results from initial activation of the QRS by conduction over the accessory pathway (Table 4-6).[7]

Causes and Clinical Significance

WPW is sometimes called *bundle of Kent syndrome,* named after Stanley Kent, a London physiologist.

WPW is more common in males than females and approximately two thirds of individuals with WPW have no associated heart disease.[3] WPW occurs in approximately 4 out of 100,000 people and is one of the most common causes of tachydysrhythmias in infants and children. Although the accessory pathway in WPW is believed to be congenital in origin, symptoms associated with preexcitation often do not appear until young adulthood.

Individuals with preexcitation syndrome are predisposed to tachydysrhythmias because there is a loss of the protective blocking mechanism provided by the AV node and because the accessory pathway provides a mechanism for reentry. Signs and symptoms associated with rapid ventricular rates may include palpitations, anxiety, weakness, dizziness, chest pain, shortness of breath, and shock.

TABLE 4-6	CHARACTERISTICS OF WOLFF-PARKINSON-WHITE (WPW) SYNDROME
Rate	Usually 60-100 beats/min if the underlying rhythm is sinus in origin
Rhythm	Regular, unless associated with atrial fibrillation
P waves	Normal and positive in lead II unless WPW is associated with atrial fibrillation
PR interval	If P waves are observed, less than 0.12 sec
QRS duration	Usually greater than 0.12 sec; slurred upstroke of the QRS complex (delta wave) may be seen in one or more leads

FIGURE **4-13**
Typical Wolff-Parkinson-White pattern showing the short PR interval, delta wave, wide QRS complex, and secondary ST and T-wave changes.

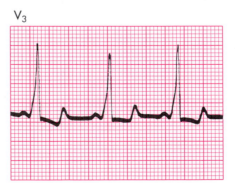

V₃

PSVT and atrial fibrillation are the two most common tachydysrhythmias seen in WPW. Atrial fibrillation and atrial flutter that occur in the presence of an accessory pathway are particularly dangerous because of the extremely rapid ventricular rate than can result from conduction of the atrial impulses directly into the ventricles. The ventricular rate can be 250 to 300 beats/min and can deteriorate into ventricular fibrillation, resulting in sudden death.[4]

Intervention

The stable but symptomatic patient with AVRT may be managed with oxygen therapy, IV access, attempts to slow or convert the rhythm with vagal maneuvers, and, if unsuccessful, administration of amiodarone. Medications used to slow AV conduction such as digoxin and verapamil should be **avoided** because they may accelerate the speed of conduction through the accessory pathway, resulting in a further increase in heart rate. If the patient presents with signs and symptoms of hemodynamic compromise because of the rapid ventricular rate, preparations should be made for synchronized cardioversion.

ATRIAL FLUTTER

Atrial flutter is an ectopic atrial rhythm in which an irritable site depolarizes regularly at an extremely rapid rate. Atrial flutter has been classified into two types. Type I atrial flutter is caused by a reentrant circuit that is localized in the right atrium. Type I atrial flutter is also called *typical* or *classical atrial flutter.* Type II atrial flutter is called *atypical* or *very rapid atrial flutter.* Patients with type II atrial flutter often develop atrial fibrillation. The precise mechanism of type II atrial flutter has not been defined.

In atrial flutter, an irritable focus within the atrium typically depolarizes at a rate of 300/min. If each impulse were transmitted to the ventricles, the ventricular rate would equal 300/min. The healthy AV node protects the ventricles from these extremely fast atrial rates.

Normally, the AV node cannot conduct faster than approximately 180 impulses/min. Thus, at an atrial rate of 300/min, every other impulse arrives at the AV node while it is still refractory. The resulting ventricular response of 150 beats/min is called 2:1 conduction. (The ratio of the atrial rate [300/min] to the ventricular rate [150/min] is 2 to 1). Conduction ratios in atrial flutter are usually even (2:1, 4:1, 6:1) but can vary. In individuals with an accessory pathway, atrial flutter may be associated with 1:1 conduction (because the AV node is bypassed), producing extremely rapid ventricular rates.

ECG Criteria

In type I atrial flutter, the atrial rate ranges from 250 to 350 beats/min. In type II atrial flutter, the atrial rate ranges from 350 to 450 beats/min. Because of this extremely rapid stimulation, waveforms are produced that resemble the teeth of a saw, or a picket fence, called "flutter" waves (Figure 4-14). Flutter waves are thought to consist of the atrial

WPW associated with atrial fibrillation may be confused with ventricular tachycardia because of its wide QRS complex; however, WPW is usually irregular; ventricular tachycardia is usually regular.

Medications such as digoxin and verapamil slow conduction over the AV node but not across the accessory pathway.

Atrial flutter with an atrial rate of 300 beats/min and a ventricular rate of 75/min = 4:1 conduction; 50/min = 6:1 conduction, etc.

Flutter waves are also referred to as *F waves.*

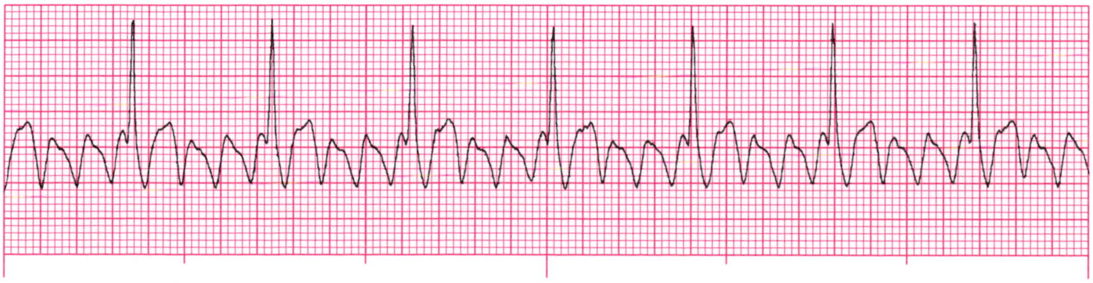

FIGURE **4-14**
Atrial flutter.

depolarization wave followed by the atrial repolarization wave (the atrial T wave) that is not often observed with other dysrhythmias. Flutter waves are best observed in leads II, III, aVF, and V_1.

Because P waves are not observed with this rhythm, the PR interval is not measurable. The QRS complex during atrial flutter is usually 0.10 sec or less because atrial flutter is a supraventricular rhythm, and the impulse is conducted normally through the AV junction and ventricles. However, if flutter waves are buried in the QRS complex or if an intraventricular conduction delay exists, the QRS will appear wide (greater than 0.10 sec).

Because conduction ratios in atrial flutter are usually even (2:1, 4:1, 6:1), the ventricular rhythm is often regular; however, variable conduction can also occur, producing an irregular ventricular rhythm (Table 4-7).

Causes and Clinical Significance

Count the patient's pulse for a full minute.

Atrial flutter is usually a paroxysmal rhythm precipitated by a PAC that may last for seconds to hours and occasionally 24 hours or more. Chronic atrial flutter is unusual because the rhythm usually reverts to sinus rhythm or atrial fibrillation, either spontaneously or with treatment.[6]

Atrial flutter is reportedly more common in men than in women (4.7 to 1).[6]

Atrial flutter may occur in conditions such as pulmonary embolism, chronic ventilatory failure, thyrotoxicosis, alcohol intoxication, ischemic heart disease, hypoxia, or digitalis or quinidine toxicity. Atrial flutter most often occurs in patients with mitral or tricuspid valve disease but may occur (rarely) in patients without cardiac disease. This dysrhythmia is common after cardiac surgery and occurs in approximately 5% of patients after acute myocardial infarction.

The severity of signs and symptoms associated with atrial flutter vary, depending on the ventricular rate, the duration of the dysrhythmia, and the patient's cardiovascular status. The more rapid the ventricular rate, the more likely the patient is to be symptomatic with this dysrhythmia. The patient may be asymptomatic and not require treatment or may experience serious signs and symptoms and complain of palpitations or skipped beats, weakness, dizziness, or chest pressure/pain.

Intervention

Vagal maneuvers will not convert atrial flutter because the reentry circuit is located in the atria not the AV node.

When atrial flutter is present with 2:1 conduction, it may be difficult to differentiate the dysrhythmia from sinus tachycardia, atrial tachycardia, AV nodal reentrant tachycardia,

TABLE 4-7	CHARACTERISTICS OF ATRIAL FLUTTER
Rate	Atrial rate 250-450 beats/min, typically 300 beats/min; ventricular rate variable—determined by AV blockade; the ventricular rate will usually not exceed 180 beats/min because of the intrinsic conduction rate of the AV junction
Rhythm	Atrial regular, ventricular regular or irregular depending on AV conduction/blockade
P waves	No identifiable P waves; saw-toothed "flutter" waves are present
PR interval	Not measurable
QRS duration	Usually less than 0.10 sec but may be widened if flutter waves are buried in the QRS complex or an intraventricular conduction delay exists

AV reentrant tachycardia, or PSVT. Vagal maneuvers may help identify the rhythm by temporarily slowing AV conduction and revealing the underlying flutter waves.

In cases of atrial flutter associated with a rapid ventricular rate, treatment is first directed toward controlling the ventricular response. If cardiac function is normal, medications such as calcium channel blockers (e.g., diltiazem, verapamil) or beta-blockers (e.g., esmolol, metoprolol, propranolol) should be used. If cardiac function is impaired, medications such as digoxin, diltiazem, or amiodarone may be used.

If the patient exhibits serious signs and symptoms (shortness of breath, chest pain, hypotension, decreased level of consciousness, acute MI, congestive heart failure) because of the rapid ventricular rate, synchronized cardioversion may be performed. Atrial flutter may convert to a sinus rhythm with as little as 25 joules, although at least 50 joules is generally recommended.

> Some cardiologists recommend an initial synchronized shock with 100 joules because it is nearly always successful in converting atrial flutter.

Radiofrequency catheter ablation for type I atrial flutter is associated with a success rate of 80% to 90%.[7]

ATRIAL FIBRILLATION (AFIB)

Atrial fibrillation (Afib) occurs because of multiple reentry circuits in the atria. This dysrhythmia may occur acutely (lasting less than 48 hours), paroxysmally (intermittent), or chronically (lasting at least 1 month). In atrial fibrillation, the atria are depolarized at a rate of 400 to 600 beats/min. These rapid impulses cause the muscles of the atria to quiver (fibrillate), resulting in ineffectual atrial contraction, a subsequent decrease in cardiac output, and loss of atrial kick.

> Atrial fibrillation is the most common sustained dysrhythmia.

ECG Criteria

In atrial fibrillation, the AV node attempts to protect the ventricles from the hundreds of impulses bombarding it per minute by blocking many of the impulses generated by the irritable sites in the atria. The ventricular rate and rhythm are determined by the degree of blocking by the AV node of these rapid impulses.

> In patients with a normal AV junction, new onset Afib is typically associated with a ventricular rate between 110 and 180 beats/min.[8]

Because of the quivering of the atrial muscle and because there is no uniform wave of atrial depolarization in atrial fibrillation, there is no P wave. Instead, the baseline is erratic (wavy) in appearance, corresponding with the atrial rate of 400 to 600 beats/min. These wavy deflections are called "fibrillatory" waves (Figure 4-15).

> Fibrillatory waves are referred to as *f waves*.

In Afib, atrial depolarization occurs very irregularly, and the ventricular response (rhythm) is usually very irregular. The ventricular rhythm associated with atrial

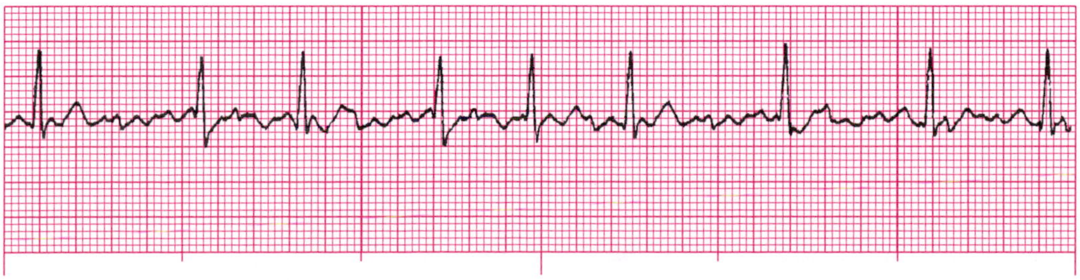

FIGURE **4-15**
Atrial fibrillation.

FIGURE **4-16**
Atrial fibrillation
with complete AV
block. Ventricular
rate is slow and
regular because of
the block.

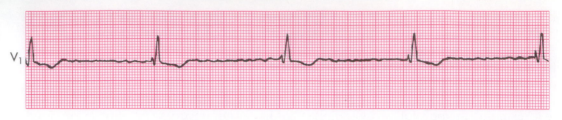

TABLE **4-8**	CHARACTERISTICS OF ATRIAL FIBRILLATION
Rate	Atrial rate usually greater than 400-600 beats/min; ventricular rate variable
Rhythm	Ventricular rhythm usually irregularly irregular
P waves	No identifiable P waves; fibrillatory waves present; erratic, wavy baseline
PR interval	Not measurable
QRS duration	Usually less than 0.10 sec but may be widened if an intraventricular conduction delay exists

The presence of an accessory pathway should be considered in Afib with a ventricular rate of more than 180 beats/min.

fibrillation is described as *irregularly irregular.* When the ventricular rate is less than 100 beats/min, atrial fibrillation is termed *controlled.* When above 100 beats/min, it is called *uncontrolled.*

Afib can occur simultaneously with complete AV block. The resulting ventricular rhythm will be slow and regular (Figure 4-16). Consider digitalis toxicity when atrial fibrillation is accompanied by a slow ventricular rate.

The PR interval is not measurable because no P waves are seen with this dysrhythmia. The duration of the QRS complex is usually 0.10 sec or less because the rhythm is supraventricular in origin, and the impulse is conducted normally through the AV junction and ventricles. However, if the impulse travels abnormally through the ventricles, the QRS will appear wide (>0.10 sec) (Table 4-8).

Causes and Clinical Significance

Count the patient's pulse for a full minute.

Atrial fibrillation is observed in about 15% of patients with acute MI; atrial flutter is much less common.[9]

Conditions commonly associated with atrial fibrillation include rheumatic heart disease, coronary artery disease, hypertension, mitral or tricuspid valve disease, congestive heart failure, pericarditis, pulmonary embolism, cardiomyopathy, and hypoxia. Other precipitants of atrial fibrillation include drugs or intoxicants (e.g., alcohol, carbon monoxide), acute or chronic pulmonary disease, enhanced vagal tone, enhanced sympathetic tone, hypokalemia, and hyperthyroidism. Paroxysmal atrial fibrillation has been associated with excessive alcohol consumption in otherwise healthy individuals ("holiday heart syndrome").[8]

Patients experiencing Afib may develop intra-atrial emboli because the atria are not contracting, and blood stagnates in the atrial chambers. This predisposes the patient to systemic emboli, particularly stroke, if the clots dislodge spontaneously or because of conversion to a sinus rhythm. It is estimated that 15% to 20% of strokes in patients without rheumatic heart disease are the result of atrial fibrillation, and the incidence is even higher for those with rheumatic heart disease.[7]

The severity of signs and symptoms associated with atrial fibrillation vary, depending on the ventricular rate, the duration of the dysrhythmia, and the patient's cardiovascular status. The more rapid the ventricular rate, the more likely the patient is to be symptomatic with this dysrhythmia.

The patient may be asymptomatic or may experience serious signs and symptoms. Atrial fibrillation with a rapid ventricular response may produce signs and symptoms that include lightheadedness, palpitations, dyspnea, chest pressure/pain, and hypotension.

Afib with a rapid ventricular response is commonly called *Afib with RVR.*

Intervention

In the stable patient with atrial fibrillation associated with a rapid ventricular rate, treatment is first directed toward controlling the ventricular response, rather than converting the dysrhythmia to a sinus rhythm. If cardiac function is normal, calcium channel blockers or beta-blockers may be used. If cardiac function is impaired, medications such as digoxin, diltiazem, or amiodarone may be used.

Medications that slow conduction through the AV node will not generally convert Afib (or atrial flutter) to a sinus rhythm because the reentry circuit is located in the atria, not the AV node, and is not affected.

To convert atrial fibrillation to sinus rhythm, Class Ia medications (procainamide), Class Ic agents (flecainide, propafenone), and/or Class III antidysrhythmics (such as amiodarone) may be used. Amiodarone is an effective medication for patients with congestive heart failure and atrial fibrillation. Although associated with a number of side effects, low-dose amiodarone appears to be well tolerated. Ibutilide (a Class III antidysrhythmic) is also used to convert atrial fibrillation to sinus rhythm but works best in new-onset atrial fibrillation.

Class Ia medications may be associated with significant side effects, including torsades de pointes (TdP).

If the patient exhibits serious signs and symptoms (shortness of breath, chest pain, hypotension, decreased level of consciousness, acute MI, congestive heart failure) because of the rapid ventricular rate, synchronized cardioversion may be considered.

Elective cardioversion may be performed in patients that fail to respond to an initial trial of medications. Anticoagulation is recommended for any patient undergoing elective cardioversion. A widely accepted practice is to begin prophylactic anticoagulation 2 to 3 weeks before and continue therapy for about 4 weeks after the procedure.

Radiofrequency catheter ablation for individuals with symptomatic atrial fibrillation refractory to medication therapy is associated with a success rate of 100%, but chronic pacemaker therapy is required if the energy is used to produce complete AV block. Newer modifications of this technique involve application of the radiofrequency energy to portions of the AV junction to modify (but not completely destroy) AV nodal conduction.[7]

A summary of atrial rhythm characteristics can be found in Table 4-9.

TABLE 4-9 ATRIAL RHYTHMS: SUMMARY OF CHARACTERISTICS

	PACs	Wandering atrial pacemaker	SVT	WPW	Atrial flutter	Atrial fibrillation
Rate	Usually within normal range but depends on underlying rhythm	Usually 60-100/min; if rate greater than 100/min, the rhythm is termed *multifocal atrial tachycardia*	150-250/min	Usually 60-100 beats/min if the underlying rhythm is sinus in origin	Atrial rate 250-450/min; typically 300/min; ventricular rate variable, determined by AV blockade	Atrial rate 400-600/min; ventricular rate variable
Rhythm	Regular with premature beats	May be irregular as pacemaker site shifts from SA node to ectopic atrial locations and AV junction	Regular	Regular, unless associated with atrial fibrillation	Atrial regular, ventricular regular or irregular	Ventricular rhythm usually irregularly irregular
P waves (lead II)	Premature, positive in lead II, one precedes each QRS, differ from sinus P waves, may be lost in preceding T wave	Size, shape, and direction may change from beat to beat	Atrial P waves may be observed that differ from sinus P waves	Normal and positive in lead II unless WPW is associated with atrial fibrillation	No identifiable P waves; saw-toothed "flutter" waves present; "sawtooth," "picket fence"	No identifiable P waves; fibrillatory waves present; erratic, wavy baseline
PR interval	May be normal or prolonged	Variable	If P waves are seen, the PRI will usually measure 0.12-0.20 sec	If P waves are observed, less than 0.12 sec	Not measurable	Not measurable
QRS	0.10 sec or less, unless abnormally conducted	Usually less than 0.10 sec	Usually less than 0.10 sec	Usually greater than 0.12 sec; delta wave may be seen in one or more leads	Usually less than 0.10 sec	Usually less than 0.10 sec
Clinical significance	Very common; presence does not imply underlying cardiac disease	Usually produces no signs and symptoms, unless associated with bradycardic rate	Rapid ventricular rate may decrease cardiac output	Extremely rapid ventricular rates possible, producing serious signs and symptoms	If accompanied by a rapid ventricular rate, there is decreased cardiac output; may deteriorate to Afib	If accompanied by a rapid ventricular rate, there is decreased cardiac output, increased stroke risk

REFERENCES

1. Crawford MV, Spence MI: *Common sense approach to coronary care,* ed 6, St Louis, 1995, Mosby.
2. Murphy JG: *Mayo clinical cardiology review,* ed 2, Philadelphia, 2000, Lippincott, Williams & Wilkins.
3. Chou T, Knilans TK: *Electrocardiography in clinical practice: adult and pediatric,* Philadelphia, 1996, WB Saunders.
4. Woods SL, Sivarajan Froelicher ES, Motzer SA: *Cardiac nursing,* ed 4, Philadelphia, 2000, Lippincott, Williams & Wilkins.
5. Touboul P, Waldo, AL: *Atrial arrhythmias: current concepts and management,* St Louis, 1990, Mosby.
6. Padrid PJ, Kowey PR, editors: *Cardiac arrhythmia: mechanisms, diagnosis, and management,* Baltimore, 1995, Williams & Wilkins.
7. Goldman L, Braunwald E: *Primary cardiology,* Philadelphia, 1998, WB Saunders.
8. Goldberger AL: *Clinical electrocardiography: a simplified approach,* ed 6, St Louis, 1999, Mosby.
9. Weil MH, Tang W, editors: *CPR: resuscitation of the arrested heart,* Philadelphia, 1999, WB Saunders.

BIBLIOGRAPHY

Berne RM, Levy MN: *Cardiovascular physiology,* ed 7, St Louis, 1997, Mosby.

Braunwauld E, Scheinman M, editors: *Arrhythmias: electrophysiologic principles,* Vol IX, Singapore, 1996, Current Medicine/Mosby.

Chou T, Knilans TK: *Electrocardiography in clinical practice: adult and pediatric,* Philadelphia, 1996, WB Saunders.

Crawford MV, Spence MI: *Common sense approach to coronary care,* ed 6, St Louis, 1995, Mosby.

Goldberger AL: *Clinical electrocardiography: a simplified approach,* ed 6, St Louis, 1999, Mosby.

Goldman L, Braunwald E: *Primary cardiology,* Philadelphia, 1998, WB Saunders.

Johnson R, Swartz MH: *A simplified approach to electrocardiography,* Philadelphia, 1986, WB Saunders.

Marriott HJL, Conover MB: *Advanced concepts in arrhythmias,* ed 3, St Louis, 1998, Mosby.

Murphy JG: *Mayo clinical cardiology review,* ed 2, Philadelphia, 2000, Lippincott, Williams & Wilkins.

Padrid PJ, Kowey PR, editors: *Cardiac arrhythmia: mechanisms, diagnosis, and management,* Baltimore, 1995, Williams & Wilkins.

Phillips RE, Feeney MK: *The cardiac rhythms: a systematic approach to interpretation,* ed 3, Philadelphia, 1990, WB Saunders.

Ryan TJ, Anderson JL, Antman EM, et al: ACC/AHA guidelines for the management of patients with acute myocardial infarction: a report of the American College of Cardiology/American Heart Association Task Force on Practice Guidelines (Committee on Management of Acute Myocardial Infarction), *J Am Coll Cardiol* 28:1328-1428, 1996.

Touboul P, Waldo AL: *Atrial arrhythmias: current concepts and management,* St Louis, 1990, Mosby.

Wagner GS: *Marriott's practical electrocardiography,* ed 9, Baltimore, 1994, Williams & Wilkins.

Woods SL, Sivarajan Froelicher ES, Motzer SA: *Cardiac nursing,* ed 4, Philadelphia, 2000, Lippincott, Williams & Wilkins.

MATCHING

_____ 1. Updated term for wandering atrial pacemaker

_____ 2. The most common preexcitation syndrome

_____ 3. Atrial rate associated with type I atrial flutter

_____ 4. Consequence of decreased ventricular filling time

_____ 5. Verapamil, diltiazem

_____ 6. Digoxin

_____ 7. ECG characteristic of a nonconducted PAC

_____ 8. Adenosine

_____ 9. Atrial rate associated with atrial fibrillation

_____ 10. Esmolol, atenolol, metoprolol, propranolol

_____ 11. Term referring to the sudden onset or cessation of a dysrhythmia

_____ 12. Ventricular rhythm may be regular or irregular, waveforms resembling teeth of a saw or picket fence before QRS

_____ 13. Early beat initiated by an irritable atrial site

_____ 14. Irregularly irregular ventricular rhythm, no identifiable P waves

_____ 15. Before elective cardioversion, prophylactic treatment with ___ is recommended for the patient in atrial fibrillation

A. 400 to 600 beats/min

B. Decreased stroke volume

C. Atrial fibrillation

D. An early P wave with no QRS following it

E. Beta-blocker

F. Multiformed atrial rhythm

G. Paroxysmal

H. Cardiac glycoside

I. 250 to 350 beats/min

J. Atrial flutter

K. Anticoagulants

L. Premature atrial complex

M. First-line medication used for most types of PSVT

N. Wolff-Parkinson-White syndrome

O. Calcium channel blocker

IDENTIFICATION AND MEASUREMENTS—PRACTICE RHYTHM STRIPS

For each of the following rhythm strips, determine the atrial and ventricular rates, measure the PR interval, QRS duration, and QT interval, and then identify the rhythm. All strips lead II unless otherwise noted.

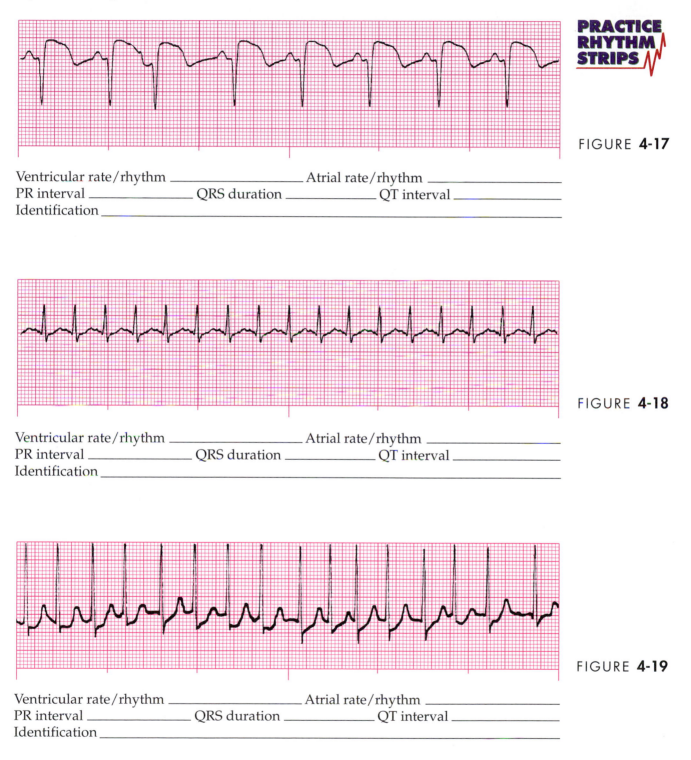

PRACTICE RHYTHM STRIPS

FIGURE **4-17**

Ventricular rate/rhythm _____ Atrial rate/rhythm _____
PR interval _____ QRS duration _____ QT interval _____
Identification _____

FIGURE **4-18**

Ventricular rate/rhythm _____ Atrial rate/rhythm _____
PR interval _____ QRS duration _____ QT interval _____
Identification _____

FIGURE **4-19**

Ventricular rate/rhythm _____ Atrial rate/rhythm _____
PR interval _____ QRS duration _____ QT interval _____
Identification _____

The rhythm strip below is from a 63-year-old female complaining of difficulty breathing. She has a history of dyspnea and CHF.

FIGURE **4-20**

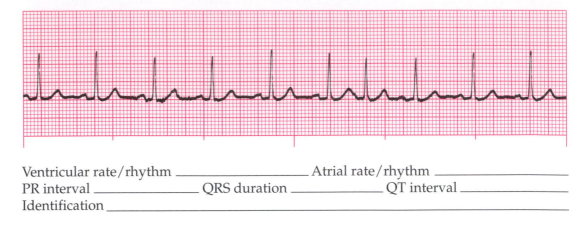

Ventricular rate/rhythm _____ Atrial rate/rhythm _____
PR interval _____ QRS duration _____ QT interval _____
Identification _____

The rhythm strip below is from a 31-year-old male with a history of "an arrhythmia." Medications include Lanoxin, quinidine, and Coumadin.

FIGURE **4-21**

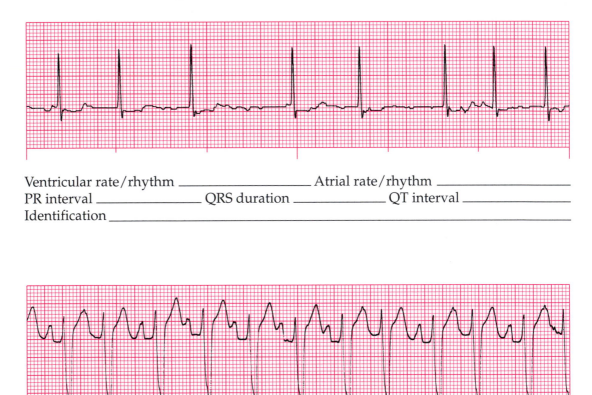

Ventricular rate/rhythm _____ Atrial rate/rhythm _____
PR interval _____ QRS duration _____ QT interval _____
Identification _____

FIGURE **4-22**

Ventricular rate/rhythm _____ Atrial rate/rhythm _____
PR interval _____ QRS duration _____ QT interval _____
Identification _____

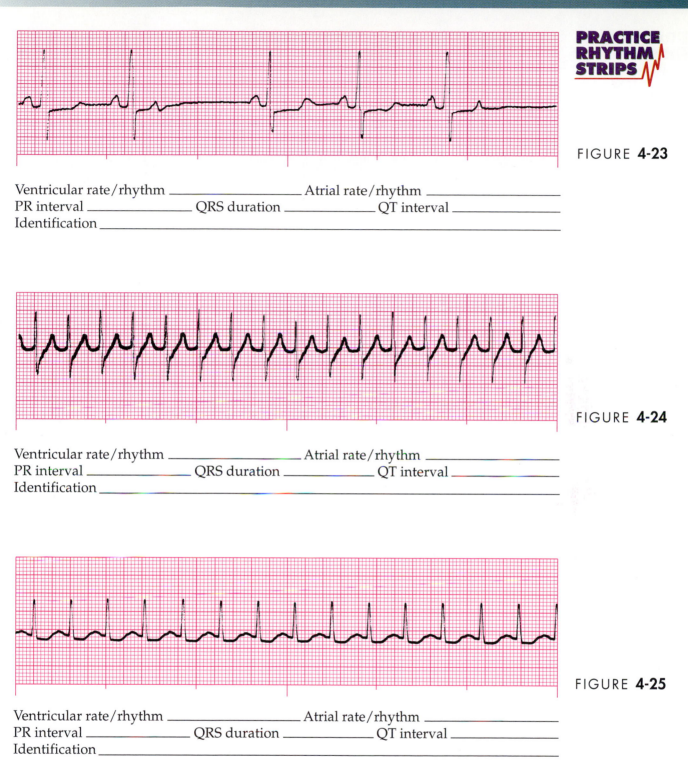

PRACTICE RHYTHM STRIPS

FIGURE **4-23**

Ventricular rate/rhythm _____ Atrial rate/rhythm _____
PR interval _____ QRS duration _____ QT interval _____
Identification _____

FIGURE **4-24**

Ventricular rate/rhythm _____ Atrial rate/rhythm _____
PR interval _____ QRS duration _____ QT interval _____
Identification _____

FIGURE **4-25**

Ventricular rate/rhythm _____ Atrial rate/rhythm _____
PR interval _____ QRS duration _____ QT interval _____
Identification _____

FIGURE **4-26**

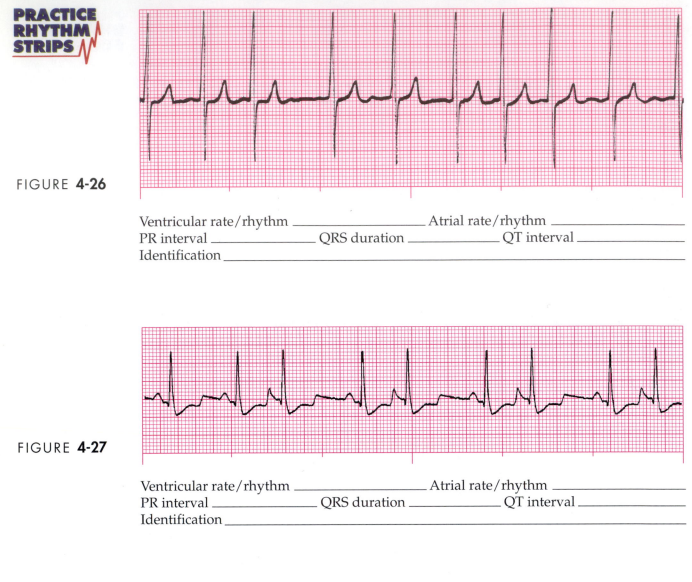

Ventricular rate/rhythm _____ Atrial rate/rhythm _____
PR interval _____ QRS duration _____ QT interval _____
Identification _____

FIGURE **4-27**

Ventricular rate/rhythm _____ Atrial rate/rhythm _____
PR interval _____ QRS duration _____ QT interval _____
Identification _____

Lead II

FIGURE **4-28**

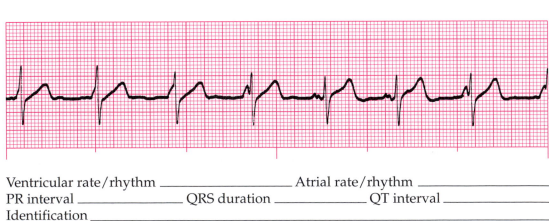

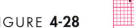

Ventricular rate/rhythm _____ Atrial rate/rhythm _____
PR interval _____ QRS duration _____ QT interval _____
Identification _____

Lead MCL₁

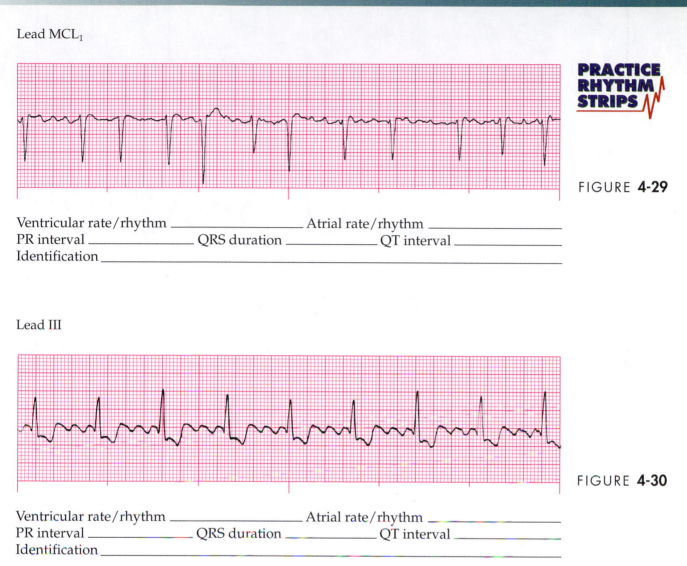

PRACTICE
RHYTHM
STRIPS

FIGURE **4-29**

Ventricular rate/rhythm _____ Atrial rate/rhythm _____
PR interval _____ QRS duration _____ QT interval _____
Identification _____

Lead III

FIGURE **4-30**

Ventricular rate/rhythm _____ Atrial rate/rhythm _____
PR interval _____ QRS duration _____ QT interval _____
Identification _____

CHAPTER 5

Junctional Rhythms

OBJECTIVES

On completion of this chapter, you will be able to:

1. Describe the ECG characteristics, possible causes, signs and symptoms, and emergency management for the following dysrhythmias that originate in the AV junction:
   a. Premature junctional complexes
   b. Junctional escape beats
   c. Junctional escape rhythm
   d. Accelerated junctional rhythm
   e. Junctional tachycardia
2. Explain the difference between premature junctional complexes and junctional escape beats.

OVERVIEW

The **AV node** is a group of specialized cells located in the lower portion of the right atrium, above the base of the tricuspid valve. The main function of the AV node is to delay the electrical impulse to allow the atria to contract and complete filling of the ventricles with blood before the next ventricular contraction.

After passing through the AV node, the electrical impulse enters the bundle of His. The bundle of His is located in the upper portion of the interventricular septum and connects the AV node with the two bundle branches. The bundle of His has pacemaker cells that are capable of discharging at a rhythmic rate of 40 to 60 beats/min. The AV node and the nonbranching portion of the **bundle of His** are called the **AV junction** (Figure 5-1). The bundle of His conducts the electrical impulse to the right and left bundle branches.

The AV junction may assume responsibility for pacing the heart if:

- The SA node fails to discharge (e.g., sinus arrest)
- An impulse from the SA node is generated but blocked as it exits the SA node (e.g., SA block)
- The rate of discharge of the SA node is slower than that of the AV junction (e.g., sinus bradycardia or the slower phase of a sinus arrhythmia)
- An impulse from the SA node is generated and is conducted through the atria but is not conducted to the ventricles (e.g., AV block)

Rhythms originating from the AV junction were formerly called *nodal rhythms* until electrophysiologic studies proved the AV node does not contain pacemaker cells, and the cells nearest the bundle of His in the AV junction are actually responsible for secondary pacing function. Rhythms originating from the AV junction are now termed **junctional dysrhythmias.**

If the AV junction paces the heart, the electrical impulse must travel in a backward **(retrograde)** direction to activate the atria. If atrial depolarization occurs before

AV node: A group of specialized cells located in the lower portion of the right atrium, above the base of the tricuspid valve.

Bundle of His: Cardiac fibers located in the upper portion of the interventricular septum; connects the AV node with the two bundle branches.

AV junction: The AV node and the nonbranching portion of the bundle of His.

Retrograde: Moving backward; moving in the opposite direction to that which is considered normal.

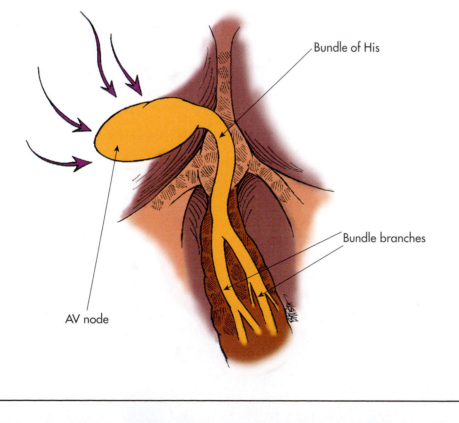

FIGURE **5-1**
AV junction.

ventricular depolarization, an inverted P wave will be seen *before* the QRS complex in leads II, III, and aVF (because the electrical impulse is traveling away from the positive electrode), and the PR interval will usually measure 0.12 sec or less. If atrial and ventricular depolarization occur simultaneously, the P wave will not be visible because it will be hidden in the QRS complex. If atrial depolarization occurs after ventricular depolarization, an inverted P wave will appear *after* the QRS complex.

The terms *upper (high), middle,* and *lower junctional beats* have been used to describe the relationship between P waves and QRS complexes previously mentioned. "The PR and RP interval, however, depends not only on the location of the pacemaker in the junction but also on the relative speed of conduction in an antegrade (forward) and retrograde (backward) direction. If the pacemaker is located in the upper portion of the AV junction but is associated with retrograde conduction delay, the P wave may appear after, instead of before, the QRS complex. Therefore, these descriptive terms may be misleading as to the actual location of the pacemaker and should no longer be used in the interpretation of the body surface ECG."[1]

PREMATURE JUNCTIONAL COMPLEXES (PJCs)

ECG Criteria

A premature junctional complex (PJC) arises from an ectopic focus within the AV junction that discharges before the next expected sinus beat. Because the impulse is conducted through the ventricles in the usual manner, the QRS complex will usually measure 0.10 sec or less. A noncompensatory (incomplete) pause often follows a PJC and represents the delay during which the SA node resets its rhythm for the next beat.

PJCs are distinguished from PACs by the P wave. A PAC typically has an upright P wave before the QRS complex in leads II, III, and aVF. A P wave may or may not be present with a PJC. If a P wave is present, it is inverted (retrograde) and may precede or follow the QRS. If the atria are stimulated first and then the ventricles, a negative (inverted) P wave will appear before the QRS in leads II, III, and aVF. The PRI will usually be less than 0.12 sec. If the electrical impulse reaches the atria and the ventricles simultaneously, there will be no visible P wave because it will be lost in the QRS complex (Table

P waves are usually positive (upright) in leads aVR and I. Inverted P waves may be observed in some, all, or none of the precordial leads.

PJCs are sometimes called premature junctional extrasystoles.

When the atria are depolarized after the ventricles, the P wave typically distorts the end of the QRS complex.

TABLE 5-1	CHARACTERISTICS OF PREMATURE JUNCTIONAL COMPLEXES (PJCs)
Rate	Usually within normal range but depends on underlying rhythm
Rhythm	Regular with premature beats
P waves	May occur before, during, or after the QRS; if visible, the P wave is inverted in leads II, III, and aVF
PR interval	If a P wave occurs before the QRS, the PR interval will usually be less than or equal to 0.12 sec; if no P wave occurs before the QRS, there will be no PR interval
QRS duration	Usually 0.10 sec or less unless an intraventricular conduction delay exists

FIGURE **5-2**
Sinus tachycardia with a PJC. This rhythm strip is from a 76-year-old female complaining of shortness of breath.

Lead II

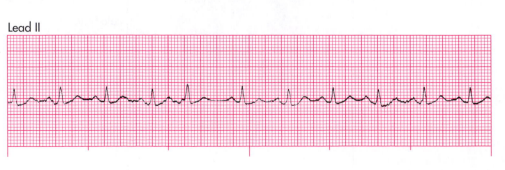

5-1). If the ventricles are stimulated first and then the atria, a negative P wave will appear *after* the QRS in leads II, III, and aVF (Figure 5-2). Therefore a PJC may produce an inverted P wave that comes before, during, or after the QRS complex.

A PJC is not an entire rhythm—it is a single beat. Therefore it is important to identify the underlying rhythm and the ectopic beat(s), i.e., "sinus bradycardia at 46 beats/min with a PJC."

Causes and Clinical Significance

PJCs are less common than either PACs or PVCs. PJCs may be caused by excessive caffeine, tobacco, or alcohol intake; valvular disease; ischemia; congestive heart failure; digitalis toxicity; increased vagal tone; acute myocardial infarction; hypoxia; electrolyte imbalance (particularly magnesium and potassium); exercise; and rheumatic heart disease.

Most individuals with PJCs are asymptomatic. However, PJCs may lead to symptoms of palpitations or the feeling of skipped beats. The sensation of skipped beats may be caused by ineffective contraction resulting from poor filling of the left ventricle during the premature beat.[2] Lightheadedness, dizziness, and other signs of decreased cardiac output may be evident if PJCs are frequent.

Intervention

PJCs do not normally require treatment. Because the rhythm is irregular, count the patient's pulse for a full minute. If PJCs occur because of ingestion of stimulants or digitalis toxicity, these substances should be withheld.

JUNCTIONAL ESCAPE BEATS/RHYTHM

ECG Criteria

A junctional escape beat originates in the AV junction and appears *late* (after the next expected sinus beat) (Table 5-2) (Figure 5-3). A junctional escape **rhythm** is several sequential junctional escape beats (Figure 5-4) (Table 5-3).

TABLE 5-2	CHARACTERISTICS OF JUNCTIONAL ESCAPE BEATS
Rate	Usually within normal range but depends on underlying rhythm
Rhythm	Regular with *late* beats
P waves	May occur before, during, or after the QRS; if visible, the P wave is inverted in leads II, III, and aVF
PR interval	If a P wave occurs before the QRS, the PR interval will usually be less than or equal to 0.12 sec; if no P wave occurs before the QRS, there will be no PR interval
QRS duration	Usually 0.10 sec or less unless an intraventricular conduction delay exists

Margin notes:

PJCs can be misdiagnosed when the P wave of a PAC is obscured by the preceding T wave.

PJCs may occur in patterns: couplets, bigeminy, trigeminy, and quadrigeminy.

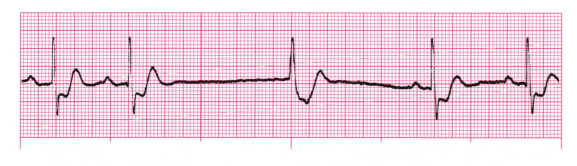

FIGURE **5-3**
Sinus rhythm at 71 beats/min with a prolonged PR interval (0.24 sec), 3.36 period of sinus arrest, and a junctional escape beat.

FIGURE **5-4**
Junctional escape rhythm. Lead II, continuous strips. **A,** Note retrograde P waves before QRS complexes. **B,** Note change in location of P waves. In the first beat, retrograde P wave is observed before the QRS. In the second beat, no P wave is observed. In the remaining beats, P wave is observed after the QRS complexes.

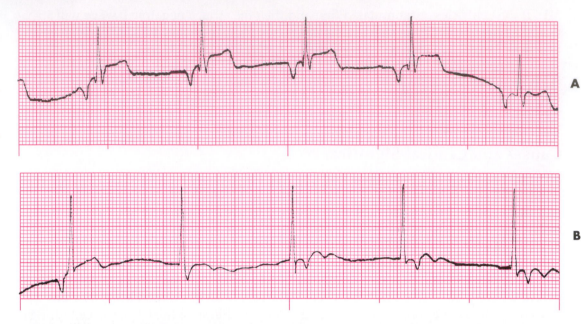

TABLE **5-3**	CHARACTERISTICS OF JUNCTIONAL ESCAPE RHYTHM
Rate	40-60 beats/min
Rhythm	Very regular
P waves	May occur before, during, or after the QRS; if visible, the P wave is inverted in leads II, III, and aVF
PR interval	If a P wave occurs before the QRS, the PR interval will usually be less than or equal to 0.12 sec; if no P wave occurs before the QRS, there will be no PR interval
QRS duration	Usually 0.10 sec or less unless an intraventricular conduction delay exists

Junctional escape beats and rhythms occur when the SA node fails to pace the heart or AV conduction fails. They occur at a very regular rate of 40 to 60 beats/min.

Causes and Clinical Significance

*A junctional escape beat is **protective**—preventing cardiac standstill.*

Junctional escape beats frequently occur during episodes of sinus arrest or following pauses of nonconducted PACs. Junctional escape beats may also be observed in healthy individuals during sinus bradycardia. A junctional rhythm may be seen in acute myocardial infarction (particularly inferior wall MI), rheumatic heart disease, valvular disease, disease of the SA node, hypoxia, increased parasympathetic tone, immediately post-cardiac surgery, and in patients taking digitalis, quinidine, beta-blockers, or calcium channel blockers.

The patient may be asymptomatic with a junctional escape rhythm or may experience signs and symptoms that may be associated with the slow heart rate and decreased cardiac output. Signs and symptoms may include weakness, chest pain or pressure, syncope, an altered level of consciousness, and hypotension.

Intervention

Atropine increases heart rate (positive chronotropic effect) by accelerating the SA node discharge rate and blocking the vagus nerve.

Treatment depends on the cause of the dysrhythmia and the patient's presenting signs and symptoms. If the dysrhythmia is caused by digitalis toxicity, this medication should be withheld. If the patient's signs and symptoms are related to the slow heart rate, atropine sulfate and/or transcutaneous pacing should be considered. Other medications that may be used in the treatment of symptomatic bradycardia include dopamine and epinephrine intravenous infusions.

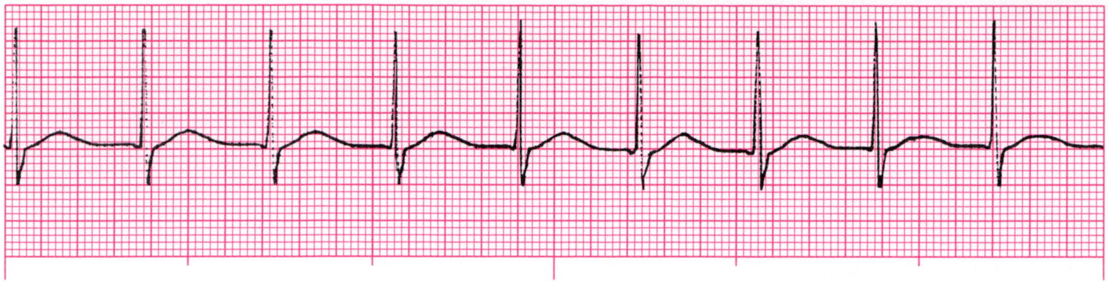

FIGURE **5-5**
Accelerated junctional rhythm.

TABLE **5-4**	CHARACTERISTICS OF ACCELERATED JUNCTIONAL RHYTHM
Rate	61-100 beats/min
Rhythm	Very regular
P waves	May occur before, during, or after the QRS; if visible, the P wave is inverted in leads II, III, and aVF
PR interval	If a P wave occurs before the QRS, the PR interval will usually be less than or equal to 0.12 sec; if no P wave occurs before the QRS, there will be no PR interval
QRS duration	Usually 0.10 sec or less unless an intraventricular conduction delay exists

ACCELERATED JUNCTIONAL RHYTHM

ECG Criteria

An accelerated junctional rhythm is an ectopic rhythm caused by enhanced automaticity of the bundle of His, resulting in a regular ventricular response at a rate of 61 to 100 beats/min (Figure 5-5). The ECG criteria for an accelerated junctional rhythm are the same as for a junctional escape rhythm. The only difference between the two rhythms is the increase in the ventricular rate (Table 5-4).

Causes and Clinical Significance

Causes of this dysrhythmia include digitalis toxicity, acute myocardial infarction, cardiac surgery, rheumatic fever, COPD, and hypokalemia. The patient may be asymptomatic with this dysrhythmia because the ventricular rate is 61 to 100 beats/min; however, the patient should be monitored closely.

Intervention

If this dysrhythmia is caused by digitalis toxicity, this medication should be withheld.

JUNCTIONAL TACHYCARDIA

ECG Criteria

Junctional tachycardia is three or more sequential premature junctional complexes occurring at a rate of more than 100 beats/min (Figure 5-6). *Paroxysmal junctional tachycardia* is a term used to describe a junctional tachycardia that starts and ends suddenly and is often precipitated by a premature junctional complex. When the ventricular rate is

AV nodal reentrant tachycardia (AVNRT) and AV reentrant tachycardia (AVRT) were discussed in Chapter 4.

TABLE **5-5**	CHARACTERISTICS OF JUNCTIONAL TACHYCARDIA
Rate	101-180 beats/min
Rhythm	Very regular
P waves	May occur before, during, or after the QRS; if visible, the P wave is inverted in leads II, III, and aVF
PR interval	If a P wave occurs before the QRS, the PR interval will usually be less than or equal to 0.12 sec; if no P wave occurs before the QRS, there will be no PR interval
QRS duration	Usually 0.10 sec or less unless an intraventricular conduction delay exists

greater than 150 beats/min, this rhythm is difficult to distinguish from atrial tachycardia and may simply be called *supraventricular tachycardia (SVT)* (Table 5-5).

Causes and Clinical Significance

Junctional tachycardia is an ectopic rhythm that originates in the pacemaker cells found in the bundle of His. This dysrhythmia is believed to be caused by enhanced automaticity and may occur because of myocardial ischemia or infarction, congestive heart failure, or digitalis toxicity.

With sustained ventricular rates of 150 beats/min or more, the patient may complain of a sudden feeling of a "racing heart" and severe anxiety. Because of the fast ventricular rate, the ventricles may be unable to fill completely, resulting in decreased cardiac output. Junctional tachycardia associated with acute myocardial infarction may increase myocardial ischemia and the frequency and severity of chest pain; extend the size of the infarction; cause congestive heart failure, hypotension, cardiogenic shock; and/or predispose the patient to ventricular dysrhythmias.

Intervention

Treatment depends on the severity of the patient's signs and symptoms. Signs and symptoms of hemodynamic compromise include shock, chest pain, hypotension, shortness of breath, pulmonary congestion, congestive heart failure, acute MI, and/or decreased level of consciousness.

Symptomatic patients with stable vital signs and normal cardiac function are treated with oxygen therapy, IV access, vagal maneuvers (coughing, bearing down) and, if unsuccessful, administration of adenosine. If adenosine administration is unsuccessful, amiodarone, a beta-blocker, or a calcium channel blocker may be used.

Symptomatic patients with impaired cardiac function may be treated with amiodarone.

A summary of all junctional rhythm characteristics can be found in Table 5-6.

TABLE 5-6	JUNCTIONAL RHYTHMS: SUMMARY OF CHARACTERISTICS				
	PJCs	Junctional escape beat	Junctional escape rhythm	Accelerated junctional rhythm	Junctional tachycardia
Rate	Usually within normal range but depends on underlying rhythm	Usually within normal range but depends on underlying rhythm	40-60 beats/min	61-100 beats/min	101-180 beats/min
Rhythm	Regular with premature beats	Regular with late beats	Regular	Regular	Regular
P waves (lead II)	May occur before, during, or after the QRS; if visible, the P wave is inverted in leads II, III, and aVF	May occur before, during, or after the QRS; if visible, the P wave is inverted in leads II, III, and aVF	May occur before, during, or after the QRS; if visible, the P wave is inverted in leads II, III, and aVF	May occur before, during, or after the QRS; if visible, the P wave is inverted in leads II, III, and aVF	May occur before, during, or after the QRS; if visible, the P wave is inverted in leads II, III, and aVF
PR interval	If P wave is present before the QRS, usually less than or equal to 0.12 sec; if no P wave occurs before the QRS, there will be no PR interval	If P wave is present before the QRS, usually less than or equal to 0.12 sec; if no P wave occurs before the QRS, there will be no PR interval	If P wave is present before the QRS, usually less than or equal to 0.12 sec; if no P wave occurs before the QRS, there will be no PR interval	If P wave is present before the QRS, usually less than or equal to 0.12 sec; if no P wave occurs before the QRS, there will be no PR interval	If P wave is present before the QRS, usually less than or equal to 0.12 sec; if no P wave occurs before the QRS, there will be no PR interval
QRS	Usually 0.10 sec or less unless an intraventricular conduction delay exists	Usually less than 0.10 sec	Usually 0.10 sec or less unless an intraventricular conduction delay exists	Usually 0.10 sec or less unless an intraventricular conduction delay exists	Usually 0.10 sec or less unless an intraventricular conduction delay exists
Clinical significance	Most individuals with PJCs are asymptomatic; lightheadedness, dizziness, and other signs of decreased cardiac output may be evident if PJCs are frequent; if the patient is taking digitalis, check digoxin level	Signs and symptoms of decreased cardiac output may be present because of underlying bradycardic rate and/or SA node dysfunction; if the patient is taking digitalis, check digoxin level	Signs and symptoms of decreased cardiac output may be present because of bradycardic rate and/or SA node dysfunction; if the patient is taking digitalis, check digoxin level	Most individuals are asymptomatic as the ventricular rate is within normal limits; if the patient is taking digitalis, check digoxin level	The more rapid the rate, the greater the incidence of symptoms caused by increased myocardial oxygen demand; signs of decreased cardiac output may be evident because of the increased rate; if the patient is taking digitalis, check digoxin level

REFERENCES

1. Chou T, Knilans TK: *Electrocardiography in clinical practice: adult and pediatric,* Philadelphia, 1996, WB Saunders.
2. Padrid PJ, Kowey PR, editors: *Cardiac arrhythmia: mechanisms, diagnosis, and management,* Baltimore, 1995, Williams & Wilkins.

BIBLIOGRAPHY

Berne RM, Levy MN: *Cardiovascular physiology,* ed 7, St Louis, 1997, Mosby.

Braunwauld E, Scheinman M, editors: *Arrhythmias: electrophysiologic principles,* Vol IX, Singapore, 1996, Current Medicine/Mosby.

Chou T, Knilans TK: *Electrocardiography in clinical practice: adult and pediatric,* Philadelphia, 1996, WB Saunders.

Crawford MV, Spence MI: *Common sense approach to coronary care,* ed 6, St Louis, 1995, Mosby.

Goldberger AL: *Clinical electrocardiography: a simplified approach,* ed 6, St Louis, 1999, Mosby.

Huszar RJ: *Basic dysrhythmias: interpretation and management,* ed 2, St Louis, 1994, Mosby.

Johnson R, Swartz MH: *A simplified approach to electrocardiography,* Philadelphia, 1986, WB Saunders.

Marriott HJL, Conover MB: *Advanced concepts in arrhythmias,* ed 3, St Louis, 1998, Mosby.

Padrid PJ, Kowey PR, editors: *Cardiac arrhythmia: mechanisms, diagnosis, and management,* Baltimore, 1995, Williams & Wilkins.

Phalen T: *The 12-lead ECG in acute myocardial infarction,* St Louis, 1996, Mosby.

Phillips RE, Feeney MK: *The cardiac rhythms: a systematic approach to interpretation,* ed 3, Philadelphia, 1990, WB Saunders.

Wagner GS: *Marriott's practical electrocardiography,* ed 9, Baltimore, 1994, Williams & Wilkins.

Woods SL, Sivarajan Froelicher ES, Motzer SA: *Cardiac nursing,* ed 4, Philadelphia, 2000, Lippincott, Williams & Wilkins.

STOP & REVIEW

MATCHING

___ 1. Impulse(s) originating from a source other than the sinoatrial node

___ 2. Name given to a dysrhythmia that originates in the AV junction with a ventricular rate between 61 to 100 beats/min

___ 3. ___ toxicity/excess is a common cause of junctional dysrhythmias.

___ 4. A beat originating from the AV junction that appears later than the next expected beat

___ 5. Location of the P wave on the ECG if atrial and ventricular depolarization occur simultaneously

___ 6. Medication that increases heart rate (positive chronotropic effect) by accelerating the SA node discharge rate and blocking the vagus nerve

___ 7. Normal duration of a QRS complex in a junctional dysrhythmia

___ 8. Characteristic of specialized cardiac cells to spontaneously initiate an electrical impulse without being stimulated from another source

___ 9. In a junctional rhythm, location of the P wave on the ECG if ventricular depolarization precedes atrial depolarization

___ 10. Normal duration of a PR interval

___ 11. A beat originating from the AV junction that appears earlier than the next expected sinus beat

___ 12. The ability of a cardiac cell to receive an electrical stimulus and propagate that impulse to an adjacent cardiac cell

___ 13. Primary waveform used to differentiate PJCs from PACs

___ 14. Normal (intrinsic) rate for the AV junction

___ 15. In a junctional rhythm, location of the P wave on the ECG if atrial depolarization precedes ventricular depolarization

A. 0.12 to 0.20 sec
B. Automaticity
C. Inverted P wave precedes the QRS complex in leads II, III, and aVF
D. Premature junctional complex (PJC)
E. 0.10 sec or less
F. 40 to 60 beats/min
G. Inverted P wave occurs after the QRS complex in leads II, III, and aVF
H. Digitalis
I. Conductivity
J. Hidden within the QRS complex (not visible)
K. Accelerated junctional rhythm
L. Atropine
M. Ectopic
N. Junctional escape beat
O. P wave

IDENTIFICATION AND MEASUREMENTS—PRACTICE RHYTHM STRIPS

For each of the following rhythm strips, determine the atrial and ventricular rates, measure the PR interval, QRS duration, and QT interval, and then identify the rhythm. All strips lead II unless otherwise noted.

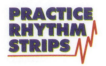

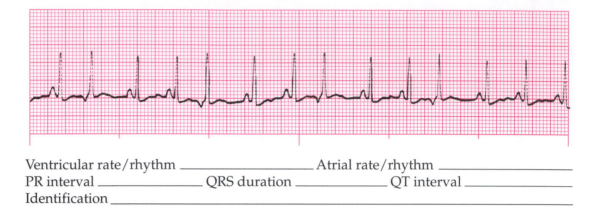

FIGURE 5-7

Ventricular rate/rhythm _____ Atrial rate/rhythm _____
PR interval _____ QRS duration _____ QT interval _____
Identification _____

The rhythm strip below is from an 88-year-old female who experienced a syncopal episode. Blood sugar 96. Medications include verapamil. History: MI 9 years ago, CVA 5 years ago, hypertension, and diabetes.

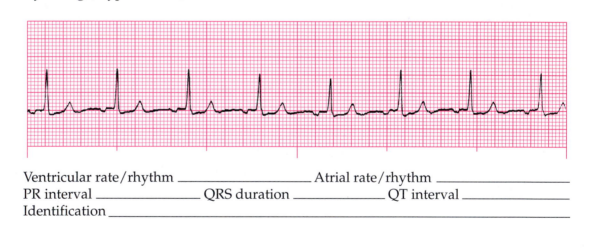

FIGURE 5-8

Ventricular rate/rhythm _____ Atrial rate/rhythm _____
PR interval _____ QRS duration _____ QT interval _____
Identification _____

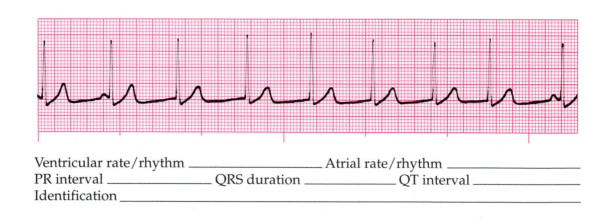

FIGURE 5-9

Ventricular rate/rhythm _____ Atrial rate/rhythm _____
PR interval _____ QRS duration _____ QT interval _____
Identification _____

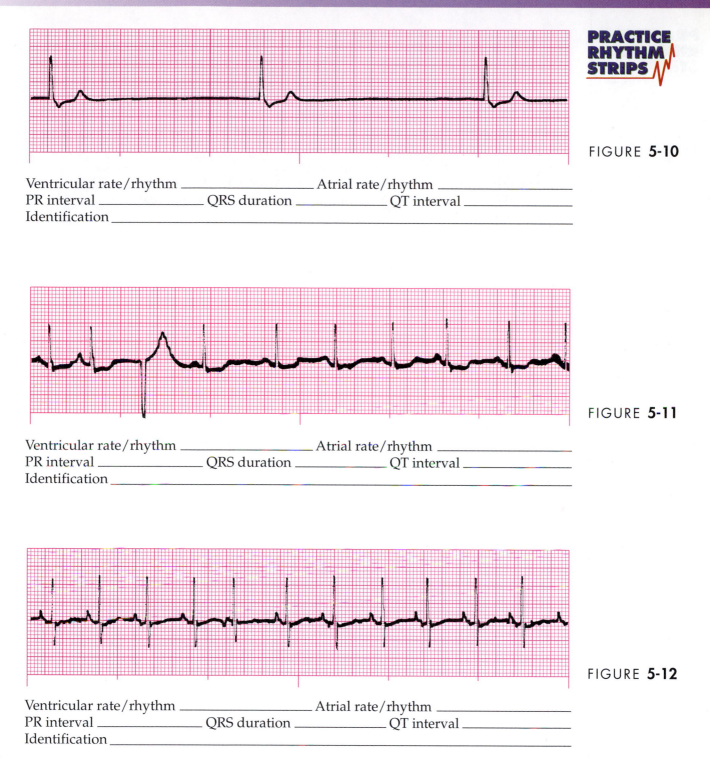

FIGURE **5-10**

Ventricular rate/rhythm _____ Atrial rate/rhythm _____
PR interval _____ QRS duration _____ QT interval _____
Identification _____

FIGURE **5-11**

Ventricular rate/rhythm _____ Atrial rate/rhythm _____
PR interval _____ QRS duration _____ QT interval _____
Identification _____

FIGURE **5-12**

Ventricular rate/rhythm _____ Atrial rate/rhythm _____
PR interval _____ QRS duration _____ QT interval _____
Identification _____

PRACTICE
RHYTHM
STRIPS

FIGURE **5-13**

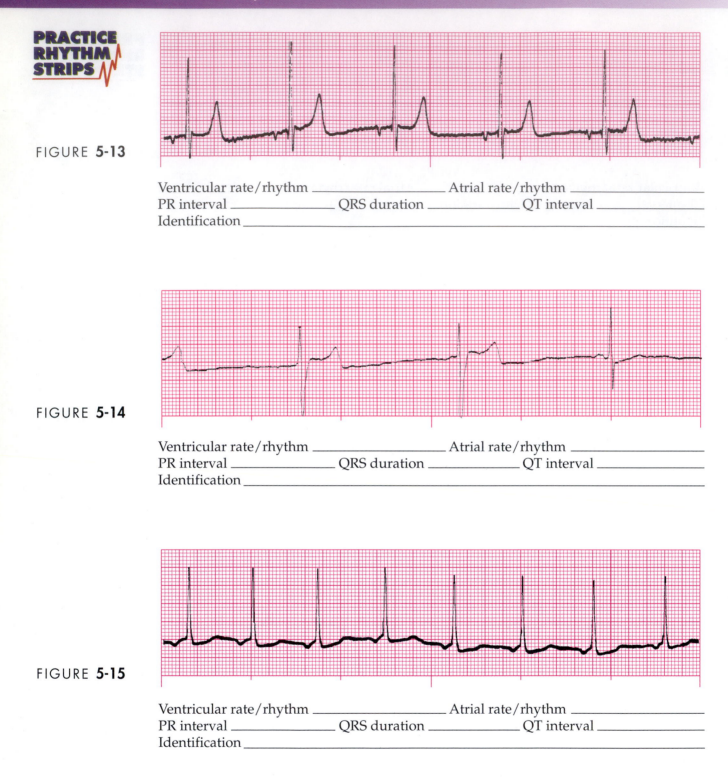

Ventricular rate/rhythm _____ Atrial rate/rhythm _____
PR interval _____ QRS duration _____ QT interval _____
Identification _____

FIGURE **5-14**

Ventricular rate/rhythm _____ Atrial rate/rhythm _____
PR interval _____ QRS duration _____ QT interval _____
Identification _____

FIGURE **5-15**

Ventricular rate/rhythm _____ Atrial rate/rhythm _____
PR interval _____ QRS duration _____ QT interval _____
Identification _____

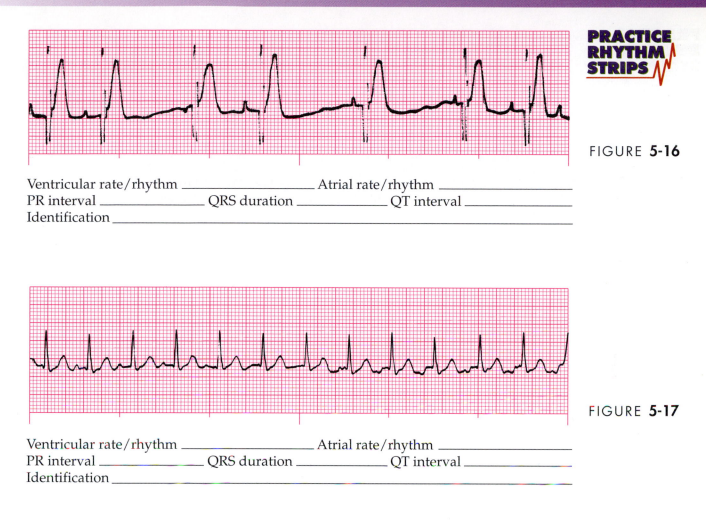

FIGURE **5-16**

Ventricular rate/rhythm _____ Atrial rate/rhythm _____
PR interval _____ QRS duration _____ QT interval _____
Identification _____

FIGURE **5-17**

Ventricular rate/rhythm _____ Atrial rate/rhythm _____
PR interval _____ QRS duration _____ QT interval _____
Identification _____

The rhythm strip below is from a 67-year-old female presenting with congestive heart failure (CHF). Pedal edema present, crackles bilaterally. She had an MI 4 years ago.

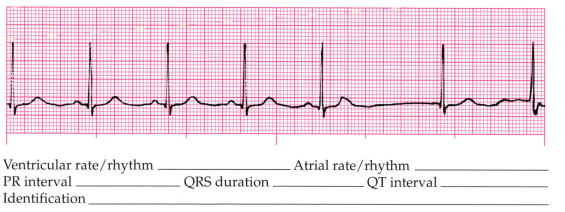

FIGURE **5-18**

Ventricular rate/rhythm _____ Atrial rate/rhythm _____
PR interval _____ QRS duration _____ QT interval _____
Identification _____

PRACTICE RHYTHM STRIPS

FIGURE **5-19**

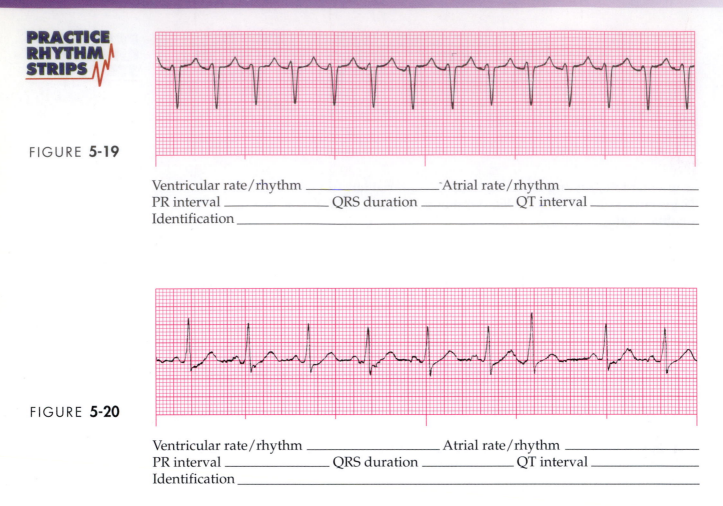

Ventricular rate/rhythm _____ Atrial rate/rhythm _____
PR interval _____ QRS duration _____ QT interval _____
Identification _____

FIGURE **5-20**

Ventricular rate/rhythm _____ Atrial rate/rhythm _____
PR interval _____ QRS duration _____ QT interval _____
Identification _____

CHAPTER 6

Ventricular Rhythms

OBJECTIVES

On completion of this chapter, you will be able to:

1. Describe the ECG characteristics, possible causes, signs and symptoms, and emergency management for the following dysrhythmias that originate in the ventricles:
   a. Premature ventricular complexes (PVCs)
   b. Ventricular escape beats
   c. Ventricular escape (idioventricular) rhythm (IVR)
   d. Accelerated idioventricular rhythm (AIVR)
   e. Ventricular tachycardia (VT)
   f. Torsades de pointes (TdP)
   g. Ventricular fibrillation (VF)
   h. Asystole
2. Explain the terms *bigeminy, trigeminy, quadrigeminy,* and *"run"* when used to describe premature complexes.
3. Explain the difference between premature ventricular complexes and ventricular escape beats.
4. Explain the terms *monomorphic* and *polymorphic ventricular tachycardia.*
5. Discuss long QT syndrome (LQTS).
6. State the purpose and procedure for defibrillation.
7. List the indications for defibrillation.
8. Explain the term *P-wave asystole.*
9. Explain the term *pulseless electrical activity.*

OVERVIEW

The ventricles are the heart's least efficient pacemaker and normally generate impulses at a rate of 20 to 40 beats/min. The ventricles may assume responsibility for pacing the heart if:

- SA node fails to discharge
- Impulse from the SA node is generated but blocked as it exits the SA node
- Rate of discharge of the SA node is slower than that of the ventricles
- Irritable site in either ventricle produces an early beat or rapid rhythm

The shape of the QRS complex is influenced by the site of origin of the electrical impulse.

Normally an electrical impulse originating in the SA node, atria, or AV junction results in simultaneous depolarization of the right and left ventricles. The resulting QRS complex is usually narrow, measuring less than 0.10 sec in duration.

If the atria are depolarized after the ventricles, retrograde P waves may be seen.

Ventricular beats and rhythms may originate from any part of the ventricles. When an ectopic site within a ventricle assumes responsibility for pacing the heart, the electrical impulse bypasses the normal intraventricular conduction pathway, and stimulation of the ventricles occurs asynchronously. As a result, ventricular beats and rhythms are typically characterized by QRS complexes that are abnormally shaped and prolonged (greater than 0.12 sec).

Because ventricular depolarization is abnormal, ventricular repolarization is also abnormal, resulting in changes in ST segments and T waves. T waves are usually in a direction opposite that of the QRS complex—if the major QRS deflection is negative, the ST segment is usually elevated and the T wave positive (upright); if the major QRS deflection is positive, the ST segment is usually depressed and the T wave is usually negative (inverted). P waves are usually not seen with ventricular dysrhythmias but if they are visible, they have no consistent relationship to the QRS complex (AV dissociation).

PREMATURE VENTRICULAR COMPLEXES (PVCs)

ECG Criteria

PVCs are also referred to as *premature ventricular extrasystoles* or *ventricular premature beats.*

A **premature ventricular complex (PVC)** arises from an irritable focus within either ventricle. PVCs may be caused by enhanced automaticity or reentry. By definition, a PVC is **premature,** occurring earlier than the next expected sinus beat. The QRS of a PVC is typically equal to or greater than 0.12 sec because the PVC depolarizes the ventricles prematurely and in an abnormal manner. The T wave is usually in the opposite direction of the QRS complex (Table 6-1).

Compensatory pause: A pause is termed *compensatory* (or *complete*) if the normal beat following a premature complex occurs when expected.

A **full compensatory pause** often follows a PVC. This occurs because the SA node is not affected by the PVC and discharges at its regular rate and rhythm, including the period during and after the PVC. "A full compensatory pause does not reliably differentiate

TABLE 6-1	CHARACTERISTICS OF PREMATURE VENTRICULAR COMPLEXES (PVCs)
Rate	Usually within normal range but depends on underlying rhythm
Rhythm	Essentially regular with premature beats; if the PVC is an interpolated PVC, the rhythm will be regular
P waves	Usually absent or, with retrograde conduction to the atria, may appear after the QRS (usually upright in the ST segment or T wave)
PR interval	None with the PVC because the ectopic beat originates in the ventricles
QRS duration	Greater than 0.12 sec, wide and bizarre, T wave frequently in opposite direction of the QRS complex

ventricular ectopy from atrial ectopy because atrial ectopy may produce a similar compensatory pattern if it does not reset the SA node. In addition, when PVCs are retrogradely conducted to the atria, as in slow sinus rates, they can reset the SA node and a full compensatory pause may not be present."[1]

To determine whether or not the pause following a premature complex is compensatory or noncompensatory, measure the distance between three normal beats. Compare the distance between three beats, one of which includes the premature complex. The pause is compensatory (or complete) if the normal beat following the premature complex occurs when expected (i.e., when the distance is the same).

A **fusion beat** (Figure 6-1) is a result of an electrical impulse from a supraventricular site (such as the SA node) discharging at the same time as an ectopic site in the ventricles. However, because fusion beats are a result of both supraventricular and ventricular depolarization, these beats do not resemble normally conducted beats, nor do they resemble true ventricular beats.

Fusion beat: A beat that occurs because of simultaneous activation of one cardiac chamber by two sites (foci).

A PVC is not an entire rhythm—it is a single beat. Therefore it is important to identify the underlying rhythm and the ectopic beat(s), i.e., "sinus tachycardia at 138 beats/min with frequent PVCs."

Types of PVCs

PVCs may occur in patterns:

- Pairs (couplets): Two sequential PVCs
- "Runs" or "bursts": Three or more sequential PVCs, known as *ventricular tachycardia (VT)*
- Bigeminal PVCs (ventricular bigeminy): Every other beat is a PVC
- Trigeminal PVCs (ventricular trigeminy): Every third beat is a PVC
- Quadrigeminal PVCs (ventricular quadrigeminy): Every fourth beat is a PVC

Uniform and Multiformed PVCs

Premature ventricular beats that look the same in the same lead and originate from the same anatomic site (focus) are called **uniform** PVCs (Figure 6-2). PVCs that appear differ-

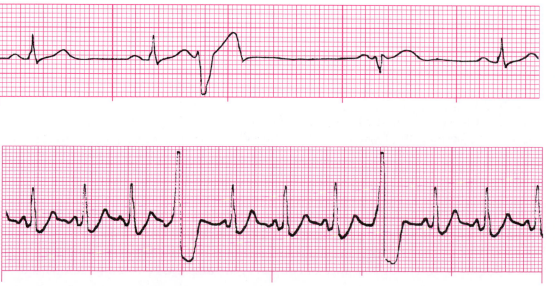

FIGURE 6-1
Sinus bradycardia with PVC (third complex from left) and fusion beat (fourth complex from left).

FIGURE 6-2
Sinus tachycardia with frequent uniform PVCs.

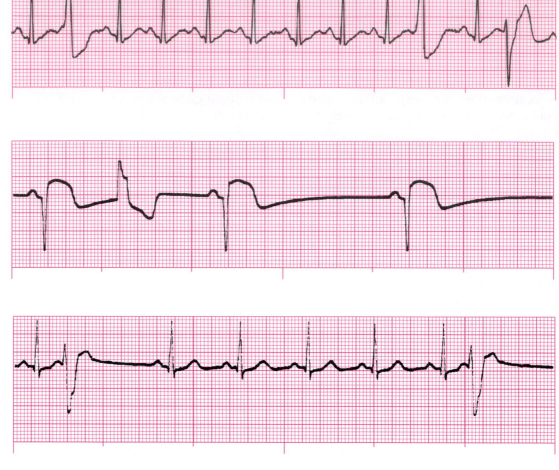

FIGURE **6-3**
Sinus tachycardia with multiform PVCs.

FIGURE **6-4**
Sinus bradycardia with an interpolated PVC and ST segment elevation.

FIGURE **6-5**
Sinus rhythm with two R-on-T PVCs.

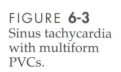 Ectopic beats from the same focus tend to have a constant coupling interval (the interval between the ectopic beat and the preceding beat of the basic rhythm).[3]

If an interpolated PVC produces a palpable pulse, frequent interpolated PVCs may cause signs and symptoms because of an increased heart rate.

ent from one another in the same lead are called **multiform** PVCs (Figure 6-3). Multiform PVCs often, but do not always, arise from different anatomic sites. The terms *unifocal* and *multifocal* are sometimes used to describe PVCs that are similar or different in appearance. Uniform PVCs are unifocal, but multiform PVCs are not necessarily multifocal.[2]

Interpolated PVCs
A PVC may occur without interfering with the normal cardiac cycle. An **interpolated PVC** (Figure 6-4) does not have a full compensatory pause—it is "squeezed" between two regular complexes and does not disturb the underlying rhythm. The PR interval of the cardiac cycle following the PVC may be longer than normal.

R-on-T PVCs
R-on-T PVCs occur when the R wave of a PVC falls on the T wave of the preceding beat (Figure 6-5). Because the T wave is vulnerable (relative refractory period) to any electrical stimulation, it is possible that a PVC occurring during this period of the cardiac cycle will precipitate VT or VF; however, VT and VF most commonly occur without a preceding R-on-T PVC, and most R-on-T PVCs do not precipitate a sustained ventricular tachydysrhythmia.[3]

Couplets may also be referred to as *two in a row* or *back-to-back PVCs*.

Paired PVCs (Couplets)
A pair of PVCs occurring in immediate succession is called a **couplet** or **paired PVCs** (Figure 6-6). The appearance of couplets indicates the ventricular ectopic site

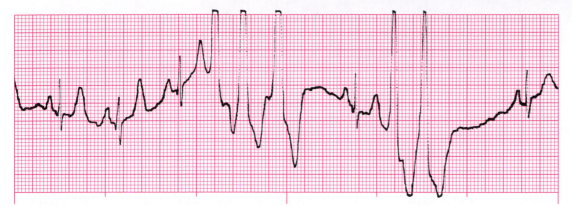

FIGURE **6-6**
Sinus rhythm with a run of VT and one episode of couplets.

BOX 6-1   COMMON CAUSES OF PVCs

- Normal variant
- Hypoxia
- Stress, anxiety
- Exercise
- Digitalis toxicity
- Acid-base imbalance
- Myocardial ischemia
- Electrolyte imbalance (hypokalemia, hypocalcemia, hypercalcemia, hypomagnesemia)
- Congestive heart failure
- Increased sympathetic tone
- Acute myocardial infarction
- Stimulants (alcohol, caffeine, tobacco)
- Medications (sympathomimetics, cyclic antidepressants, phenothiazines)

---

is extremely irritable. Three or more PVCs occurring in immediate succession at a rate of more than 100 beats/min is considered a "salvo," "run," or "burst" of ventricular tachycardia.

Causes and Clinical Significance

PVCs can occur in healthy persons with apparently normal hearts and for no apparent cause. Ventricular ectopy has been recorded in more than half of normal persons undergoing ambulatory ECG monitoring. The incidence of PVCs increases with age.

PVCs may occur because of hypoxia, stress, an increase in catecholamines, stimulants (alcohol, caffeine, tobacco), acid-base imbalance, electrolyte imbalance, digitalis toxicity, medications (epinephrine, dopamine, phenothiazines, isoproterenol), ischemia, myocardial infarction, or congestive heart failure (Box 6-1).

PVCs can occur at rest or may be associated with exercise. In normal individuals, premature ventricular beats may increase, decrease, or be completely suppressed by exercise.[2]

PVCs may or may not produce palpable pulses. Patients experiencing PVCs may be asymptomatic or complain of palpitations, a "racing heart," skipped beats, or chest or

PVCs are the most common dysrhythmia in healthy individuals and in those with organic heart disease.

Patients often describe premature beats as "flip-flops."

As with all cardiac dysrhythmias, it is important to *treat the patient, not the monitor.*

neck discomfort. These symptoms may be caused by the greater than normal contractile force of the postectopic beats or the feeling that the heart has stopped during the long pause after the premature complexes.[4] If the PVCs are frequent, signs of decreased cardiac output may be present.

Studies have shown that the presence of frequent PVCs 7 to 10 days after an MI is associated with a fivefold increase in the risk of symptomatic or fatal dysrhythmias during follow-up.[5]

Intervention

Routine use of medications to treat PVCs is no longer recommended.

Treatment of PVCs depends on the cause, patient's signs and symptoms, and on the clinical situation. Most patients experiencing PVCs do not require treatment with antidysrhythmic medications. There is no evidence that suppression of PVCs reduces mortality, particularly in patients with no structural heart disease.[6] "The use of prophylactic lidocaine is no longer recommended. Although prophylactic lidocaine reduces the incidence of VF, it is associated in many series with an increase in cardiac death, possibly because it abolishes ventricular escape rhythms in patients who may also be prone to bradycardia."[7] Treatment of PVCs seen in the setting of acute MI should be directed at ensuring adequate oxygenation, relief of pain, and rapid identification and correction of hypoxia, heart failure, and electrolyte or acid-base abnormalities.

VENTRICULAR ESCAPE BEATS/RHYTHM

ECG Criteria

A **ventricular escape beat** (Figure 6-7) is a ventricular ectopic beat that occurs after a pause in which the supraventricular pacemakers failed to initiate an impulse. Ventricu-

TABLE 6-2	CHARACTERISTICS OF VENTRICULAR ESCAPE BEATS
Rate	Usually within normal range but depends on underlying rhythm
Rhythm	Essentially regular with late beats; the ventricular escape beat occurs after the next expected sinus beat
P waves	Usually absent or, with retrograde conduction to the atria, may appear after the QRS (usually upright in the ST segment or T wave)
PR interval	None with the ventricular escape beat because the ectopic beat originates in the ventricles
QRS duration	Greater than 0.12 sec, wide and bizarre, T wave frequently in opposite direction of the QRS complex

FIGURE **6-7** Ventricular escape beat following a nonconducted premature atrial complex (PAC).

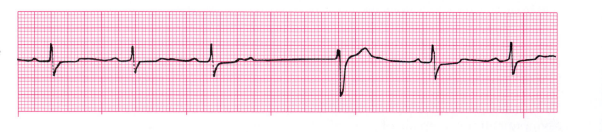

lar escape beats are wide, the QRS measuring 0.12 sec or greater, and occur *late* in the cardiac cycle, appearing after the next expected sinus beat (Table 6-2). The ventricular escape beat is a *protective* mechanism, protecting the heart from more extreme slowing or even asystole. A ventricular escape or **idioventricular rhythm (IVR)** exists when three or more sequential ventricular escape beats occur at a rate of 20 to 40 beats/min (Figure 6-8) (Table 6-3).

The ventricular rate in IVR is between 20 to 40 beats/min, the intrinsic firing rate of the ventricles. The QRS complexes seen in IVR are wide and bizarre because the impulses originate in the ventricles (bypassing the normal conduction pathway). When the ventricular rate slows to a rate of less than 20 beats/min, some refer to the rhythm as an agonal rhythm or "dying heart."

Causes and Clinical Significance

IVR may occur when the SA node and the AV junction fail to initiate an electrical impulse, when the rate of discharge of the SA node or AV junction becomes less than the inherent ventricular rate, or when impulses generated by a supraventricular site are blocked. IVR may also occur because of myocardial infarction, digitalis toxicity, or metabolic imbalances.

Because the ventricular rate associated with this rhythm is slow (20 to 40 beats/min) with a loss of atrial kick, the patient may experience severe hypotension, weakness, disorientation, lightheadedness, or loss of consciousness because of decreased cardiac output.

A ventricular escape beat is **protective**—preventing cardiac standstill.

When this rhythm is in its terminal stages, the complexes may lose some of their form and become irregular.

TABLE 6-3	CHARACTERISTICS OF VENTRICULAR ESCAPE (IDIOVENTRICULAR) RHYTHM	
Rate	20-40 beats/min	
Rhythm	Essentially regular	
P waves	Usually absent or, with retrograde conduction to the atria, may appear after the QRS (usually upright in the ST segment or T wave)	
PR interval	None	
QRS duration	Greater than 0.12 sec, T wave frequently in opposite direction of the QRS complex	

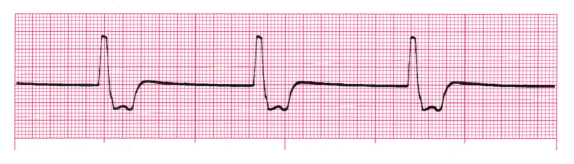

FIGURE **6-8**
Idioventricular rhythm (IVR).

Intervention

Lidocaine should be *avoided* in the management of this rhythm because lidocaine may abolish ventricular activity, possibly causing asystole in a patient with an idioventricular rhythm. If the patient is symptomatic because of the slow rate and/or loss of atrial kick, atropine may be ordered in an attempt to block the vagus nerve and stimulate the SA node to overdrive the ventricular rhythm, or transcutaneous pacing may be attempted. If the patient is pulseless despite the appearance of organized electrical activity on the cardiac monitor (a clinical situation termed *pulseless electrical activity*), management should include CPR, oxygen administration and endotracheal intubation, IV access, and an aggressive search for the underlying cause of the situation.

ACCELERATED IDIOVENTRICULAR RHYTHM (AIVR)

ECG Criteria

Some cardiologists consider the ventricular rate range of AIVR to be 41 to 120 beats/min.

An **accelerated idioventricular rhythm (AIVR)** exists when three or more sequential ventricular escape beats occur at a rate of 41 to 100 beats/min (Figure 6-9). P waves are usually absent but, with retrograde conduction to the atria, may appear after the QRS (usually upright in the ST segment or T wave). The ventricular rhythm is essentially regular with a QRS that is greater than 0.12 sec in duration. The T wave is frequently in an opposite direction of the QRS complex (Table 6-4).

Causes and Clinical Significance

AIVR can be mistaken for VT if the ventricular rate is not counted and the patient assessed.

AIVR is usually considered a benign escape rhythm that appears when the sinus rate slows and disappears when the sinus rate speeds up. AIVR is often seen during the first 12 hours of a myocardial infarction and is particularly common after successful reperfusion therapy. AIVR is seen in both anterior and inferior MI and in 90% of patients during the first 24 hours after reperfusion.[2] AIVR has been reported in 10% to 40% of patients with acute MI,[8] in patients with digitalis toxicity, subarachnoid hemorrhage, and in patients with rheumatic and hypertensive heart disease.

TABLE 6-4	CHARACTERISTICS OF ACCELERATED IDIOVENTRICULAR RHYTHM (AIVR)
Rate	41-100 beats/min
Rhythm	Essentially regular
P waves	Usually absent or, with retrograde conduction to the atria, may appear after the QRS (usually upright in the ST segment or T wave)
PR interval	None
QRS duration	Greater than 0.12 sec, T wave frequently in opposite direction of the QRS complex

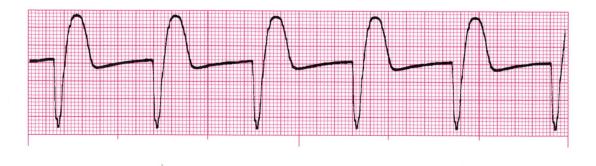

FIGURE 6-9 Accelerated idioventricular rhythm (AIVR).

Intervention

If the patient is asymptomatic, no treatment is necessary. If the patient is symptomatic because of the loss of atrial kick, atropine may be ordered in an attempt to block the vagus nerve and stimulate the SA node to overdrive the ventricular rhythm, or transcutaneous pacing may be attempted. Medications to suppress the ventricular rhythm should be avoided because this rhythm is protective and often transient, spontaneously resolving on its own.

AIVR is also called *nonparoxysmal VT* or *idioventricular tachycardia.*

VENTRICULAR TACHYCARDIA (VT)

ECG Criteria

Ventricular tachycardia (VT) (Figure 6-10) exists when three or more PVCs occur in immediate succession at a rate greater than 100 beats/min. VT may occur as a short run lasting less than 30 seconds (nonsustained) but more commonly persists for more than 30 seconds (sustained). VT may occur with or without pulses, and the patient may be stable or unstable with this rhythm.

Ventricular tachycardia, like PVCs, may originate from an ectopic focus in either ventricle. In VT, the QRS complex is wide and bizarre. P waves, if visible, bear no relationship to the QRS complex. The ventricular rhythm is usually regular but may be slightly irregular. When the QRS complexes of VT are of the same shape and amplitude, the rhythm is termed **monomorphic VT** (Table 6-5). When the QRS complexes of VT vary in shape and amplitude, the rhythm is termed **polymorphic VT.**

Monomorphic VT with a ventricular rate greater than 200 beats/min is called *ventricular flutter* by some cardiologists.[2]

Monomorphic: Having the same shape.

Polymorphic: Varying in shape.

Causes and Clinical Significance

Sustained monomorphic VT is often associated with underlying heart disease, particularly myocardial ischemia, and rarely occurs in patients without underlying structural heart disease. The most common cause of sustained monomorphic VT in American adults is coronary artery disease with prior myocardial infarction.[3] Other causes of VT

TABLE 6-5	CHARACTERISTICS OF MONOMORPHIC VENTRICULAR TACHYCARDIA
Rate	101-250 beats/min
Rhythm	Essentially regular
P waves	May be present or absent; if present, they have no set relationship to the QRS complexes, appearing between the QRSs at a rate different from that of the VT
PR interval	None
QRS duration	Greater than 0.12 sec; often difficult to differentiate between the QRS and T wave

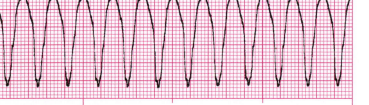

FIGURE **6-10**
Monomorphic ventricular tachycardia (VT).

include cardiomyopathy, cyclic antidepressant overdose, digitalis toxicity, valvular heart disease, mitral valve prolapse, trauma (e.g., myocardial contusion, invasive cardiac procedures), acid-base imbalance, electrolyte imbalance (e.g., hypokalemia, hyperkalemia, hypomagnesemia), and increased production of catecholamines (e.g., cocaine abuse).[2]

The term *cyclic antidepressants* is used in this text because different types of these medications exist (e.g., tricyclics, quadricyclics, etc.)

Signs and symptoms associated with this dysrhythmia vary. Syncope may occur because of an abrupt onset of VT. The patient's only warning symptom may be a brief period of lightheadedness. In victims of sudden cardiac death, VT deteriorating to VF was the rhythm observed in most cases.[9-12]

VT at a rate of 101-125 beats/min is generally better tolerated than that of VT at a higher rate.

Signs and symptoms of hemodynamic compromise related to the tachycardia may include shock, chest pain, hypotension, shortness of breath, pulmonary congestion, congestive heart failure, acute myocardial infarction, and/or a decreased level of consciousness.

Intervention

VT does not usually respond to vagal maneuvers.

Treatment is based on the patient's presentation. *Stable* but symptomatic patients are treated with oxygen therapy, IV access, and administration of ventricular antidysrhythmics to suppress the rhythm.

If the patient's potassium level is low, consider administration of potassium and magnesium.

Unstable patients (usually a sustained heart rate of 150 beats/min or more) whose signs and symptoms are a result of the rapid heart rate are treated with administration of oxygen, IV access, consideration of the use of medications, sedation (if awake and time permits) followed by electrical therapy. CPR should be initiated for the pulseless patient in VT until a defibrillator is available.

A supraventricular tachycardia with an intraventricular conduction delay may be difficult to distinguish from ventricular tachycardia. It should be remembered that VT is considered a potentially life-threatening dysrhythmia. *When unclear whether a regular, wide-QRS tachycardia is VT or SVT with an intraventricular conduction delay, treat the rhythm as ventricular tachycardia until proven otherwise.*

POLYMORPHIC VENTRICULAR TACHYCARDIA

Polymorphic VT that occurs in the presence of a long QT interval is called *torsades de pointes.*

Polymorphic ventricular tachycardia (VT) refers to a rapid ventricular dysrhythmia with beat-to-beat changes in the shape and amplitude of the QRS complexes. Polymorphic VT can be further divided into two classifications based on its association with a normal or prolonged QT interval as follows:

1. Long QT syndrome (LQTS)
   a. Acquired (iatrogenic)
   b. Congenital (idiopathic)
2. Normal QT

The term *QT interval* is used regardless of whether the QRS complex begins with a Q or R wave.

The QT interval is measured from the beginning of the QRS complex to the end of the T wave. In the absence of a Q wave, the QT interval is measured from the beginning of the R wave to the end of the T wave. The QT interval represents total ventricular activity—the time from ventricular depolarization (activation) to repolarization (recovery).

The duration of the QT interval varies according to age, gender, and particularly heart rate. As the heart rate increases, the QT interval decreases. As the heart rate decreases, the QT interval increases. Because of the variability of the QT interval with the heart rate, it can be measured more accurately if it is corrected (adjusted) for the patient's heart rate. The corrected QR interval is noted as QTc. Many clinical studies do not consider the QT interval abnormally long unless the QT interval corrected for the heart rate exceeds 0.44 sec.

To more rapidly, but less accurately, determine the QT interval, measure the interval between two consecutive R waves (R-R interval) and divide the number by two. Measure the QT interval. If the measured QT interval is less than half the R-R interval, it is probably normal. A QT interval that is approximately half the R-R interval is considered "borderline." A QT interval that is more than half the R-R interval is considered "prolonged."

"The normal QT type of polymorphic VT has a pattern similar to that of TdP. However, unlike TdP it is not related to sinus bradycardia, preceding pauses, or electrolyte abnormalities. It is important to distinguish between long QT syndrome and normal QT because they have different mechanisms and treatments."[13] Standard antidysrhythmic medications are administered in the management of normal QT polymorphic VT.

Polymorphic VT that occurs in the presence of a normal QT interval is simply referred to as *polymorphic VT.*

Long QT Syndrome (LQTS)

Long QT syndrome (LQTS) is an abnormality of the heart's electrical system. The mechanical function of the heart is entirely normal. The electrical problem is thought to be caused by defects in cardiac ion channels that affect repolarization. These electrical defects predispose affected persons to TdP that leads to syncope and may result in sudden cardiac death.

LQTS may be acquired or inherited. The acquired form of LQTS is more common and usually caused by medications that prolong the QT interval. Inherited LQTS is caused by mutations of genes that encode the cardiac ion channels and is estimated to be present in 1 in 7000 persons in the United States. Inherited LQTS may cause as many as 3000 unexpected deaths in children and young adults per year.[14] Inherited LQTS is sometimes, but not always, associated with deafness. LQTS occurs in all races and ethnic groups although the relative frequency in each group is not yet known because no systematic screening of different groups has been attempted.[14]

About one third of individuals who have LQTS never exhibit symptoms. A lack of symptoms does not exclude an individual or family from having LQTS. The usual symptoms of LQTS include syncope or sudden death, typically occurring during physical activity or emotional upset. The syncopal episodes are often misdiagnosed as the common faint (vasovagal event) or a seizure. Actual seizures are uncommon in LQTS, but epilepsy is one of the common errors in diagnosis.

Symptoms most commonly begin in preteen to teenage years but may be present from a few days of age to middle age.

Cases in which LQTS should be considered include a sudden loss of consciousness during physical exertion or during emotional excitement, sudden and unexplained loss of consciousness during childhood and teenage years, a family history of unexplained syncope, any young person that has an unexplained cardiac arrest, and epilepsy in children. Common triggers of LQTS include swimming, running, being startled (an alarm clock, a loud horn, a ringing phone), anger, crying, test taking, and other stressful situations.

The diagnosis of LQTS is commonly suspected or made from the ECG. Beta-blockers are frequently used in the management of patients with LQTS and are effective in about

90% of affected patients. New information regarding the genetics of the syndrome suggests that a subset of patients might be treated with other medications, instead of or in addition to beta-blockers.

Children and young adults should have an ECG as part of their evaluation for an unexplained loss of consciousness episode.

Torsades de Pointes (TdP)

ECG Criteria

Torsades de pointes (TdP) is a dysrhythmia intermediary between ventricular tachycardia and ventricular fibrillation[2] and is a type of polymorphic VT associated with a prolonged QT interval. *Torsades de pointes* is French for "twisting of the points," which describes the QRS that changes in shape, amplitude, and width and appears to "twist" around the isoelectric line, resembling a spindle (Figure 6-11). The singular form, *torsade de pointes*, refers to one episode (several [5 to 10] "pointes").[15] The plural form, *torsades de pointes*, refers to more than one episode or to a prolonged attack.[13]

A typical cycle consists of 5 to 20 QRS complexes.

TdP has a ventricular rate typically between 200 to 250 beats/min but may range from 150 to 300 beats/min.[2] This dysrhythmia is characterized by two or more cycles of QRS complexes with alternating polarity (the QRS complexes twist from upright to negative or negative to upright and back) (Table 6-6).

Causes and Clinical Significance

TdP may be precipitated by slow heart rates and is associated with medications or electrolyte disturbances that prolong the QT interval. A prolonged QT interval indicates a

FIGURE **6-11**
Torsades de pointes (TdP). This rhythm strip is from a 77-year-old male 3 days post-MI. Chief complaint at the onset of this episode was chest pain. Past medical history of previous MI and abdominal aortic aneurysm repair. Lidocaine was given and the patient was defibrillated several times without success. Lab work revealed a serum potassium (K+) level of 2.0. K+ was administered IV. Patient converted to a sinus rhythm with next defibrillation.

TABLE **6-6** CHARACTERISTICS OF TORSADES DE POINTES (TDP)	
Rate	150-300 beats/min, typically 200-250 beats/min
Rhythm	May be regular or irregular
P waves	None
PR interval	None
QRS duration	Greater than 0.12 sec; gradual alteration in amplitude and direction of the QRS complexes

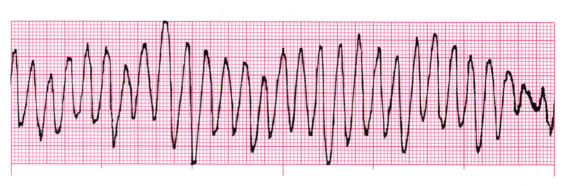

TABLE 6-7 CAUSES OF ACQUIRED LONG QT SYNDROME

Classification	Generic name	Trade name
Pharmacologic agents		
Antibiotics	Erythromycin	E-Mycin, EES, EryPeds
Antifungal		(and others)
medications	Trimethoprim and	Bactrim, Septra
	sulfamethoxazole	
Antihistamines	Pentamidine	Pentam intravenous
	Ketoconazole	Nizoral
	Fluconazole	Diflucan
Cardiac	Itraconazole	Sporanox
medications	Terfenidine	Seldane
	Astemizole	Hismanal
	Diphenhydramine	Benadryl
	Quinidine	Quinidine, Quinidex,
		Duraquin, Quinaglute
	Procainamide	Pronestyl, Procan SR
Diuretics	Disopyramide	Norpace
Gastrointestinal	Amiodarone	Cordarone
medications	Sotalol	Betapace
Psychotropic	Bepridil	Vascor
medications	Indapamide	Lozol
	Cisapride	Propulsid
	Amitriptyline	Elavil
	Desipramine	Norpramin, Pertofrane
	Phenothiazines and	Compazine, Stelazine,
	derivatives	Thorazine, Mellaril,
		Etrafon, Trilafon
	Haloperidol	Haldol
	Risperidone	Risperdal
Liquid-protein diets		
Hypothyroidism		
Central nervous system disease—subarachnoid hemorrhage		
Organophosphate insecticides		
Electrolyte abnormalities—hypokalemia, hypomagnesemia, hypocalcemia		

lengthened relative refractory period (vulnerable period) that puts the ventricles at risk for TdP. A prolonged QT interval may be congenital or acquired. Causes of acquired QT interval prolongation are listed in Table 6-7. Lengthening of the QT interval may be the only warning sign suggesting impending TdP.

Symptoms associated with TdP are usually related to the decreased cardiac output that occurs because of the fast ventricular rate. Patients may complain of palpitations, light-headedness, or may experience a syncopal episode or seizures. TdP may be initiated by a PVC and may occasionally terminate spontaneously and recur after several seconds or minutes or may deteriorate to VF.

Intervention

Obtaining a 12-lead ECG may be helpful in identifying TdP because the rhythm may appear to be monomorphic VT in one lead but present the pattern typical of TdP in another.[2] Treatment of TdP includes discontinuation of type IA antidysrhythmics (if drug induced), correction of electrolyte abnormalities, and any one of the following interven-

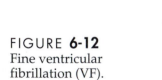 Magnesium is contraindicated in patients with renal failure.

tions: overdrive pacing, magnesium, isoproterenol, lidocaine, or phenytoin. Defibrillation may be necessary for termination of sustained episodes of TdP.

Ventricular Fibrillation (VF)

ECG Criteria

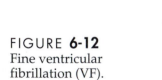 The rate of the undulations varies between 150 and 500/min.[2]

Ventricular fibrillation (VF) is a chaotic rhythm that originates in the ventricles. In VF, there is no organized depolarization of the ventricles. The ventricular myocardium quivers and, as a result, there is no effective myocardial contraction and no pulse. The resulting rhythm is irregularly irregular with chaotic deflections that vary in shape and amplitude. No normal-looking waveforms are visible (Table 6-8).

VF with low amplitude waves (less than 3 mm) is frequently called "fine" ventricular fibrillation (Figure 6-12). Waves that are more easily visible are described as "coarse" (greater than 3 mm) (Figure 6-13).

Causes and Clinical Significance

"Approximately 85% of ambulatory out-of-hospital cardiac arrests in adults over 30 years of age are related to pulseless VT or VF, most often caused by myocardial ischemia." In patients who are known to have ischemic heart disease and whose ECGs are continuously monitored, cardiac arrest is most often due to VT. In the setting of progres-

TABLE 6-8	CHARACTERISTICS OF VENTRICULAR FIBRILLATION (VF)
Rate	Cannot be determined because there are no discernible waves or complexes to measure
Rhythm	Rapid and chaotic with no pattern or regularity
P waves	Not discernible
PR interval	Not discernible
QRS duration	Not discernible

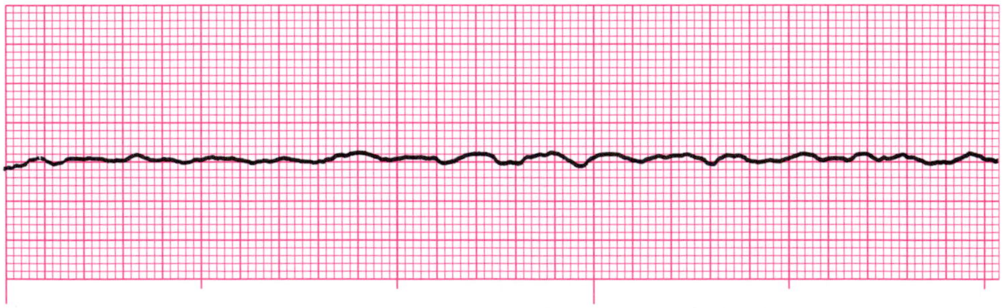

FIGURE **6-12**
Fine ventricular fibrillation (VF).

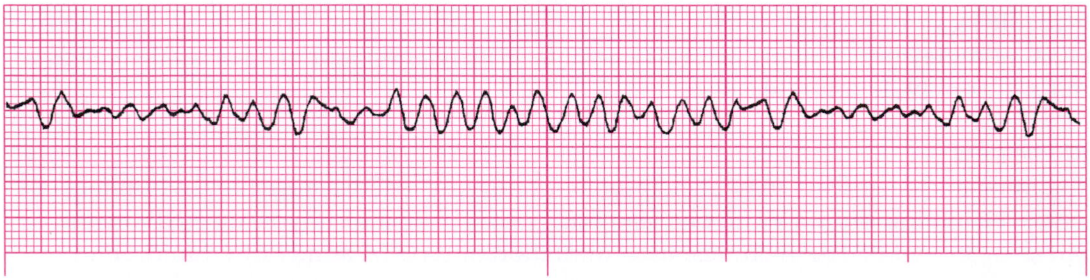

FIGURE **6-13**
Coarse ventricular fibrillation (VF).

sive myocardial ischemia, VT typically deteriorates into VF within an interval of three minutes. For this reason, first responders detect VF as the predominant rhythm after they arrive on the scene."[17]

The patient in VF is unresponsive, apneic, and pulseless. Extrinsic factors that enhance the vulnerability of the myocardium to fibrillate include increased sympathetic nervous system activity, vagal stimulation, metabolic abnormalities (e.g., hypokalemia, hypomagnesemia), antidysrhythmics and other medications (e.g., psychotropics, digitalis, sympathomimetics), and environmental factors (e.g., electrocution). Intrinsic factors include hypertrophy, ischemia, myocardial failure, enhanced AV conduction (e.g., bypass tracts, "fast" AV node), abnormal repolarization, and bradycardia.[18]

> Because artifact can mimic VF, *always* check the patient's pulse before beginning treatment for VF.

Intervention

CPR should be initiated for the patient in VF until a defibrillator is available. On arrival of the defibrillator, unsynchronized shocks should be delivered (Box 6-2), an endotracheal tube should be placed, IV access established, and medications administered per current resuscitation guidelines.

> For each minute of untreated VF, the success of defibrillation decreases by approximately 10%.[19]

It has been demonstrated that patients whose initial fibrillation amplitudes were greater than 0.2 mV (2 mm) had a significantly greater likelihood of resuscitation and that this amplitude declined over time.[20] Factors influencing fibrillation amplitude include electrode size, location, resistance of the chest wall to current, the shape of the chest, and skin condition.[17]

A return of spontaneous circulation is more frequently associated with *early* defibrillation of VF.[17] Defibrillation later in the course of VF is more likely to result in asystole or pulseless electrical activity.[20]

BOX 6-2 **ELECTRICAL THERAPY: DEFIBRILLATION (UNSYNCHRONIZED COUNTERSHOCK)**

DESCRIPTION AND PURPOSE
The purpose of defibrillation is to produce momentary asystole. The shock attempts to completely depolarize the myocardium and provide an opportunity for the natural pacemaker centers of the heart to resume normal activity. Defibrillation is a random delivery of energy—the discharge of energy is not related to the cardiac cycle.

INDICATIONS
- Pulseless VT
- Ventricular fibrillation
- Sustained torsades de pointes
- Undue delay in delivery of synchronized cardioversion

PROCEDURE
1. Apply conductive material to the defibrillator paddles (gel) or chest wall (disposable defibrillator pads). Remove nitroglycerin paste/patches from the patient's chest if present.
2. Turn on the defibrillator.
3. Select the appropriate energy level for the clinical situation/dysrhythmia.
4. Place the defibrillator paddles (or self-adhesive defib pads) on the patient's chest. If using manual defibrillator paddles, apply firm pressure.
5. Charge the paddles and recheck the ECG rhythm.
6. LOOK (360 degrees) to be sure the area is clear. Call "Clear"!
7. Depress both discharge buttons simultaneously to deliver the shock.
8. Reassess the ECG rhythm.

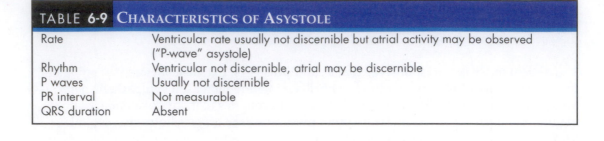

TABLE 6-9	CHARACTERISTICS OF ASYSTOLE
Rate	Ventricular rate usually not discernible but atrial activity may be observed ("P-wave" asystole)
Rhythm	Ventricular not discernible, atrial may be discernible
P waves	Usually not discernible
PR interval	Not measurable
QRS duration	Absent

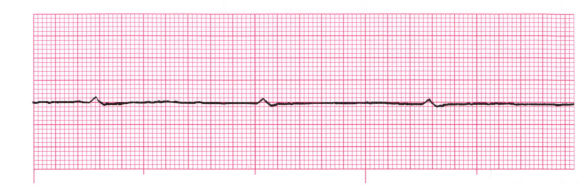

FIGURE **6-14**
"P-wave"
asystole.

ASYSTOLE (CARDIAC STANDSTILL)

ECG Criteria

Asystole is a total absence of ventricular electrical activity (Figure 6-14); thus there is no ventricular rate or rhythm, no pulse, and no cardiac output. Some atrial electrical activity may be evident. If atrial electrical activity is present, the rhythm is called "P-wave" asystole (Table 6-9).

Causes and Clinical Significance

In infants and children, asystole or idioventricular bradycardia is the initial rhythm associated with cardiopulmonary collapse in over 90% of cases.[18]

Asystole may occur because of extensive myocardial damage (possibly from ischemia or infarction), hypoxia, hypokalemia, hyperkalemia, hypothermia, acidosis, drug overdose, ventricular aneurysm, acute respiratory failure, or traumatic cardiac arrest. Ventricular asystole may occur temporarily following termination of a tachydysrhythmia by medication administration, defibrillation, or synchronized cardioversion.

Intervention

If unclear as to whether a rhythm is fine ventricular fibrillation or asystole, treat the rhythm as VF.

Treatment of asystole includes confirmation of the absence of a pulse, immediate CPR, confirmation of the rhythm in two leads, endotracheal intubation, IV access, consideration of the possible causes of the rhythm, consideration of early initiation of transcutaneous pacing, and medication therapy.

PULSELESS ELECTRICAL ACTIVITY (PEA)

ECG Criteria

Pulseless electrical activity (PEA) is a clinical situation, not a specific dysrhythmia. PEA exists when organized electrical activity (other than VT) is observed on the cardiac monitor, but the patient's pulse cannot be palpated (Figure 6-15).

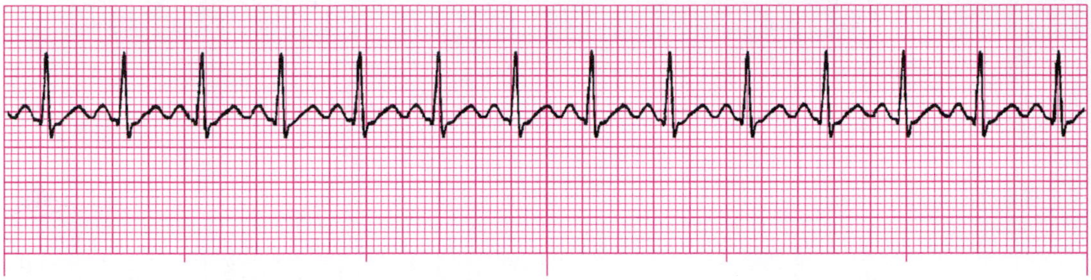

FIGURE **6-15**
Sinus tachycardia. However, if no pulse is associated with the rhythm, the clinical situation is termed *pulseless electrical activity (PEA).*

BOX **6-3**	PATCH-4-MD

Possible causes of PEA:
Pulmonary embolism
Acidosis
Tension pneumothorax
Cardiac tamponade
Hypovolemia (most common cause)
Hypoxia
Heat/cold (hypo-/hyperthermia)
Hypo-/hyperkalemia (and other electrolytes)
Myocardial infarction
Drug overdose/accidents (cyclic antidepressants, calcium channel blockers, beta-blockers, digoxin)

Causes and Clinical Significance

Many conditions may cause PEA. The acronym PATCH-4-MD (Box 6-3) can be used as an aid in memorizing many of the possible causes of PEA. The most common cause of PEA is hypovolemia. The second most common cause is myocardial contractile failure, usually as a result of extensive ischemic or metabolic injury.[21] PEA has a poor prognosis unless the underlying cause can be rapidly identified and appropriately managed. "Irrespective of PEA etiology, the more normal the ECG complex and the shorter the time from cardiac arrest, the higher is the likelihood of successful resuscitation or survival. Conversely, the more abnormal the ECG complex, the longer time from cardiac arrest, the lower the likelihood of successful resuscitation or survival."[22]

Intervention

Treatment of PEA includes CPR, endotracheal intubation, IV access, an aggressive search for possible causes of the situation, and medications per current resuscitation guidelines.

A summary of all ventricular rhythm characteristics can be found in Table 6-10.

TABLE 6-10   VENTRICULAR RHYTHMS: SUMMARY OF CHARACTERISITCS

	PVCs	Ventricular escape beat	IVR	AIVR	Monomorphic VT	TdT	VF	Asystole
Rate	Usually within normal range but depends on underlying rhythm	Usually within normal range, but depends on underlying rhythm	20-40 beats/min	41-100 beats/min	101-250 beats/min	150-300 beats/min	Not discernible	None
Rhythm	Regular with premature beats	Regular with *late* beats	Essentially regular	Essentially regular	Usually regular	Irregular	Chaotic	None
P waves (lead II)	Usually absent or, with retrograde conduction to the atria, may appear after the QRS (usually upright in the ST segment or T wave)	Usually absent or, with retrograde conduction to the atria, may appear after the QRS (usually upright in the ST segment or T wave)	Usually absent or, with retrograde conduction to the atria, may appear after the QRS (usually upright in the ST segment or T wave)	Usually absent or, with retrograde conduction to the atria, may appear after the QRS (usually upright in the ST segment or T wave)	May be present or absent; if present, have no set relationship to the QRS complexes, appearing between the QRSs at a rate different from that of the VT	Independent or none	Absent	Atrial activity may be observed ("P-wave" asystole)
PR interval	None	None	None	None	None	None	None	None
QRS	>0.12 sec	>0.12 sec	>0.12 sec	>0.12 sec	>0.12 sec	>0.12 sec	Not discernible	Absent
Clinical significance	PVCs may or may not produce palpable pulses; may be asymptomatic or complain of palpitations, a "racing heart," skipped beats, or chest or neck discomfort	A *protective mechanism*, protecting the heart from more extreme slowing or even asystole	Possible severe hypotension, weakness, disorientation, lightheadedness, or loss of consciousness because of decreased cardiac output resulting from slow rate	Usually asymptomatic; however, possible dizziness, lightheadedness, or other signs of hemodynamic compromise may result from loss of atrial kick	Possible palpitations, shortness of breath, chest pain, or discomfort; loss of consciousness, especially if VT is prolonged or sustained	Possible palpitations, syncope, and/or dizziness	Unresponsive, apneic, and pulseless	Unresponsive, apneic, and pulseless

REFERENCES

1. Crawford MV, Spence MI: *Common sense approach to coronary care*, ed 6, St Louis, 1995, Mosby.
2. Chou T, Knilans TK: *Electrocardiography in clinical practice: adult and pediatric*, Philadelphia, 1996, WB Saunders.
3. Goldberger AL: *Clinical electrocardiography: a simplified approach*, ed 6, St Louis, 1999, Mosby.
4. Kinney MR, Packa DR, editors: *Andreoli's comprehensive cardiac care*, ed 8, St Louis, 1996, Mosby.
5. Callans DJ, Josephson ME: Ventricular tachycardias in the setting of coronary artery disease. In Zipes DP, Jalife J, editors: *Cardiac electrophysiology: from cell to bedside*, Philadelphia, 1995, WB Saunders.
6. Goldman L, Braunwald E: *Primary cardiology*, Philadelphia, 1998, WB Saunders.
7. Crawford MH, editor: *Current diagnosis and treatment in cardiology*, Norwalk, 1995, Appleton & Lange.
8. Murphy JG: *Mayo clinical cardiology review*, ed 2, Philadelphia, 2000, Lippincott, Williams & Wilkins.
9. Panidis IP, Morganroth J: Holter monitoring and sudden cardiac death, *Cardiovasc Rev Rep* 5(3):283; 287-290; 297-299; 303-304, 1984.
10. Olshausen KV, Witt T, Pop T, Treese N, Bethge KP, Meyer J: Sudden cardiac death while wearing a Holter monitor, *Am J Cardiol* 67(5):381-386, 1991.
11. Milner PG, Platia EV, Reid PR, Griffith LS: Ambulatory electrocardiographic recordings at the time of fatal cardiac arrest, *Am J Cardiol* 56(10):588-592, 1985.
12. Panidis IP, Morganroth J: Sudden death in hospitalized patients: cardiac rhythm disturbances detected by ambulatory electrocardiographic monitoring, *J Am Coll Cardiol* 2(5):798-805, 1983.
13. Marriott HJL, Conover MB: *Advanced concepts in arrhythmias*, ed 3, St Louis, 1998, Mosby.
14. Vincent GM: *Long QT syndrome, Cardiology clinics*, Vol 18, Number 2, Philadelphia, 2000, WB Saunders.
15. Conover MB: *Understanding electrocardiography*, ed 7, St Louis, 1996, Mosby.
16. Weil MH, Tang W, editors: *CPR: resuscitation of the arrested heart*, Philadelphia, 1999, WB Saunders.
17. Paradis NA, Halperin HR, Nowak RM, editors: *Cardiac arrest: the science and practice of resuscitation medicine*, Baltimore, 1996, Williams & Wilkins.
18. Eisenberg MS, Horwood BT, Cummins RO, et al: Cardiac arrest and resuscitation. A tale of 29 cities, *Ann Emerg Med* 19:179-186, 1990.
19. Weaver WD, Cobb LA, Dennis D, et al: Amplitude of ventricular fibrillation waveform and outcome after cardiac arrest, *Ann Intern Med* 102:53-55, 1985.
20. Weil MH, Tang W, editors: *CPR: resuscitation of the arrested heart*, Philadelphia, 1999, WB Saunders.
21. Aufderheide TP: In Paradis NA, Halperin HR, Nowak RM, editors: *Cardiac arrest: the science and practice of resuscitation medicine*, Baltimore, 1996, Williams & Wilkins.

BIBLIOGRAPHY

Berne RM, Levy MN: *Cardiovascular physiology*, ed 7, St Louis, 1997, Mosby.
Braunwauld E, Scheinman M, editors: *Arrhythmias: electrophysiologic principles*, Vol IX, Singapore, 1996, Current Medicine/Mosby.
Callans DJ, Josephson ME: Ventricular tachycardias in the setting of coronary artery disease. In Zipes DP, Jalife J, editors: *Cardiac electrophysiology: from cell to bedside*, Philadelphia, 1995, WB Saunders.
Chou T, Knilans TK: *Electrocardiography in clinical practice: adult and pediatric*, Philadelphia, 1996, WB Saunders Company.
Crawford MH, editor: *Current diagnosis and treatment in cardiology*, Norwalk, 1995, Appleton & Lange.
Crawford MV, Spence MI: *Common sense approach to coronary care*, ed 6, St Louis, 1995, Mosby.
Goldberger AL: *Clinical electrocardiography: a simplified approach*, ed 6, St Louis, 1999, Mosby.
Goldman L, Braunwald E: *Primary cardiology*, Philadelphia, 1998, WB Saunders.

Gordon T, Kannel WB: Premature mortality from coronary heart disease: the Framingham study, *JAMA* 215:1617, 1971

Huszar RJ: *Basic dysrhythmias: interpretation and management,* ed 2, St Louis, 1994, Mosby.

Johnson R, Swartz MH: *A simplified approach to electrocardiography,* Philadelphia, 1986, WB Saunders.

Kahn, MG: *Cardiac drug therapy,* ed 5, London, 2000, Harcourt Publishers Limited.

Kinney MR, Packa DR, editors: *Andreoli's comprehensive cardiac care,* ed 8, St Louis, 1996, Mosby.

Marriott HJL, Conover MB: *Advanced concepts in arrhythmias,* ed 3, St Louis, 1998, Mosby.

Padrid PJ, Kowey PR, editors: *Cardiac arrhythmia: mechanisms, diagnosis, and management,* Baltimore, 1995, Williams & Wilkins.

Paradis NA, Halperin HR, Nowak RM, editors: *Cardiac arrest: the science and practice of resuscitation medicine,* Baltimore, 1996, Williams & Wilkins.

Phalen T: *The 12-lead ECG in acute myocardial infarction,* St Louis, 1996, Mosby.

Phillips RE, Feeney MK: *The cardiac rhythms: a systematic approach to interpretation,* ed 3, Philadelphia, 1990, WB Saunders.

Wagner GS: *Marriott's practical electrocardiography,* ed 9, Baltimore, 1994, Williams & Wilkins.

Woods SL, Sivarajan Froelicher ES, Motzer SA: *Cardiac nursing,* ed 4, Philadelphia, 2000, Lippincott, Williams & Wilkins.

STOP & REVIEW

MATCHING

___ 1. Two sequential PVCs

___ 2. Medication that should be avoided in the management of IVR or AIVR

___ 3. Pattern in which every other beat is an ectopic beat

___ 4. Clinical situation in which organized electrical activity (other than VT) is observed on the cardiac monitor, but the patient is pulseless

___ 5. Essentially regular ventricular rhythm with a ventricular rate of 40 beats/min or less

___ 6. Type of PVC that occurs between two normal beats and does not interrupt the underlying rhythm

___ 7. Absence of electrical activity on the cardiac monitor

___ 8. Medication used in the management of torsades de pointes

___ 9. Essentially regular ventricular rhythm with a ventricular rate of 41 to 100 beats/min

___ 10. Name given a PVC falling on the T wave of the preceding beat

___ 11. PVCs of similar configuration in the same lead

___ 12. Pattern in which every third beat is an ectopic beat

___ 13. Ventricular beat that occurs later than the next expected sinus beat; protective mechanism

___ 14. Medications associated with prolongation of the QT interval and precipitation of torsades de pointes

___ 15. Essentially regular ventricular rhythm with a ventricular rate of more than 100 beats/min

A. R-on-T phenomenon
B. Asystole
C. Trigeminy
D. Ventricular tachycardia
E. Ventricular escape beat
F. Uniform
G. Bigeminy
H. Accelerated idioventricular rhythm
I. Pulseless electrical activity
J. Ventricular escape rhythm
K. Lidocaine
L. Magnesium sulfate
M. Quinidine, procainamide
N. Couplet
O. Interpolated

IDENTIFICATION AND MEASUREMENTS—PRACTICE RHYTHM STRIPS

For each of the following rhythm strips, determine the atrial and ventricular rates, measure the PR interval, QRS duration, and QT interval, and then identify the rhythm. All strips lead II unless otherwise noted.

PRACTICE RHYTHM STRIPS

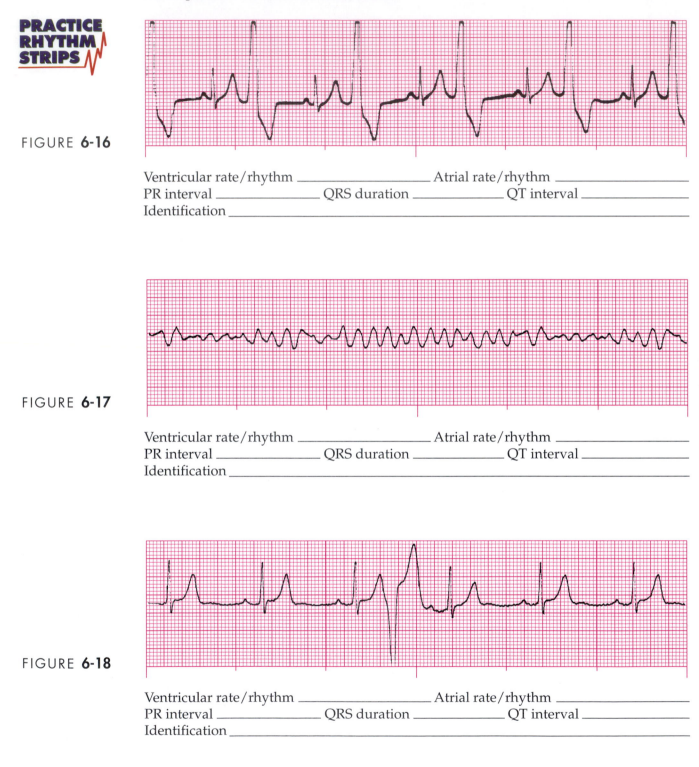

FIGURE **6-16**

Ventricular rate/rhythm _____ Atrial rate/rhythm _____
PR interval _____ QRS duration _____ QT interval _____
Identification _____

FIGURE **6-17**

Ventricular rate/rhythm _____ Atrial rate/rhythm _____
PR interval _____ QRS duration _____ QT interval _____
Identification _____

FIGURE **6-18**

Ventricular rate/rhythm _____ Atrial rate/rhythm _____
PR interval _____ QRS duration _____ QT interval _____
Identification _____

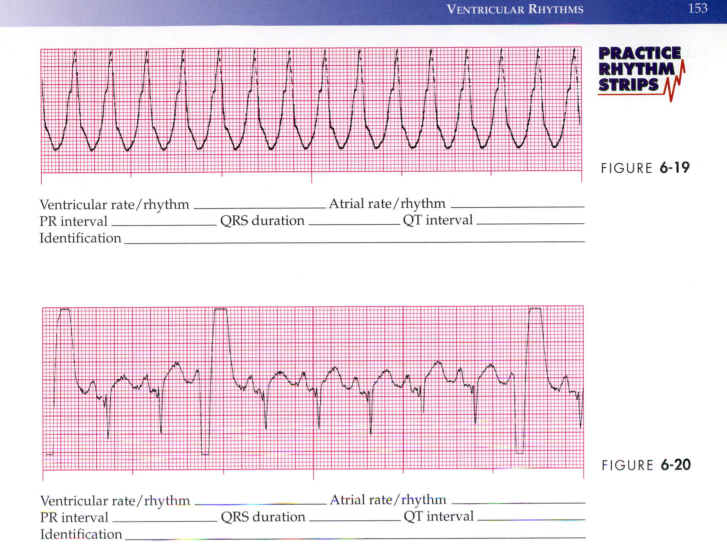

PRACTICE
RHYTHM
STRIPS

FIGURE **6-19**

Ventricular rate/rhythm _____ Atrial rate/rhythm _____
PR interval _____ QRS duration _____ QT interval _____
Identification _____

FIGURE **6-20**

Ventricular rate/rhythm _____ Atrial rate/rhythm _____
PR interval _____ QRS duration _____ QT interval _____
Identification _____

The rhythm strip below is from a 2-year-old female kicked in the head by a horse (traumatic cardiac arrest). Lead III.

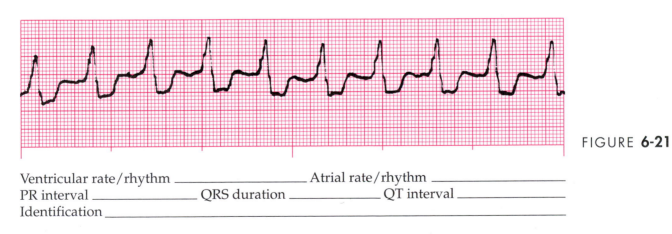

FIGURE **6-21**

Ventricular rate/rhythm _____ Atrial rate/rhythm _____
PR interval _____ QRS duration _____ QT interval _____
Identification _____

**PRACTICE
RHYTHM
STRIPS**

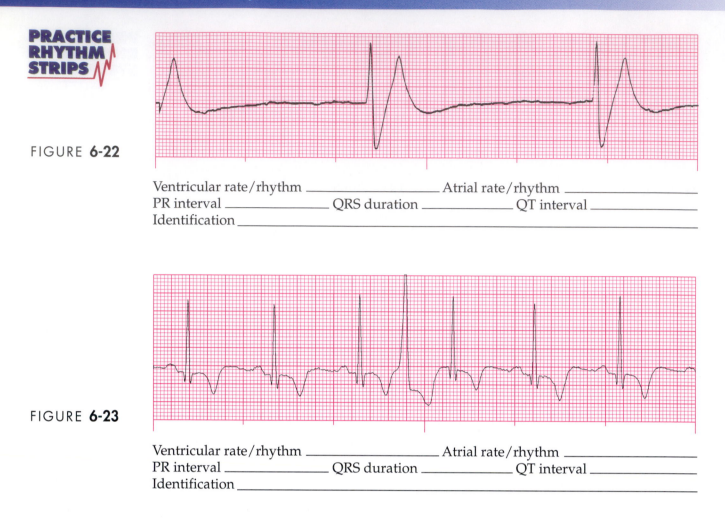

FIGURE **6-22**

Ventricular rate/rhythm _____ Atrial rate/rhythm _____
PR interval _____ QRS duration _____ QT interval _____
Identification _____

FIGURE **6-23**

Ventricular rate/rhythm _____ Atrial rate/rhythm _____
PR interval _____ QRS duration _____ QT interval _____
Identification _____

The rhythm strip below is from a 19-year-old male who walked into the emergency department after ingesting a number of unknown medications (per patient) in a suicide attempt. He became unresponsive 5 minutes after his arrival. Initial rhythms before the onset of this dysrhythmia were monomorphic VT and then complete AV block. After a brief episode of the rhythm below, the patient again converted to a complete AV block. Drug screen was negative. A transvenous pacemaker was inserted, and the patient was admitted to CCU.

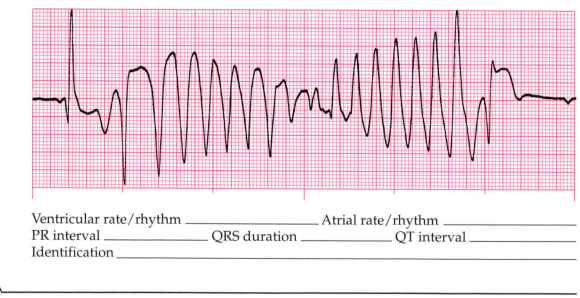

FIGURE **6-24**

Ventricular rate/rhythm _____ Atrial rate/rhythm _____
PR interval _____ QRS duration _____ QT interval _____
Identification _____

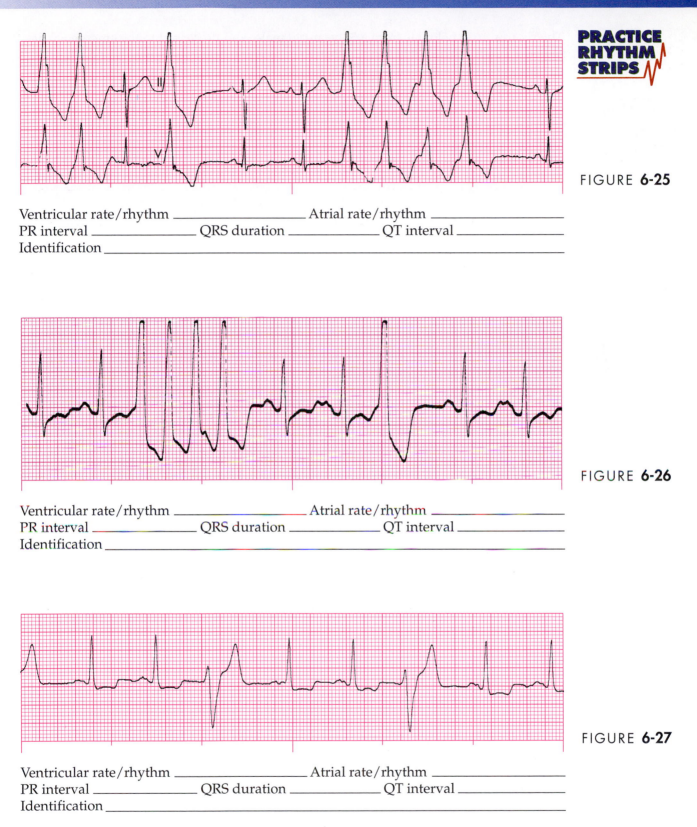

FIGURE **6-25**

Ventricular rate/rhythm _____ Atrial rate/rhythm _____
PR interval _____ QRS duration _____ QT interval _____
Identification _____

FIGURE **6-26**

Ventricular rate/rhythm _____ Atrial rate/rhythm _____
PR interval _____ QRS duration _____ QT interval _____
Identification _____

FIGURE **6-27**

Ventricular rate/rhythm _____ Atrial rate/rhythm _____
PR interval _____ QRS duration _____ QT interval _____
Identification _____

PRACTICE RHYTHM STRIPS

The rhythm strip below is from a 37-year-old male who presented to the emergency department with seizures. He had a history of a 3-day methamphetamine binge. The rhythm converted with diltiazem (Cardizem).

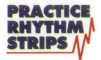

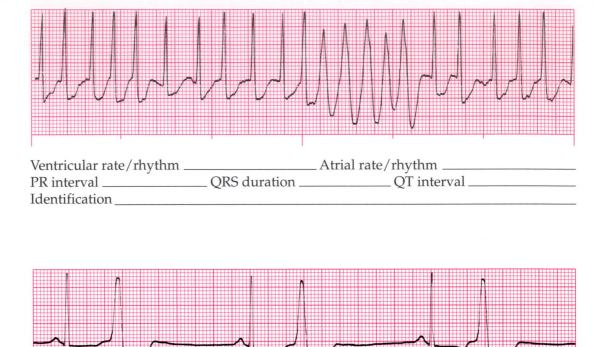

FIGURE **6-28**

Ventricular rate/rhythm _____ Atrial rate/rhythm _____
PR interval _____ QRS duration _____ QT interval _____
Identification _____

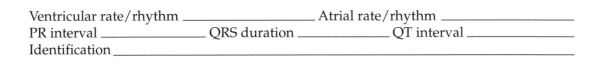

FIGURE **6-29**

Ventricular rate/rhythm _____ Atrial rate/rhythm _____
PR interval _____ QRS duration _____ QT interval _____
Identification _____

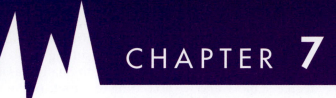

CHAPTER **7**

Atrioventricular (AV) Blocks

OBJECTIVES

On completion of this chapter, you will be able to:

Describe the ECG characteristics, possible causes, signs and symptoms, and emergency management for the following dysrhythmias:
- First-degree AV block
- Second-degree AV block, type I
- Second-degree AV block, type II
- Second-degree AV block, 2:1 conduction
- Complete AV block

OVERVIEW

AV junction: The AV node and the bundle of His.

The **AV junction** is an area of specialized conduction tissue that provides the electrical links between the atrium and ventricle. If a delay or interruption in impulse conduction occurs within the AV node, bundle of His, or His-Purkinje system, the resulting dysrhythmia is called an *atrioventricular (AV) block*. AV blocks have been traditionally classified in two ways—according to the degree of block and/or according to the site of the block.

Depolarization and repolarization are slow in the AV node, making this area vulnerable to blocks in conduction (AV blocks).

Remember that the PR interval reflects depolarization of the right and left atria (P wave) and the spread of the impulse through the AV node, bundle of His, right and left bundle branches, and the Purkinje fibers. The PR interval is the key to differentiating the *type* of AV block. The key to differentiating the *level* (location) of the block is the width of the

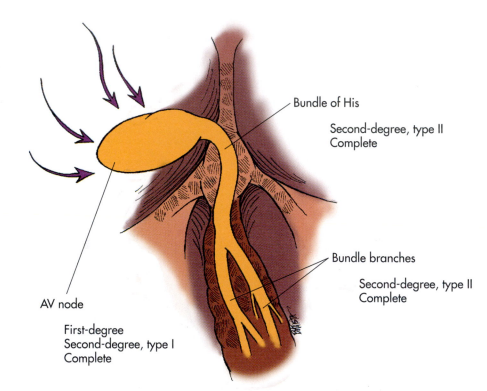

FIGURE **7-1**
Locations of AV block.

TABLE **7-1** CLASSIFICATION OF AV BLOCKS			
Degree of block	Incomplete blocks		First-degree AV block
			Second-degree AV block, type I
			Second-degree AV block, type II
			Second-degree AV block, 2:1 conduction
	Complete block		Complete (third-degree) AV block
Site of block	AV node		First-degree AV block
			Second-degree AV block, type I
			Complete (third-degree) AV block
	Infranodal (subnodal)	Bundle of His	Second-degree AV block, type II (uncommon)
			Complete (third-degree) AV block
		Bundle branches	Second-degree AV block, type II (more common)
			Complete (third-degree) AV block

QRS complex and, in second- and third-degree (complete) AV blocks, the rate of the escape rhythm.

In first-degree AV block, impulses from the SA node to the ventricles are *delayed* (not blocked). First-degree AV block usually occurs at the AV node (Figure 7-1). With second-degree AV blocks, there is an *intermittent* disturbance in conduction of impulses between the atria and ventricles. The site of block in second-degree AV block type I is typically at the AV node. The site of block in second-degree AV block type II is the bundle of His or, more commonly, the bundle branches. In complete or third-degree AV block, the AV junction does not conduct any impulses between the atria and ventricles. The site of block in a complete AV block may be the AV node or, more commonly, the bundle of His or bundle branches.

The clinical significance of an AV block depends on the degree (severity) of the block, the rate of the escape pacemaker (junctional vs. ventricular), and the patient's response to that ventricular rate (Table 7-1).

FIRST-DEGREE AV BLOCK

ECG Criteria

A PR interval of normal duration (0.12 to 0.20 sec) indicates the electrical impulse was conducted normally through the atria, AV node, bundle of His, bundle branches, and Purkinje fibers. In first-degree AV block, all components of the ECG tracing are usually within normal limits except the PR interval. This is because electrical impulses flow normally from the SA node through the atria, but there is a delay in impulse conduction, most commonly at the level of the AV node. Despite its name, in first-degree AV block, the sinus impulse is not *blocked* (all sinus beats are conducted)—impulses are *delayed* for the same period before they are conducted to the ventricles. This delay in AV conduction results in a PR interval that is more than 0.20 sec in duration and constant (Table 7-2).

In first-degree AV block, each P wave is followed by a QRS complex (1:1 relationship). The QRS duration is usually 0.10 sec or less unless an intraventricular conduction delay exists (Figure 7-2).

The PR interval is usually between 0.21 and 0.48 sec. Occasionally, a PR interval greater than 0.8 sec may be seen.[1] However, PR intervals as long as 1 sec or more have been reported.[2]

TABLE 7-2 CHARACTERISTICS OF FIRST-DEGREE AV BLOCK	
Rate	Usually within normal range but depends on underlying rhythm
Rhythm	Regular
P waves	Normal in size and shape, one positive (upright) P wave before each QRS in leads II, III, and aVF
PR interval	Prolonged (greater than 0.20 sec) but constant
QRS duration	Usually 0.10 sec or less unless an intraventricular conduction delay exists

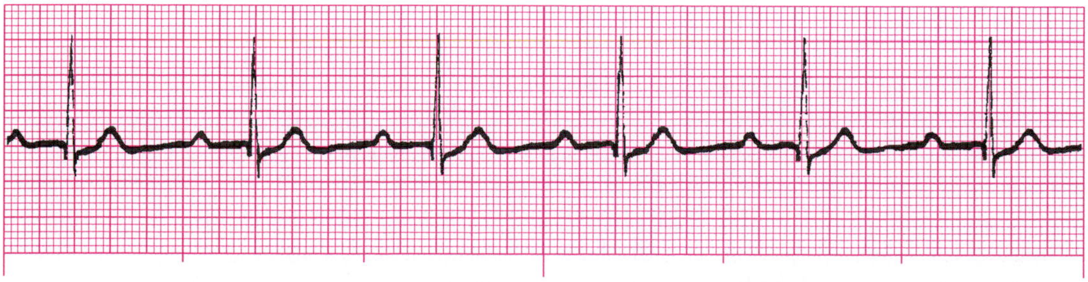

FIGURE **7-2**
Sinus rhythm at 60 beats/min with a first-degree AV block.

First-degree AV block is not a dysrhythmia itself but a condition describing the consistent prolonged PR interval viewed on the ECG rhythm strip. If a cardiac rhythm fits the criteria for sinus bradycardia even though the PR interval is prolonged and constant, the rhythm is identified as "sinus bradycardia at 40 beats/min with a first-degree AV block."

Causes and Clinical Significance

First-degree AV block may be a normal finding in individuals with no history of cardiac disease, especially in athletes. First-degree AV block may also occur because of ischemia or injury to the AV node or junction, medication therapy (e.g., quinidine, procainamide, beta-blockers, calcium channel blockers, digitalis, and amiodarone), rheumatic heart disease, hyperkalemia, acute myocardial infarction (often inferior wall MI), or increased vagal tone. Approximately 5% to 10% of patients with acute myocardial infarction have first-degree AV block at some point during the peri-infarct period.[3]

Intervention

The patient with a first-degree AV block is often asymptomatic; however, marked first-degree AV block can lead to symptoms even in the absence of higher degrees of AV block.[5] First-degree AV block that occurs with acute myocardial infarction should be monitored closely.

SECOND-DEGREE AV BLOCKS

Overview

Two types of second-degree AV blocks based on jugular pulse tracings were first described by an early 20th century European physician named Wenckebach. In 1924, a German electrocardiographer named Mobitz identified the same dysrhythmias previously identified by Wenckebach. Mobitz termed the rhythms type I (later called Mobitz I) and type II (later known as Mobitz II).

When some, but not all, atrial impulses are blocked from reaching the ventricles, second-degree AV block results. Because the SA node is generating impulses in a normal manner, each P wave will occur at a regular interval across the rhythm strip (all P waves will plot through on time), although not every P wave will be followed by a QRS complex. This suggests that the atria are being depolarized normally, but not every impulse is being conducted to the ventricles. As a result, more P waves than QRS complexes are visible on the ECG rhythm strip.

Second-degree AV block is classified as type I or type II, depending on the location of the block above (type I) or below (type II) the bundle of His.

Second-Degree AV Block, Type I (Wenckebach, Mobitz Type I)

ECG Criteria

The conduction delay in second-degree AV block type I (Figure 7-3) usually occurs at the level of the AV node. In this type of second-degree AV block, impulses generated by the SA node take longer and longer to conduct through the AV node, appearing on the ECG as lengthening PR intervals. The lengthening PR intervals eventually result in a P wave that falls during the refractory period of the ventricles. Because the ventricles are refractory, the sinus impulse is blocked. The blocked sinus impulse appears on the ECG as a P wave with no QRS after it (dropped beat). Thus the atria are depolarized (represented by the P wave), but the AV junction fails to conduct the impulse from the atria to the ventricles (reflected on the ECG by the absence of a QRS complex). The QRS usu-

Mild prolongation of the PR interval may be a normal variant, occurring especially with physiologic sinus bradycardia during rest or sleep.[4]

In second-degree AV block types I and II, the ventricular rhythm (R-R interval) is irregular.

Second-degree AV block type I is also known as Mobitz type I or Wenckebach. The Wenckebach pattern is the progressive lengthening of the PR interval followed by a P wave with no QRS complex.

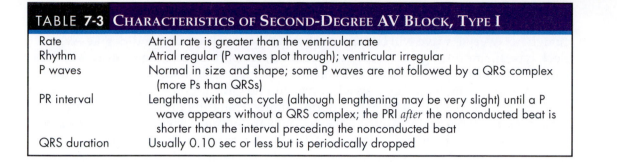

TABLE 7-3	CHARACTERISTICS OF SECOND-DEGREE AV BLOCK, TYPE I
Rate	Atrial rate is greater than the ventricular rate
Rhythm	Atrial regular (P waves plot through); ventricular irregular
P waves	Normal in size and shape; some P waves are not followed by a QRS complex (more Ps than QRSs)
PR interval	Lengthens with each cycle (although lengthening may be very slight) until a P wave appears without a QRS complex; the PRI *after* the nonconducted beat is shorter than the interval preceding the nonconducted beat
QRS duration	Usually 0.10 sec or less but is periodically dropped

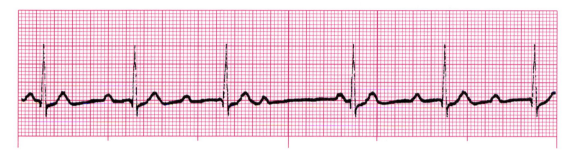

FIGURE **7-3**
Second-degree
AV block, type I.

ally measures 0.10 sec or less unless an intraventricular conduction delay exists. Because QRS complexes are periodically dropped, the ventricular rhythm is irregular. The cycle then begins again. The repetition of this cyclic pattern is called "grouped beating" (Table 7-3).

Causes and Clinical Significance

Second-degree AV block type I is caused by conduction delay within the AV node and is most commonly associated with AV nodal ischemia secondary to occlusion of the right coronary artery.[6] Second-degree AV block type I may also occur because of increased parasympathetic tone or the effects of medication (e.g., digitalis, beta-blockers, verapamil). When associated with an acute inferior wall myocardial infarction, this dysrhythmia is usually transient, resolving within 48 to 72 hours as the effects of parasympathetic stimulation disappear. Second-degree AV block type I may progress to a complete AV block, although the risk of progression to this type of AV block is low.[4]

Second-degree AV block type I may be seen in up to 10% of patients with acute MI.[3]

Intervention

The patient with this dysrhythmia is usually asymptomatic because the ventricular rate often remains nearly normal, and cardiac output is not significantly affected. If the patient is symptomatic and the dysrhythmia is a result of medications, these substances should be withheld. If the heart rate is slow and serious signs and symptoms (low blood pressure, shortness of breath, congestive heart failure, chest pain, pulmonary congestion, decreased level of consciousness) occur because of the slow rate, atropine and/or temporary pacing should be considered. When this dysrhythmia occurs in conjunction with acute myocardial infarction, the patient should be observed for increasing AV block.

Second-Degree AV Block, Type II (Mobitz Type II)

ECG Criteria

The conduction delay in second-degree AV block type II occurs below the AV node, either at the bundle of His or, more commonly, at the level of the bundle branches. This type of block is more serious than second-degree AV block type I and frequently progresses to complete AV block.

Second-degree AV block type II is also called *Mobitz type II AV block.*

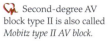

Because the SA node is generating impulses in a normal manner, each P wave occurs at a regular interval across the rhythm strip (all P waves will plot through on time), although not every P wave will be followed by a QRS complex. In second-degree AV block type II, impulses generated by the SA node are conducted to the ventricles at the same rate (appearing on the ECG as a constant PR interval) until an impulse is suddenly blocked—appearing on the ECG as a P wave with no QRS after it (dropped beat) (Figure 7-4). The PR interval is usually within normal limits or slightly prolonged. Because QRS complexes are periodically dropped, the ventricular rhythm is irregular. If the block occurs in the bundle of His (uncommon), the QRS will remain narrow. If the block occurs below the bundle of His (more common), the QRS will be more than 0.10 sec in duration (Table 7-4).

Causes and Clinical Significance

The bundle branches receive their primary blood supply from the left coronary artery. Thus disease of the left coronary artery or an anterior myocardial infarction is usually associated with blocks that occur within the bundle branches. Second-degree AV block type II may also occur because of acute myocarditis or other types of organic heart disease. The patient's response to this dysrhythmia is usually related to the ventricular rate. If the ventricular rate is within normal limits, the patient may be asymptomatic. More commonly, the ventricular rate is significantly slowed and serious signs and symptoms result (low blood pressure, shortness of breath, congestive heart failure, pulmonary congestion, decreased level of consciousness) because of the slow rate and decreased cardiac output.

Patients with type II second-degree AV block are often symptomatic, have a compromised prognosis, and commonly progress to complete AV block.[7]

Intervention

Second-degree AV block type II may rapidly progress to complete AV block without warning. If the patient is symptomatic, transcutaneous pacing should be instituted until transvenous pacemaker insertion can be accomplished.

Second-degree AV block type II usually indicates the need for a permanent pacemaker.

TABLE 7-4	CHARACTERISTICS OF SECOND-DEGREE AV BLOCK, TYPE II
Rate	Atrial rate is greater than the ventricular rate; ventricular rate is often slow
Rhythm	Atrial regular (P waves plot through); ventricular irregular
P waves	Normal in size and shape; some P waves are not followed by a QRS complex (more Ps than QRSs)
PR interval	Within normal limits or slightly prolonged but constant for the conducted beats; there may be some shortening of the PR interval that follows a nonconducted P wave
QRS duration	Usually 0.10 sec or greater, periodically absent after P waves

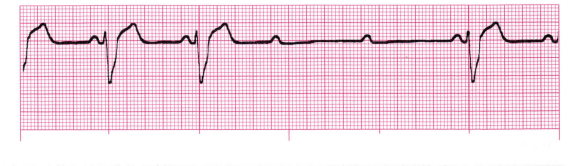

FIGURE **7-4**
Second-degree
AV block, type II.

Second-Degree AV Block, 2:1 Conduction (2:1 AV Block)

ECG Criteria

When two conducted P waves occur *consecutively*, the PR intervals of the consecutive beats should be compared to identify either type I or type II second-degree AV block. If two P waves occur for every one QRS complex (2:1 conduction), the decision as to what to term the rhythm is based on the width of the QRS complex.

A 2:1 AV conduction pattern associated with a narrow QRS complex (0.10 sec or less) usually represents a form of second-degree AV block, type I (Figure 7-5). A 2:1 AV conduction pattern associated with wide QRS complexes (greater than 0.10 sec) is usually associated with a delay in conduction below the bundle of His—thus it is usually a type II block (Figure 7-6).

The terms *high-grade* or *advanced* second-degree AV block may be used to describe two or more consecutive P waves that are not conducted. For example, in 3:1 block, every third P wave is conducted; in 4:1 block, every fourth P wave is conducted. In cases of advanced AV block, it may be difficult to determine the type of second-degree block because the block may involve either a type I or type II mechanism. If the PR interval varies and its length is inversely related to the interval between the P wave and its preceding R wave, the rhythm is most likely a second-degree block, type I.[8] If the PR interval is constant for all conducted beats, the rhythm is most likely a second-degree AV block, type II (Table 7-5).

Second-degree AV block with 2:1 conduction may be caused by block within the AV node (type I) or more distal block within the His-Purkinje system (type II).[6]

TABLE 7-5	CHARACTERISTICS OF SECOND-DEGREE AV BLOCK, 2:1 CONDUCTION
Rate	Atrial rate is twice the ventricular rate
Rhythm	Atrial regular (P waves plot through); ventricular regular
P waves	Normal in size and shape; every other P wave is followed by a QRS complex (more Ps than QRSs)
PR interval	Constant
QRS duration	Within normal limits if the block occurs above the bundle of His (probably type I); wide if the block occurs below the bundle of His (probably type II); absent after every other P wave

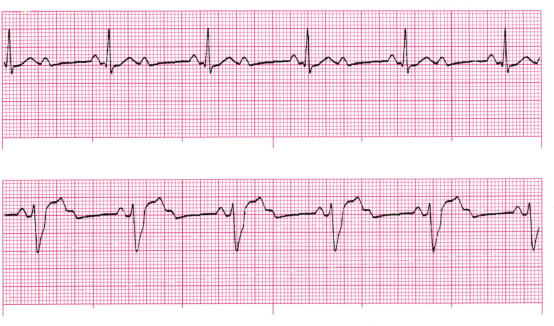

FIGURE 7-5
Second-degree AV block, 2:1 conduction, probably type I.

FIGURE 7-6
Second-degree AV block, 2:1 conduction, probably type II.

Causes and Clinical Significance

The causes and clinical significance of second-degree AV block with 2:1 conduction are those of type I or type II block previously described. Clinically, conduction usually improves in response to exercise or administration of atropine or catecholamines in type I AV block. In type II AV block, conduction typically worsens with exercise or administration of atropine or catecholamines.

COMPLETE AV BLOCK

ECG Criteria

Complete AV block is also called *third-degree AV block.*

Complete AV block is a form of AV dissociation.

First- and second-degree AV blocks are types of *incomplete blocks* because the AV junction conducts at least some impulses to the ventricles.[4] With *complete AV block,* the atria and ventricles beat independently of each other. Impulses generated by the sinoatrial node are blocked before reaching the ventricles. The block may occur at the AV node, bundle of His, or bundle branches. A secondary pacemaker (either junctional or ventricular) stimulates the ventricles; therefore, the QRS may be narrow or wide, depending on the location of the escape pacemaker and the condition of the intraventricular conduction system (Table 7-6).

Narrow QRS indicates a junctional pacemaker; wide QRS indicates a ventricular pacemaker.

Complete AV block associated with an inferior myocardial infarction is thought to be the result of a block above the bundle of His and often occurs after progression from first-degree AV block or second-degree AV block, type I. The resulting rhythm is usually sta-

TABLE 7-6	CHARACTERISTICS OF COMPLETE AV BLOCK
Rate	Atrial rate is greater than the ventricular rate; the ventricular rate is determined by the origin of the escape rhythm
Rhythm	Atrial regular (P waves plot through); ventricular regular; there is no relationship between the atrial and ventricular rhythms
P waves	Normal in size and shape
PR interval	None—the atria and ventricles beat independently of each other; thus there is no true PR interval
QRS duration	Narrow or wide, depending on the location of the escape pacemaker and the condition of the intraventricular conduction system; narrow indicates junctional pacemaker; wide indicates ventricular pacemaker

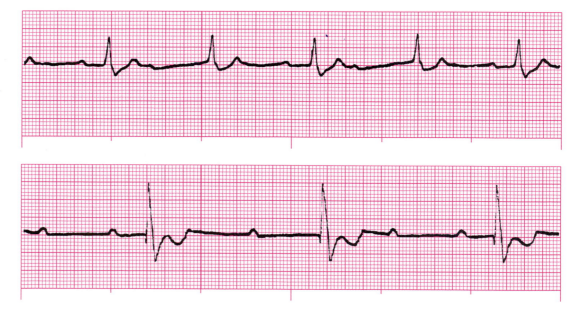

FIGURE **7-7**
Complete AV block with a junctional escape pacemaker (QRS 0.08 to 0.10 sec).

FIGURE **7-8**
Complete AV block with a ventricular escape pacemaker (QRS 0.12 to 0.14 sec).

ble, and the escape pacemaker is usually junctional with narrow QRS complexes and a ventricular rate of more than 40 beats/min (Figure 7-7).

Complete AV block associated with an anterior MI is usually preceded by second-degree AV block type II or an intraventricular conduction delay (e.g., right or left bundle branch block). The resulting rhythm is usually unstable, and the escape pacemaker is usually ventricular with wide QRS complexes and a ventricular rate of less than 40 beats/min (Figure 7-8).

Causes and Clinical Significance

Complete AV block has an incidence of 5.8% in the early period of acute MI and is nearly twice as common with inferior/posterior infarctions compared with anterior infarction.[6] When associated with an inferior MI, complete AV block often resolves on its own within a week. Complete AV block associated with an anterior MI may develop suddenly and without warning, usually 12 to 24 hours after the onset of acute ischemia.

Generally, complete AV block with narrow QRS complexes (junctional escape pacemaker with a ventricular rate of more than 40 beats/min) is a more stable rhythm that a complete AV block with wide QRS complexes (ventricular pacemaker with a ventricular rate that is usually less than 40 beats/min) because the ventricular escape pacemaker is usually slower and less consistent.[4]

Complete AV block that occurs with an acute anterior MI is often an indication for insertion of a permanent pacemaker.

Intervention

The patient's signs and symptoms will depend on the origin of the escape pacemaker (junctional vs. ventricular) and the patient's response to a slower ventricular rate.

If the QRS is narrow and the patient is symptomatic, initial management consists of atropine and/or transcutaneous pacing. If the QRS is wide and the patient is symptomatic, transcutaneous pacing should be instituted while preparations are made for insertion of a transvenous pacemaker.

Table 7-7 will help you learn to recognize the differences between second- and third-degree AV blocks. First, determine if the ventricular rhythm is regular or irregular. Next, look at the PR intervals. Based on this information, you should be able to identify the rhythm strips in this chapter.

A summary of AV block characteristics can be found in Table 7-8.

TABLE 7-7 AV BLOCKS: QUICK SUMMARY		
	Second-degree AV block, type I	Second-degree AV block, type II
Ventricular rhythm	Irregular	Irregular
PR interval	Progressively lengthening	Constant
QRS width	Usually narrow	Usually wide
	Second-degree AV block, 2:1 conduction	Complete (third-degree) AV block
Ventricular rhythm	Regular	Regular
PR interval	Constant	None—no relationship between P waves and QRS complexes
QRS width	May be narrow or wide	May be narrow or wide

TABLE 7-8 ATRIOVENTRICULAR BLOCKS: SUMMARY OF CHARACTERISTICS

	First-degree	Second-degree, type I	Second-degree, type II	Second-degree, 2:1 conduction	Complete (third-degree)
Rate	Usually within normal range but depends on underlying rhythm	Atrial rate > ventricular; both often within normal limits	Atrial rate is greater than the ventricular rate; ventricular rate often slow	Atrial rate > ventricular rate	Atrial rate > ventricular rate; ventricular rate determined by origin of escape rhythm
Rhythm	Atrial regular; ventricular regular	Atrial regular; ventricular irregular	Atrial regular, ventricular irregular	Atrial regular, ventricular regular	Atrial regular, ventricular regular
P waves (lead II)	Normal, one P wave precedes each QRS	Normal in size and shape; some P waves are not followed by a QRS complex (more Ps than QRSs)	Normal in size and shape; some P waves are not followed by a QRS complex (more Ps than QRSs)	Normal in size and shape; every other P wave is not followed by a QRS complex (more Ps than QRSs)	Normal in size and shape; some P waves are not followed by a QRS complex (more Ps than QRSs)
PR interval	>0.20 sec and constant	Lengthens with each cycle until a P wave appears without a QRS	Normal or slightly prolonged but constant for conducted beats	Constant	None—the atria and ventricles beat independently of each other; thus there is no true PR interval
QRS	Usually <0.10 sec unless an intraventricular conduction delay exists	Usually <0.10 sec unless an intraventricular conduction delay exists	Usually >0.10 sec, periodically absent after P waves	Within normal limits if block above bundle of His (probably type I); wide if block below bundle of His (probably type II); absent after every other P wave	Narrow or wide, depending on location of escape pacemaker and condition of intraventricular conduction
Clinical significance	Patient often asymptomatic, but first-degree AV block that occurs with acute MI should be monitored closely for increasing heart block	Usually asymptomatic	May rapidly progress to complete AV block without warning	Signs and symptoms will depend on the origin of escape pacemaker and patient's response to ventricular rate	Signs and symptoms will depend on the origin of escape pacemaker and patient's response to ventricular rate

REFERENCES

1. Kahn MG: *Rapid ECG interpretation,* Philadelphia, 1997, WB Saunders.
2. Rusterholz AP, Marriott HJL: How long can the P-R interval be? *Am J Noninvasive Cardiol* 8:11-13, 1994.
3. Murphy JG: *Mayo clinical cardiology review,* ed 2, Philadelphia, 2000, Lippincott, Williams & Wilkins.
4. Goldberger AL: *Clinical electrocardiography: a simplified approach,* ed 6, St Louis, 1999, Mosby.
5. Barold SS: Indications for permanent cardiac pacing in first-degree AV block: class I, II, or III? *PACE* 19:747-751, 1996.
6. Padrid PJ, Kowey PR, editors: *Cardiac arrhythmia: mechanisms, diagnosis, and management,* Baltimore, 1995, Williams & Wilkins.
7. Dhingra RC, Denes P, Wu D, Chuquimia R, Rosen KM: The significance of second-degree atrioventricular block and bundle branch block: observations regarding site and type of block, *Circulation* 49:638-646, 1974.
8. Chou T, Knilans TK: *Electrocardiography in clinical practice: adult and pediatric,* Philadelphia, 1996, WB Saunders.

BIBLIOGRAPHY

Chou T, Knilans TK: *Electrocardiography in clinical practice: adult and pediatric,* Philadelphia, 1996, WB Saunders.

Crawford MV, Spence MI: *Common sense approach to coronary care,* ed 6, St Louis, 1995, Mosby.

Goldberger AL: *Clinical electrocardiography: a simplified approach,* ed 6, St Louis, 1999, Mosby.

Goldman L, Braunwald E: *Primary cardiology,* Philadelphia, 1998, WB Saunders.

Johnson R, Swartz MH: *A simplified approach to electrocardiography,* Philadelphia, 1986, WB Saunders.

Kahn MG: *Cardiac drug therapy,* ed 5, London, 2000, Harcourt Publishers Limited.

Kahn MG: *Rapid ECG interpretation,* Philadelphia, 1997, WB Saunders.

Kinney MR, Packa DR, editors: *Andreoli's comprehensive cardiac care,* ed 8, St Louis, 1996, Mosby.

Marriott HJL, Conover MB: *Advanced concepts in arrhythmias,* ed 3, St Louis, 1998, Mosby.

Murphy JG, *Mayo clinical cardiology review,* ed 2, Philadelphia, 2000, Lippincott, Williams & Wilkins.

Padrid PJ, Kowey PR, editors: *Cardiac arrhythmia: mechanisms, diagnosis, and management,* Baltimore, 1995, Williams & Wilkins.

Paradis NA, Halperin HR, Nowak RM, editors: *Cardiac arrest: the science and practice of resuscitation medicine,* Baltimore, 1996, Williams & Wilkins.

Phillips RE, Feeney MK: *The cardiac rhythms: a systematic approach to interpretation,* ed 3, Philadelphia, 1990, WB Saunders.

Wagner GS: *Marriott's practical electrocardiography,* ed 9, Baltimore, 1994, Williams & Wilkins.

Woods SL, Sivarajan Froelicher ES, Motzer SA: *Cardiac nursing,* ed 4, Philadelphia, 2000, Lippincott, Williams & Wilkins.

MATCHING

___ 1. PR interval pattern in second-degree AV block, type I

___ 2. A ___ escape rhythm with a complete AV block, usually has a ventricular rate of 40 beats/min or less

___ 3. AV block that often progresses to a complete AV block without warning

___ 4. Location of the block in a second-degree AV block, type II

___ 5. Second-degree AV block type I is most commonly associated with an ___ myocardial infarction

___ 6. Normal duration of the PR interval

___ 7. AV block characterized by regular P-P intervals, regular R-R intervals, and a PR interval with no consistent value or pattern

___ 8. Common location of the block in a second-degree AV block, type I

___ 9. PR interval pattern in second-degree AV block, type II

___ 10. Location of the block in a complete AV block

___ 11. Ventricular rhythm pattern in second-degree AV block, types I and II

___ 12. AV block characterized by a PR interval greater than 0.20 sec and one P wave for each QRS complex

___ 13. Ventricular rhythm pattern in second-degree AV block 2:1 conduction and complete AV block

___ 14. A ___ escape rhythm with a complete AV block, usually has a narrow QRS and a ventricular rate of 40 to 60 beats/min

___ 15. Second-degree AV block type II is most commonly associated with an ___ myocardial infarction

A. Constant
B. First-degree AV block
C. Complete AV block
D. AV node, bundle of His, or bundle branches
E. Progressive lengthening
F. Irregular
G. Inferior wall
H. Second-degree AV block, type II
I. Ventricular
J. Anterior wall
K. Bundle of His or bundle branches
L. Junctional
M. 0.12 to 0.20 sec
N. AV node
O. Regular

IDENTIFICATION AND MEASUREMENTS—PRACTICE RHYTHM STRIPS

For each of the following rhythm strips, determine the atrial and ventricular rates, measure the PR interval, QRS duration, and QT interval, and then identify the rhythm. All strips lead II unless otherwise noted.

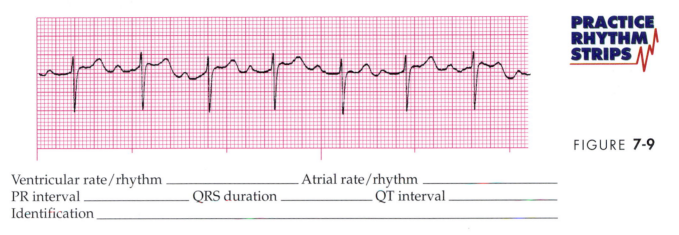

PRACTICE RHYTHM STRIPS

FIGURE **7-9**

Ventricular rate/rhythm _____ Atrial rate/rhythm _____
PR interval _____ QRS duration _____ QT interval _____
Identification _____

The rhythm strip below is from a 77-year-old female who stated she felt fine. She stopped at a blood pressure machine in Wal-Mart, and the machine would not read her pulse rate. She subsequently went to her physician's office and then to the emergency department.

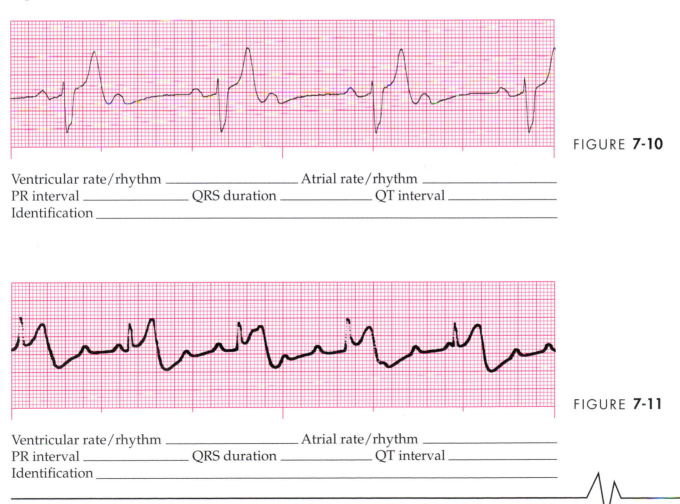

FIGURE **7-10**

Ventricular rate/rhythm _____ Atrial rate/rhythm _____
PR interval _____ QRS duration _____ QT interval _____
Identification _____

FIGURE **7-11**

Ventricular rate/rhythm _____ Atrial rate/rhythm _____
PR interval _____ QRS duration _____ QT interval _____
Identification _____

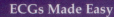

PRACTICE
RHYTHM
STRIPS

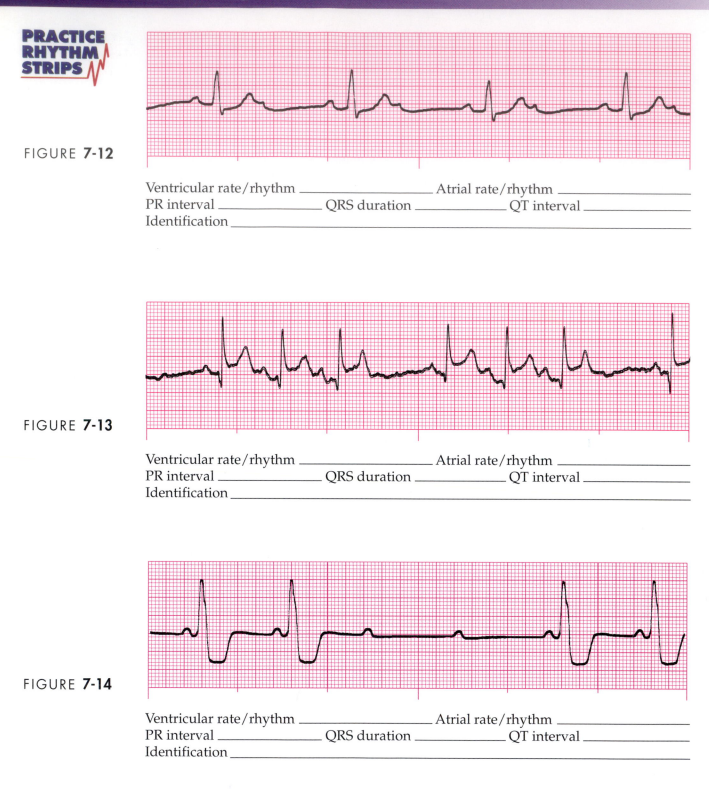

FIGURE **7-12**

Ventricular rate/rhythm _____ Atrial rate/rhythm _____
PR interval _____ QRS duration _____ QT interval _____
Identification _____

FIGURE **7-13**

Ventricular rate/rhythm _____ Atrial rate/rhythm _____
PR interval _____ QRS duration _____ QT interval _____
Identification _____

FIGURE **7-14**

Ventricular rate/rhythm _____ Atrial rate/rhythm _____
PR interval _____ QRS duration _____ QT interval _____
Identification _____

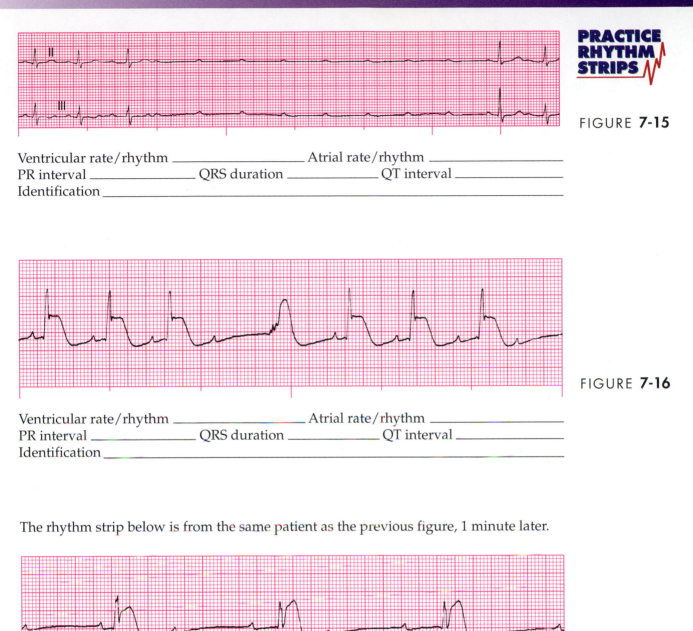

FIGURE **7-15**

Ventricular rate/rhythm _____ Atrial rate/rhythm _____
PR interval _____ QRS duration _____ QT interval _____
Identification _____

FIGURE **7-16**

Ventricular rate/rhythm _____ Atrial rate/rhythm _____
PR interval _____ QRS duration _____ QT interval _____
Identification _____

The rhythm strip below is from the same patient as the previous figure, 1 minute later.

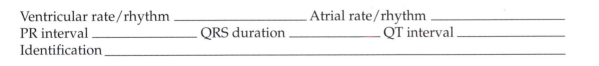
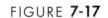

FIGURE **7-17**

Ventricular rate/rhythm _____ Atrial rate/rhythm _____
PR interval _____ QRS duration _____ QT interval _____
Identification _____

CHAPTER 8

Pacemaker Rhythms

OBJECTIVES

On completion of this chapter, you will be able to:

1. Define the following terms: *sensitivity, capture, asynchronous, synchronous, threshold.*
2. Identify the components of a pacemaker system.
3. Describe a unipolar and bipolar pacing electrode.
4. Explain the differences between fixed-rate and demand pacemakers.
5. Describe the primary pacing modes.
6. Identify the cardiac chamber(s) stimulated by different pacing methods.
7. Describe the appearance of a typical pacemaker spike on the ECG.
8. Describe the appearance of the waveform on the ECG produced as a result of:
   a. Atrial pacing
   b. Ventricular pacing
9. Describe the benefits of AV sequential pacing.
10. Identify the primary indications for pacemaker therapy.
11. List three contraindications for transcutaneous pacing.
12. Identify the complications of pacing.
13. List three types of pacemaker malfunction.

PACEMAKER TERMINOLOGY

A wave: Atrial paced event; the atrial stimulus or the point in the intrinsic atrial depolarization (P wave) at which atrial sensing occurs; analogous to the P wave of intrinsic waveforms.

AA interval: Interval between two consecutive atrial stimuli, with or without an interceding ventricular event; analogous to the P-P interval of intrinsic waveforms.

Asynchronous pacemaker: (Fixed-rate) pacemaker that continuously discharges at a preset rate regardless of the patient's intrinsic activity.

Atrial pacing: Pacing system with a lead attached to the right atrium designed to correct abnormalities in the SA node (sick sinus syndrome).

Automatic interval: Period, expressed in milliseconds, between two consecutive paced events in the same cardiac chamber without an intervening sensed event (e.g., AA interval, VV interval); also known as the demand interval, basic interval, or pacing interval.

AV interval: In dual-chamber pacing, the length of time between an atrial sensed or atrial paced event and the delivery of a ventricular pacing stimulus; analogous to the P-R interval of intrinsic waveforms; also called the *artificial* or *electronic* PR interval.

AV sequential pacemaker: Pacemaker that stimulates first the atrium, then the ventricle, mimicking normal cardiac physiology; a type of dual-chamber pacemaker.

Base rate: Rate at which the pulse generator paces when no intrinsic activity is detected; expressed in pulses/minute (ppm).

Bipolar lead: Pacing lead with two electrical poles that are external from the pulse generator; the negative pole is located at the extreme distal tip of the pacing lead; the positive pole is located several millimeters proximal to the negative electrode; the stimulating pulse is delivered through the negative electrode.

Capture: Ability of a pacing stimulus to successfully depolarize the cardiac chamber that is being paced; with one-to-one capture, each pacing stimulus results in depolarization of the appropriate chamber.

Demand (synchronous) pacemaker: Pacemaker that discharges only when the patient's heart rate drops below the preset rate for the pacemaker.

Dual-chamber pacemaker: Pacemaker that stimulates the atrium and ventricle; dual-chamber pacing is also called *physiologic pacing.*

Escape interval: Time measured between a sensed cardiac event and the next pacemaker output.

Fusion beat: In pacing, the ECG waveform that results when an intrinsic depolarization and a pacing stimulus occur simultaneously, and both contribute to depolarization of that cardiac chamber.

Hysteresis: Programmable feature in some demand pacemakers that allows programming of a longer escape interval between the intrinsic complex and the first paced event; the longer escape interval allows intrinsic beats an opportunity to inhibit the pacemaker.

Inhibition: Pacemaker response in which the output pulse is suppressed (inhibited) when an intrinsic event is sensed.

Interval: Period, measured in milliseconds, between any two designated cardiac events; in pacing, intervals are more useful than rate, because pacemaker timing is based on intervals.

Intrinsic: Inherent; naturally occurring.

Milliampere (mA): Unit of measure of electrical current needed to elicit depolarization of the myocardium.

Output: Electrical stimulus delivered by the pulse generator, usually defined in terms of pulse amplitude (volts) and pulse width (milliseconds).

Pacemaker: Artificial pulse generator that delivers an electrical current to the heart to stimulate depolarization.

Pacemaker spike: Vertical line on the ECG that indicates the pacemaker has discharged.

Pacemaker syndrome: Adverse clinical signs and symptoms that limit a patient's everyday functioning and occur in the setting of an electrically normal pacing system; common signs and symptoms include weakness, fatigue, dizziness, near or full syncope, cough, chest pain, hypotension, dyspnea, and congestive heart failure; pacemaker syndrome is most commonly associated with a loss of AV synchrony (e.g., VVI pacing) but may also occur because of an inappropriate AV interval or inappropriate rate modulation.

Pacing interval: Period, expressed in milliseconds, between two consecutive paced events in the same cardiac chamber without an intervening sensed event (e.g., AA interval, VV interval); also known as the *demand interval, basic interval,* or *automatic interval.*

Pacing system analyzer (PSA): External testing and measuring device capable of pacing the heart during pacemaker implantation; used to determine appropriate pulse generator settings for the individual patient (e.g., pacing threshold, lead impedance, pulse amplitude).

Parameter: Value that can be measured and sometimes changed, either indirectly or directly; in pacing, parameter refers to a value that influences the function of the pacemaker (e.g., sensitivity, amplitude, mode).

Pulse generator: Power source that houses the battery and controls for regulating a pacemaker.

Rate modulation: Ability of a pacemaker to increase the pacing rate in response to physical activity or metabolic demand; some type of physiologic sensor is used by the pacemaker to determine the need for an increased pacing rate; also called *rate adaptation* or *rate response.*

R wave: In pacing, R wave refers to the entire QRS complex denoting an intrinsic ventricular event.

RV interval: Period from the intrinsic ventricular event and the ventricular-paced event that follows; the pacemaker's escape interval.

Sensing: Ability of a pacemaker to recognize and respond to intrinsic electrical activity; the pacemaker's response to sensed activity depends on its programmed mode and parameters.

Threshold: Minimum level of electrical current needed to consistently depolarize the myocardium.

Unipolar lead: Pacing lead with a single electrical pole at the distal tip of the pacing lead (negative pole) through which the stimulating pulse is delivered; in a permanent pacemaker with a unipolar lead, the positive pole is the pulse generator case.

V-A interval: In dual-chamber pacing, the interval between a sensed or ventricular-paced event and the next atrial-paced event.

V-V interval: Interval between two ventricular-paced events.

V wave: Ventricular-paced event; the ventricular stimulus or the point in the intrinsic ventricular depolarization (R wave) during which ventricular sensing occurs.

Ventricular pacing: Pacing system with a lead attached in the right ventricle.

PACEMAKER SYSTEMS

Overview

A **pacemaker** is an artificial pulse generator that delivers an electrical current to the heart to stimulate depolarization. Pacemaker systems are usually named according to where the electrodes are located and the route the electrical current takes to the heart. A pacemaker system (Figure 8-1) consists of a **pulse generator** (power source) and pacing lead(s). The pulse generator houses a battery and electronic circuitry to sense and analyze the patient's **intrinsic** rhythm and the timing circuitry for pacing stimulus output.[1] The pacing lead is an insulated wire used to carry an electrical impulse from the pacemaker to the patient's heart and back to the pacemaker. The exposed portion of the pacing lead is called an *electrode,* which is placed in direct contact with the heart.

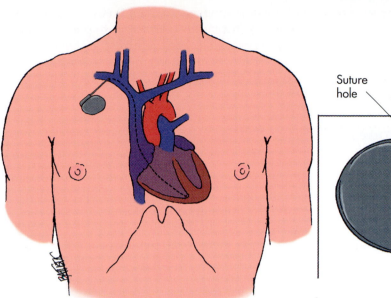

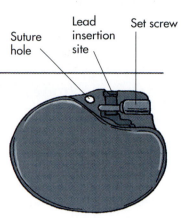

FIGURE **8-1**
Permanent pace-
maker.

Permanent Pacemakers

A permanent pacemaker is implanted in the body, usually under local anesthesia. The pacemaker's circuitry is housed in a hermetically sealed case made of titanium that is air-tight and impermeable to fluid. The electrode of a permanent pacemaker may be placed transvenously or surgically and, once the electrode is in place, the pulse genera-tor is usually implanted into the subcutaneous tissue of the anterior thorax just below the right or left clavicle. The electrode is then connected to the pulse generator. "The pa-tient's handedness, occupation, and hobbies determine whether the pacemaker is im-planted on the right or left side. In general, the nondominant side is chosen to minimize interference with the patient's daily activities."[2] Lithium batteries, with an average life of 8 to 12 years, are almost exclusively used in modern pacemakers.

Battery life depends on many factors, including how the pacemaker is pro-grammed and the percent-age of time it paces.[2]

Indications
Common indications for insertion of a permanent pacemaker include permanent or in-termittent complete AV block, permanent or intermittent second-degree AV block type II, and sinus node dysfunction, including sick sinus syndrome that may be manifested as severe sinus bradycardia, bradycardia-tachycardia syndrome, sinus arrest, or sinus block.

Temporary Pacemakers

Temporary pacing can be accomplished through transvenous, epicardial, or transcuta-neous means. Transvenous pacemakers stimulate the endocardium of the right atrium or ventricle (or both) by means of an electrode introduced into a central vein. Epicardial pacing is the placement of pacing leads directly onto or through the epicardium under direct visualization. Transcutaneous pacing (TCP) delivers pacing impulses to the heart using electrodes placed on the patient's thorax. TCP is also called *temporary external pac-ing* or *noninvasive pacing* and is covered later in this chapter.

The pulse generator of a temporary pacemaker is located externally.

Indications
Indications for emergent temporary pacing include hemodynamically significant brady-cardia (blood pressure <80 mm Hg systolic, change in mental status, pulmonary edema,

During overdrive pacing, the heart is paced briefly (seconds) at a rate faster than the rate of the tachycardia. The pacemaker is then stopped to allow return of the heart's intrinsic pacemaker.

angina); bradycardia with escape rhythms unresponsive to drug therapy; **overdrive pacing** of tachycardia—supraventricular or ventricular—refractory to pharmacologic therapy or electrical countershock; and bradyasystolic cardiac arrest. Prophylactic pacing, in the setting of acute myocardial infarction, is indicated in symptomatic sinus node dysfunction, second-degree AV block type II, complete AV block, and new left, right, or alternating bundle branch block.

Pacemaker Electrodes

Unipolar Electrodes

There are two types of pacemaker electrodes—unipolar and bipolar. A unipolar electrode (Figure 8-2) has one pacing electrode that is located at its distal tip. The negative electrode is in contact with the heart, and the pulse generator (located outside the heart) functions as the positive electrode. The **pacemaker spikes** produced by a unipolar electrode are often large because of the distance between the positive and negative electrodes.

Bipolar Electrodes

The spike produced by a bipolar electrode is often small and difficult to see.

A bipolar pacemaker electrode contains a positive and negative electrode at the distal tip of the pacing lead wire. Most temporary transvenous pacemakers have bipolar electrodes. A permanent pacemaker may have either a bipolar or a unipolar electrode.

Pacemaker Modes

Fixed-Rate (Asynchronous) Pacemakers

A **fixed-rate pacemaker** continuously discharges at a preset rate (usually 70 to 80/min) regardless of the patient's heart rate. An advantage of the fixed-rate pacemaker is its simple circuitry, reducing the risk of pacemaker failure. However, this type of pacemaker does not sense the patient's own cardiac rhythm. This may result in competition between the patient's cardiac rhythm and that of the pacemaker. Ventricular tachycardia or ventricular fibrillation may be induced if the pacemaker were to fire during the T wave (vulnerable period) of a preceding patient beat. Fixed-rate pacemakers are not often used today.

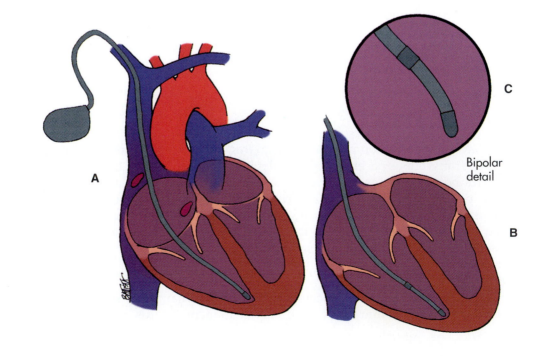

C

Bipolar detail

A

B

FIGURE **8-2**
Unipolar **(A)** and bipolar pacemaker electrodes **(B, C)**.

Demand (Synchronous, Noncompetitive) Pacemakers

A **demand pacemaker** discharges only when the patient's heart rate drops below the pacemaker's preset (base) rate. For example, if the demand pacemaker's pulse generator were preset at a rate of 70 impulses/min, it would sense the patient's heart rate and allow electrical impulses to flow from the pacemaker through the pacing lead to stimulate the heart only when the rate fell below 70 beats/min. Demand pacemakers can be programmable or nonprogrammable. The voltage level and impulse rate are preset at the time of manufacture in nonprogrammable pacemakers.

Pacemaker Identification Codes

The Intersociety Commission on Heart Disease (ICHD), now referred to as North American British Generic (NBG), developed an international identification code in 1974 to assist in identifying a pacemaker's preprogrammed pacing, sensing, and response functions. This coding system traditionally consisted of three letters. In 1980, the system was modified to add two additional functions (letters) (Table 8-1).

The first three letters are used for antibradycardia functions. The *first letter* of the code identifies the heart chamber (or chambers) paced (stimulated). The options available are:

   O, none
   A, atrium
   V, ventricle
   D, dual (both atrium and ventricle)

A pacemaker used to pace only a single chamber is represented by either *A* (atrial) or *V* (ventricular). A pacemaker capable of pacing in both chambers is represented by *D* (dual).

The *second letter* identifies the chamber of the heart where patient-initiated (intrinsic) electrical activity is sensed by the pacemaker. The letter designations for the second letter are the same as the designations for the first.

The *third letter* indicates how the pacemaker will respond when it senses patient-initiated electrical activity:

   O, no sensing
   T, a pacemaker stimulus is *triggered* in response to a sensed event
   I, sensing of intrinsic impulses *inhibits* the pacemaker from producing a stimulus
   D, dual (a combination of triggered pacing and inhibition)

The fourth and fifth letters are not commonly used, except for the letter *R* in the fourth position, which indicates that the pacemaker is a rate-responsive device.[2]

Commonly encountered pacing modes are VVI, DVI, DDD, and DDDR.

TABLE 8-1 PACEMAKER CODES

Chamber paced (first letter)	Chamber sensed (second letter)	Response to sensing (third letter)	Programmable functions (fourth letter)	Antitachycardia functions (fifth letter)
O = None	O = None (fixed-rate pacemaker)	O = None (fixed-rate pacemaker)	O = None	O = None
A = Atrium	A = Atrium	T = Triggers pacing	P = Simple programmability (rate and/or output)	P = Pacing (antitachycardia)
V = Ventricle	V = Ventricle	I = Inhibits pacing	M = Multiprogrammable	S = Shock
D = Dual chamber (atrium and ventricle)	D = Dual chamber (atrium and ventricle)	D = Dual (triggers and inhibits pacing)	C = Communication	D = Dual (pacing and shock)
			R = Rate responsive	

The *fourth letter* is most often used in permanent pacing and identifies the availability of rate responsiveness and the number of reprogrammable functions available:

O, the pacemaker is not programmable or rate responsive (most commonly found on devices manufactured before mid-1970s)

P, simple programmability where the pacemaker is limited to one or two programmable parameters (e.g., such as rate or output)

M, multiprogrammability (i.e., more than two variables can be altered)

C, capability of transmitting and/or receiving data for informational or programming purposes

R, rate responsiveness, denoting the pacemaker's ability to automatically adjust its rate to meet the body's needs caused by increased physical activity

The *fifth letter* indicates the presence of one or more active antitachycardia functions and indicates how the pacemaker will respond to tachydysrhythmias:

O, the device has no antitachycardia functions

P, the device is capable of antitachycardia pacing

S, the device is capable of delivering synchronized and unsynchronized countershocks

D, the device is capable of antitachycardia pacing, synchronized and unsynchronized countershocks

When the SA node is diseased, the body loses its ability to physiologically adjust the heart rate in response to physical or emotional stressors. Rate-responsive pacemakers contain an artificial sensor (or more than one sensor) that detects physiologic changes and adjusts the heart rate accordingly. When the patient's activity increases, the sensor becomes the regulator of the patient's heart rate. The sensor detects a signal indicating a need for a rate faster than the pacemaker's base rate and instructs the pacemaker to provide electrical stimuli (output) at the sensor-indicated rate. The patient's physician determines the pacemaker's base rate and the upper sensor-driven rate of the device.

Metabolic parameters and non-metabolic markers can be used to assess the body's physiologic demands. For example, vibration sensors detect body movement, impedance sensors detect respiratory rate and minute ventilation, and special sensors on the pacing electrode can detect central venous temperature, right atrial pressure, pH, and catecholamine levels, among other parameters.

Single-Chamber Pacemakers

A pacemaker that paces a single heart chamber (either the atrium or ventricle) has one lead placed in the heart. Atrial pacing is achieved by placing the pacing electrode in the right atrium. Stimulation of the atria produces a pacemaker spike on the ECG, followed by a P wave (Figure 8-3). Atrial pacing may be used when the SA node is diseased or damaged, but conduction through the AV junction and ventricles is normal. This type of pacemaker is ineffective if an AV block develops because it cannot pace the ventricles.

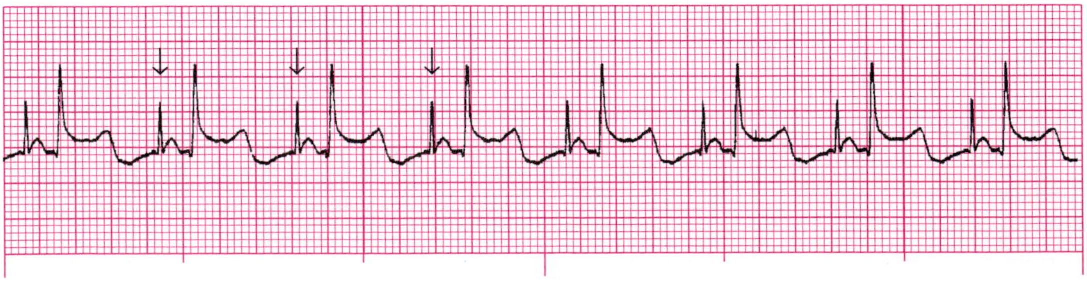

Most, if not all, pacemakers currently manufactured have a communicating ability.

A pacemaker's rate responsiveness may also be referred to as *rate modulation* or *rate adaptation*.

Implantable cardioverter defibrillators (ICDs) use the features designated by the fifth letter in the management of tachydysrhythmias.

Single-chamber or dual-chamber pacemakers can be rate responsive.

The two most common types of sensors are an activity sensor and a minute ventilation sensor.

It may be difficult to see the P wave on the ECG during atrial pacing.

FIGURE 8-3 Atrial pacing. (*Arrows*, pacer spikes.)

Ventricular pacing is accomplished by placing the pacing electrode in the right ventricle. Stimulation of the ventricles produces a pacemaker spike on the ECG, followed by a wide QRS, resembling a ventricular ectopic beat (Figure 8-4). The QRS complex is wide because a paced impulse does not follow the normal conduction pathways in the heart.

A single-chamber ventricular pacemaker can pace the ventricles but cannot coordinate pacing with the patient's intrinsic atrial rate. This results in asynchronous contraction of the atrium and ventricle (AV asynchrony). Because of this loss of AV synchrony, a ventricular demand pacemaker is rarely used in a patient with an intact SA node. Conversely, a ventricular demand pacemaker may be used for the patient with chronic atrial fibrillation.

The **ventricular demand (VVI) pacemaker** is a common type of pacemaker. With this device, the pacemaker electrode is placed in the right ventricle *(V)*; the ventricle is sensed *(V)* and the pacemaker is inhibited *(I)* when spontaneous ventricular depolarization occurs within a preset interval. When spontaneous ventricular depolarization does not occur within this preset interval, the pacemaker fires and stimulates ventricular depolarization at a preset rate.

Because a VVI pacemaker does not sense or pace atrial activity, P waves can appear anywhere in the cardiac cycle, with no relation to the QRS complexes. A disadvantage of VVI pacing is its fixed rate, regardless of the patient's level of physical activity.

Dual-Chamber Pacemakers

A pacemaker that paces both the atrium and ventricle has a two-lead system placed in the heart—one lead is placed in the right atrium, the other in the right ventricle. This type of pacemaker is called a *dual-chamber pacemaker.* An **AV sequential pacemaker** is an example of a dual-chamber pacemaker. The AV sequential pacemaker stimulates the right atrium and right ventricle sequentially (stimulating first the atrium, then the ventricle), mimicking normal cardiac physiology and thus preserving the atrial contribution to ventricular filling (atrial kick) (Figure 8-5).

> Most single-chamber pacemakers are attached to the right ventricle.

> Dual-chamber pacing is also called *physiologic pacing.*

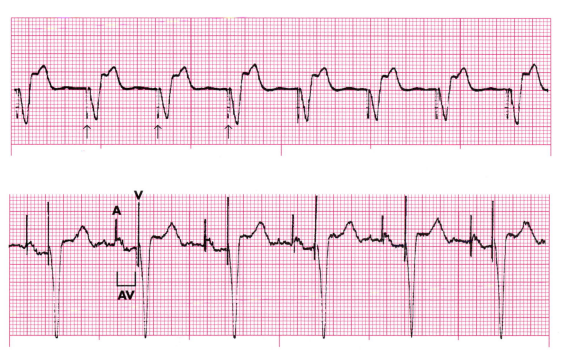

FIGURE **8-4**
Ventricular pacing. (*Arrows,* pacer spikes.)

FIGURE **8-5**
AV sequential pacing. *A,* atrial pacing; *V,* ventricular pacing; *AV,* AV interval.

The dual-chamber pacemaker may also be called a *DDD pacemaker*, indicating that both the atrium and ventricle are paced *(D)*, both chambers are sensed *(D)*, and the pacemaker has both a triggered and inhibited mode of response *(D)*. When spontaneous atrial depolarization does not occur within a preset interval, the atrial pulse generator fires and stimulates atrial depolarization at a preset rate. The pacemaker is programmed to wait—simulating the normal delay in conduction through the AV node (the PR interval). The "artificial" or "electronic" PR interval is referred to as an *AV interval.* If spontaneous ventricular depolarization does not occur within a preset interval, the pacemaker fires and stimulates ventricular depolarization at a preset rate.

The presence of a dual-chamber pacemaker does not necessarily mean that the pacemaker is in DDD mode. Dual-chamber pacemakers can be programmed to VVI mode, depending on patient need (e.g., the development of chronic atrial fibrillation).[1]

Current Research

Dual-site atrial pacing (also referred to as *biatrial pacing*) involves the use of pacemaker leads that are directed to stimulate both the right and left atria. This configuration, which is still being investigated, is being evaluated as a possible means of reducing episodes of atrial fibrillation in conjunction with antidysrhythmic medication therapy.

Biventricular pacing involves stimulating both the right and left ventricles. By stimulating both ventricular chambers, it is thought that this type of pacing will improve the efficiency of the heart's pumping action. This type of pacing is still being studied and may be of particular benefit to people with heart failure.

TRANSCUTANEOUS PACING (TCP)

Indications

Transcutaneous pacing is recommended as the initial pacing method of choice in emergency cardiac care because it is effective, quick, safe, and is the least invasive pacing technique currently available.

TCP is indicated for significant bradycardias unresponsive to atropine therapy or when atropine is not immediately available. TCP may be used as a "bridge" until transvenous pacing can be accomplished or the cause of the bradydysrhythmia is reversed (as in cases of drug overdose or hyperkalemia). TCP may be considered in asystolic cardiac arrest (less than 10 minutes in duration) and witnessed asystolic arrest.

Technique

The adhesive pacing electrodes should be applied to clean, dry skin.

Anterior-posterior electrode positioning is preferred because this position causes less stimulation of the pectoral muscles and does not interfere with ECG electrode or defibrillator paddle placement.

Transcutaneous pacing involves attaching two large pacing electrodes (approximately 8 to 10 cm in diameter) to the skin surface of the patient's outer chest wall. The pacing pads used during TCP function as a bipolar pacing system. The electrical signal exits from the negative terminal on the machine (and subsequently the negative electrode) and passes through the chest wall to the heart. Depolarization of the myocardium requires an electric current strong enough to overcome the resistance of the chest wall.

The anterior (negative) chest electrode is placed to the left of the sternum, halfway between the xiphoid process and left nipple (Figure 8-6). In female patients, the anterior electrode should be positioned under the left breast. The posterior (positive) electrode is placed on the left posterior thorax directly behind the anterior electrode. The electrodes

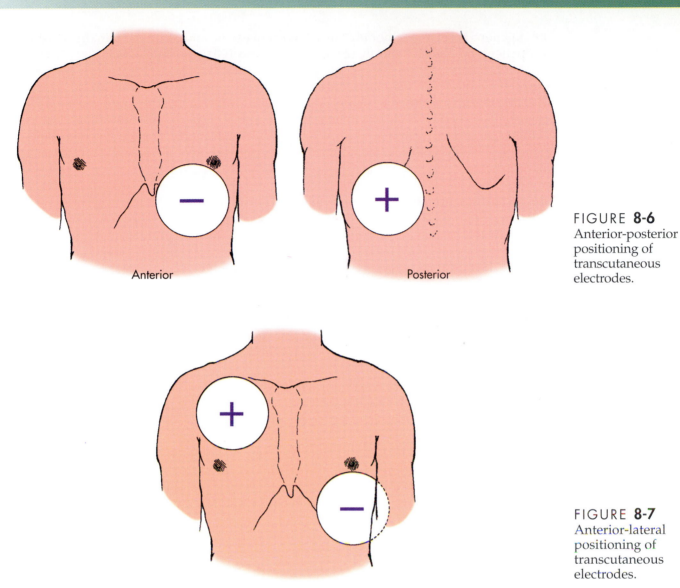

should fit completely on the patient's torso, have a minimum of 1 to 2 inches of space between electrodes, and should not overlap bony prominences of the sternum, spine, or scapula.

Studies have evaluated the importance of electrode positioning during TCP and found that, in normal volunteers, electrode placement was not crucial if the anterior electrode was of negative polarity.[3] However, electrode placement may be more significant in the critically ill patient.

If the anterior-posterior electrode position is contraindicated, the anterior-lateral position may be used. The anterior (negative) electrode is placed on the left anterior thorax, just lateral to the left nipple in the midaxillary line. The posterior (positive) electrode is placed on the right anterior upper thorax in the subclavicular area (Figure 8-7).

TCP is initiated by connecting the patient to an ECG monitor, obtaining a rhythm strip, and verifying the presence of a paceable rhythm. The pacing cable should be connected to the adhesive electrodes on the patient and to the pulse generator. After turning on the power to the pulse generator, the pacing rate should be set. In a patient with a pulse, the rate is generally set at a nonbradycardic rate between 60 and 80 beats/min. In an asystolic patient, the rate is typically set between 80 and 100 beats/min.

Chest compressions can be performed during pacing without risk of injury to the healthcare provider.

After the rate has been regulated, the stimulating current (output or milliamperes) is set. In a patient with a pulse, the current is increased slowly but steadily until capture is achieved. Sedation or analgesia may be needed to minimize the discomfort associated with this procedure (common with currents of 50 mA or more). For the asystolic patient, it is reasonable to set the current to maximal output and then decrease the output if capture is achieved.

If electrical capture is achieved without mechanical capture, the patient should be treated according to current resuscitation guidelines for pulseless electrical activity.

The cardiac monitor should be observed for **electrical** capture, usually evidenced by a wide QRS and broad T wave. In some patients, electrical capture is less obvious—indicated only as a change in the shape of the QRS. **Mechanical** capture is evaluated by assessing the patient's right upper extremity or right femoral pulses. Assessment of pulses on the patient's left side should be avoided to help minimize confusion between the presence of an actual pulse and skeletal muscle contractions caused by the pacemaker. Once capture is achieved, continue pacing at an output level slightly higher (approximately 2 mA) than the threshold of initial electrical capture. The patient's blood pressure and level of consciousness should also be assessed. Monitor the patient closely and record the ECG rhythm.

If defibrillation is necessary, the defibrillation paddles should be placed 2 to 3 cm (3/4 to 1 inch) away from the pacemaker electrodes to prevent arcing. Some pacemaker models should be turned off or disconnected before defibrillating.

Documentation should include the date and time pacing was initiated (including baseline and pacing rhythm strips), the current required to obtain capture, the pacing rate selected, the patient's responses to electrical and mechanical capture, medications administered during the procedure, and the date and time pacing was terminated.

Contraindications for TCP

Adult pacing electrodes should not be trimmed or modified in any way because such modifications may alter current distribution.

- Children weighing less than 15 kg (33 lb) unless pediatric pacing electrodes are used
- Flail chest
- Bradycardia in the setting of severe hypothermia
- Bradyasystolic cardiac arrest of more than 20 minutes in duration (relative contraindication)

TABLE 8-2 PATIENT RESPONSES TO CURRENT WITH TRANSCUTANEOUS PACING	
Output mA*	Response
20	Prickly sensation on skin
30	Slight thump on chest
40	Definite thump on chest
50	Coughing
60	Diaphragm pacing and coughing
70	Coughing and knock on chest
80	More uncomfortable than 70 mA
90	Strong, painful knock on chest
100	Leaves bed because of pain

*Responses with Zoll-NTP
From Flynn JB: *Introduction to critical care skills*, St Louis, 1993, Mosby.

Limitations of TCP

The primary limitation of TCP is patient discomfort that is proportional to the intensity of skeletal muscle contraction and the direct electrical stimulation of cutaneous nerves (Table 8-2). The degree of discomfort varies with the device used and the stimulating current required to achieve capture. Increased chest wall muscle mass, chronic obstructive pulmonary disease (COPD), or pleural effusions may require increased stimulating current.[4]

PACEMAKER MALFUNCTION

Failure to Pace

Failure to pace is a pacemaker malfunction that occurs when the pacemaker fails to deliver an electrical stimulus or when it fails to deliver the correct number of electrical stimulations per minute. Failure to pace is recognized on the ECG as an absence of pacemaker spikes (even though the patient's intrinsic rate is less than that of the pacemaker) and a return of the underlying rhythm for which the pacemaker was implanted. Patient signs and symptoms may include syncope, chest pain, bradycardia, and hypotension.

> Failure to pace is also referred to as *failure to fire.*

Causes of failure to pace include battery failure, fracture of the pacing lead wire, displacement of the electrode tip, pulse generator failure, a broken or loose connection between the pacing lead and the pulse generator, electromagnetic interference, and/or the sensitivity setting set too high.

Treatment may include adjusting the sensitivity setting, replacing the pulse generator battery, replacing the pacing lead, replacing the pulse generator unit, tightening connections between the pacing lead and pulse generator, performing an electrical check, and/or removing the source of electromagnetic interference.

Failure to Capture

Capture is successful depolarization of the atria and/or ventricles by an artificial pacemaker and is obtained after the pacemaker electrode is properly positioned in the heart. Failure to capture is the inability of the pacemaker stimulus to depolarize the myocardium and is recognized on the ECG by visible pacemaker spikes not followed by P waves (if the electrode is located in the atrium) or QRS complexes (if the electrode is located in the right ventricle) (Figure 8-8). Patient signs and symptoms may include fatigue, bradycardia, and hypotension.

Causes of failure to capture include battery failure, fracture of the pacing lead wire, displacement of pacing lead wire (common cause), perforation of the myocardium

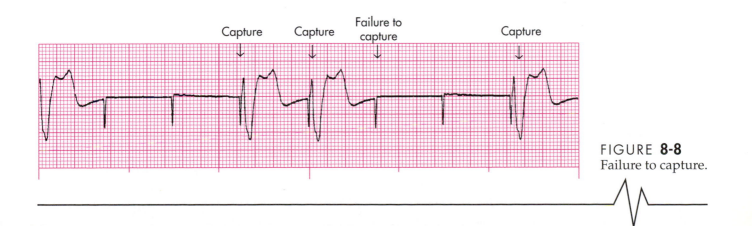

FIGURE **8-8**
Failure to capture.

by a lead wire, edema or scar tissue formation at the electrode tip, output energy (mA) set too low (common cause), and/or increased stimulation threshold because of medications, electrolyte imbalance, or increased fibrin formation on the catheter tip.

Treatment may include repositioning the patient, slowly increasing the output setting (mA) until capture occurs or the maximum setting is reached, replacing the pulse generator battery, replacing or repositioning of the pacing lead, or surgery.

Failure to Sense (Undersensing)

Sensitivity is the extent to which a pacemaker recognizes intrinsic electrical activity. Failure to sense occurs when the pacemaker fails to recognize spontaneous myocardial depolarization (Figure 8-9). This pacemaker malfunction is recognized on the ECG by pacemaker spikes that follow too closely behind the patient's QRS complexes (earlier than the programmed escape interval). Because pacemaker spikes occur when they should not, this type of pacemaker malfunction may result in pacemaker spikes that fall on T waves (R-on-T phenomenon) and/or competition between the pacemaker and the patient's own cardiac rhythm. The patient may complain of palpitations or skipped beats. R-on-T phenomenon may precipitate VT or VF.

Causes of failure to sense include battery failure, fracture of pacing lead wire, displacement of the electrode tip (most common cause), decreased P wave or QRS voltage, circuitry dysfunction (generator unable to process QRS signal), increased sensing threshold from edema or fibrosis at the electrode tip, antidysrhythmic medications, severe electrolyte disturbances, and myocardial perforation.

Treatment may include increasing the sensitivity setting, replacing the pulse generator battery, and/or replacing or repositioning the pacing lead.

Oversensing

Oversensing is a pacemaker malfunction that results from inappropriate sensing of extraneous electrical signals. Atrial sensing pacemakers may inappropriately sense ventricular activity; ventricular sensing pacemakers may misidentify a tall, peaked intrinsic T wave as a QRS complex. Oversensing is recognized on the ECG as pacemaker spikes at a rate slower than the pacemaker's preset rate (paced QRS complexes that come later than the pacemaker's preset escape interval) or no paced

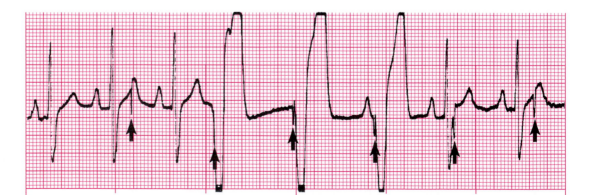

FIGURE **8-9**
Failure to sense.

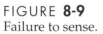

beats even though the pacemaker's preset rate is greater than the patient's intrinsic rate.

The patient with a pacemaker should avoid strong electromagnetic fields such as those associated with welding equipment or a magnetic resonance imaging (MRI) machine. Treatment includes adjustment of the pacemaker's sensitivity setting or possible insertion of a bipolar lead if oversensing is caused by unipolar lead dysfunction.

PACEMAKER COMPLICATIONS

Complications of Transcutaneous Pacing

Complications of transcutaneous pacing include pain from electrical stimulation of the skin and muscles, failure to recognize that the pacemaker is not capturing, and failure to recognize the presence of underlying treatable VF. Tissue damage, including third-degree burns, has been reported in pediatric patients with improper or prolonged transcutaneous pacing. Prolonged pacing has been associated with pacing threshold changes, leading to capture failure.

Complications of Temporary Transvenous Pacing

Complications of temporary transvenous pacing include bleeding, infection, pneumothorax, cardiac dysrhythmias, myocardial infarction, lead displacement, fracture of the pacing lead, hematoma at the insertion site, perforation of the right ventricle with or without pericardial tamponade, and perforation of the inferior vena cava, pulmonary artery, or coronary arteries because of improper placement of the pacing lead.

Complications of Permanent Pacing

Complications of permanent pacing associated with the implantation procedure include bleeding, local tissue reaction, pneumothorax, cardiac dysrhythmias, air embolism, and thrombosis. Long-term complications of permanent pacing may include infection, electrode displacement, congestive heart failure, fracture of the pacing lead, pacemaker-induced dysrhythmias, externalization of the pacemaker generator, and perforation of the right ventricle with or without pericardial tamponade.

ANALYZING PACEMAKER FUNCTION ON THE ECG

Identify the Intrinsic Rate and Rhythm

- Are P waves present? At what rate?
- Are QRS complexes present? At what rate?

Is There Evidence of Paced Activity?

- If paced atrial activity is present, evaluate the paced interval.
- Using calipers or paper, measure the distance between two consecutively paced atrial beats.
- Determine the rate and regularity of the paced interval.
- If paced ventricular activity is present, evaluate the paced interval.
- Using calipers or paper, measure the distance between two consecutively paced ventricular beats.
- Determine the rate and regularity of the paced interval.

Evaluate the Escape Interval

Escape interval: Time measured between the last beat of the patient's own rhythm and the first paced beat.

- Compare the escape interval to the paced interval measured earlier. The paced interval and escape interval should measure the same.

Analyze the Rhythm Strip

- Analyze the rhythm strip for failure to capture, failure to sense, oversensing, and failure to pace.

REFERENCES

1. Gibler WB: *Emergency cardiac care,* St Louis, 1994, Mosby.
2. Woods SL, Sivarajen Froelicher ES, Motzer SA: *Cardiac nursing,* ed 4, Philadelphia, 2000, Lippincott, Williams & Wilkins.
3. Falk RH, Ngai S: External cardiac pacing: influence of electrode placement, *Crit Care Med* 14:11, 1986.
4. Crawford MV, Spence MI: *Common sense approach to coronary care,* ed 6, St Louis, 1995, Mosby.

BIBLIOGRAPHY

Chou T, Knilans TK: *Electrocardiography in clinical practice: adult and pediatric,* Philadelphia, 1996, WB Saunders.

Crawford MV, Spence MI: *Common sense approach to coronary care,* ed 6, St Louis, 1995, Mosby.

Gibler WB: *Emergency cardiac care,* St Louis, 1994, Mosby.

Goldberger AL: *Clinical electrocardiography: a simplified approach,* ed 6, St Louis, 1999, Mosby.

Goldman L, Braunwald E: *Primary cardiology,* Philadelphia, 1998, WB Saunders.

Kahn MG: *Rapid ECG interpretation,* Philadelphia, 1997, WB Saunders.

Kinney MR, Packa DR, editors: *Andreoli's comprehensive cardiac care,* ed 8, St Louis, 1996, Mosby.

Marriott HJL, Conover MB: *Advanced concepts in arrhythmias,* ed 3, St Louis, 1998, Mosby.

Padrid PJ, Kowey PR, editors: *Cardiac arrhythmia: mechanisms, diagnosis, and management,* Baltimore, 1995, Williams & Wilkins.

Paradis NA, Halperin HR, Nowak RM, editors: *Cardiac arrest: the science and practice of resuscitation medicine,* Baltimore, 1996, Williams & Wilkins.

Woods SL, Sivarajan Froelicher ES, Motzer SA: *Cardiac nursing,* ed 4, Philadelphia, 2000, Lippincott, Williams & Wilkins.

MATCHING

___ 1. Pacemaker that discharges only when the patient's heart rate drops below the preset rate for the pacemaker

___ 2. The time measured between a sensed cardiac event and the next pacemaker output

___ 3. The ECG waveform that results when an intrinsic depolarization and a pacing stimulus occur simultaneously and both contribute to depolarization of that cardiac chamber

___ 4. Rate at which the pulse generator of a pacemaker paces when no intrinsic activity is detected; expressed in pulses per minute

___ 5. Pacemaker response in which the output pulse is suppressed when an intrinsic event is sensed

___ 6. In dual-chamber pacing, the interval between a sensed or ventricular-paced event and the next atrial-paced event

___ 7. Ability of a pacing stimulus to successfully depolarize the cardiac chamber that is being paced

___ 8. Ability of a pacemaker to increase the pacing rate in response to physical activity or metabolic demand

___ 9. A vertical line on the ECG that indicates the pacemaker has discharged

___ 10. A pacing system with a lead attached to the right atrium, designed to correct abnormalities in the SA node (sick sinus syndrome)

___ 11. The power source that houses the battery and controls for regulating a pacemaker

___ 12. Period, expressed in milliseconds, between two consecutively paced events in the same cardiac chamber without an intervening sensed event

___ 13. In dual-chamber pacing, the length of time between an atrial-sensed or atrial-paced event and the delivery of a ventricular pacing stimulus; analogous to the P-R interval of intrinsic waveforms

___ 14. Electrical stimulus delivered by a pacemaker's pulse generator

___ 15. Pacemaker that stimulates the atrium and ventricle

A. Atrial pacing
B. Pacemaker spike
C. Rate modulation
D. A-V interval
E. Capture
F. Dual-chamber pacemaker
G. Fusion beat
H. Escape interval
I. Output
J. Demand pacemaker
K. V-A interval
L. Base rate
M. Inhibition
N. Pulse generator
O. Pacing interval

IDENTIFICATION AND MEASUREMENTS—PRACTICE RHYTHM STRIPS

For each of the following rhythm strips, determine the presence of atrial- and ventricular-paced activity, the paced interval rate, and then identify the rhythm. All strips lead II unless otherwise noted.

PRACTICE RHYTHM STRIPS

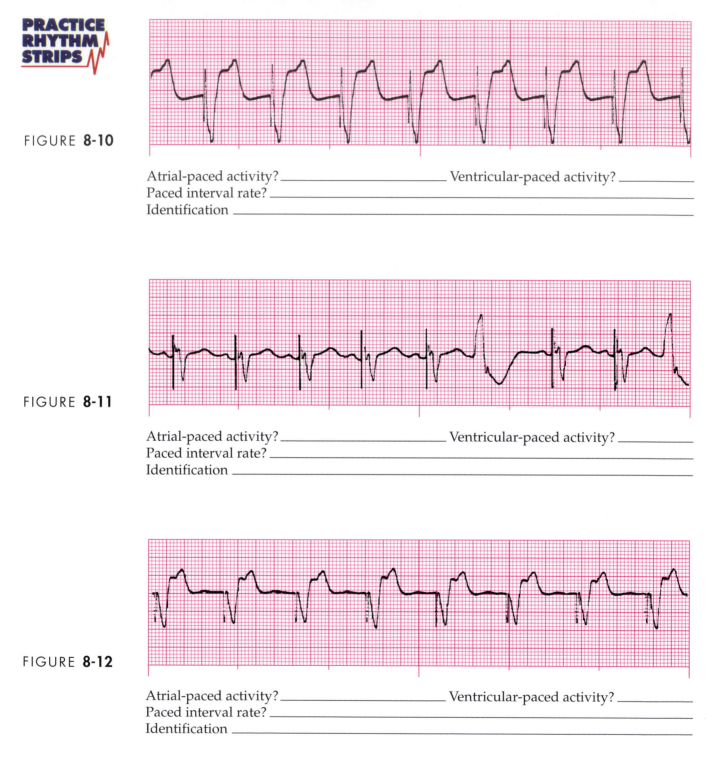

FIGURE 8-10

Atrial-paced activity? _____ Ventricular-paced activity? _____
Paced interval rate? _____
Identification _____

FIGURE 8-11

Atrial-paced activity? _____ Ventricular-paced activity? _____
Paced interval rate? _____
Identification _____

FIGURE 8-12

Atrial-paced activity? _____ Ventricular-paced activity? _____
Paced interval rate? _____
Identification _____

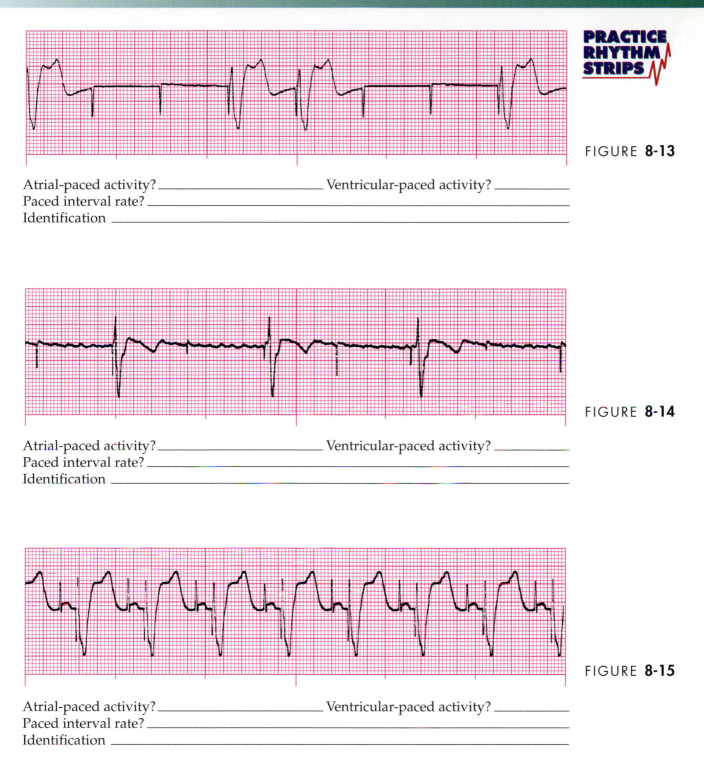

PRACTICE RHYTHM STRIPS

FIGURE **8-13**

Atrial-paced activity? _____ Ventricular-paced activity? _____
Paced interval rate? _____
Identification _____

FIGURE **8-14**

Atrial-paced activity? _____ Ventricular-paced activity? _____
Paced interval rate? _____
Identification _____

FIGURE **8-15**

Atrial-paced activity? _____ Ventricular-paced activity? _____
Paced interval rate? _____
Identification _____

PRACTICE RHYTHM STRIPS

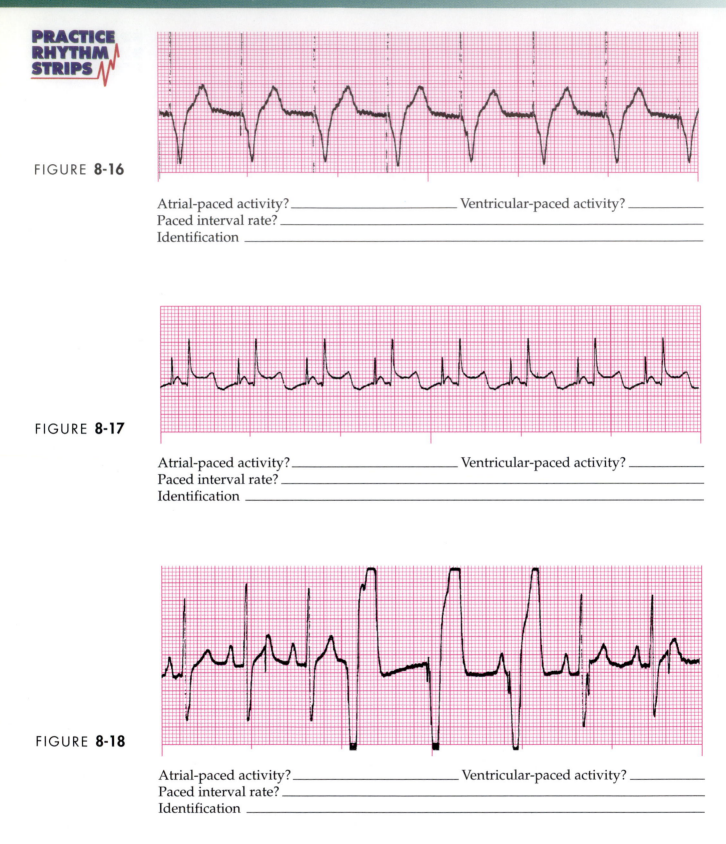

FIGURE **8-16**

Atrial-paced activity? _____ Ventricular-paced activity? _____
Paced interval rate? _____
Identification _____

FIGURE **8-17**

Atrial-paced activity? _____ Ventricular-paced activity? _____
Paced interval rate? _____
Identification _____

FIGURE **8-18**

Atrial-paced activity? _____ Ventricular-paced activity? _____
Paced interval rate? _____
Identification _____

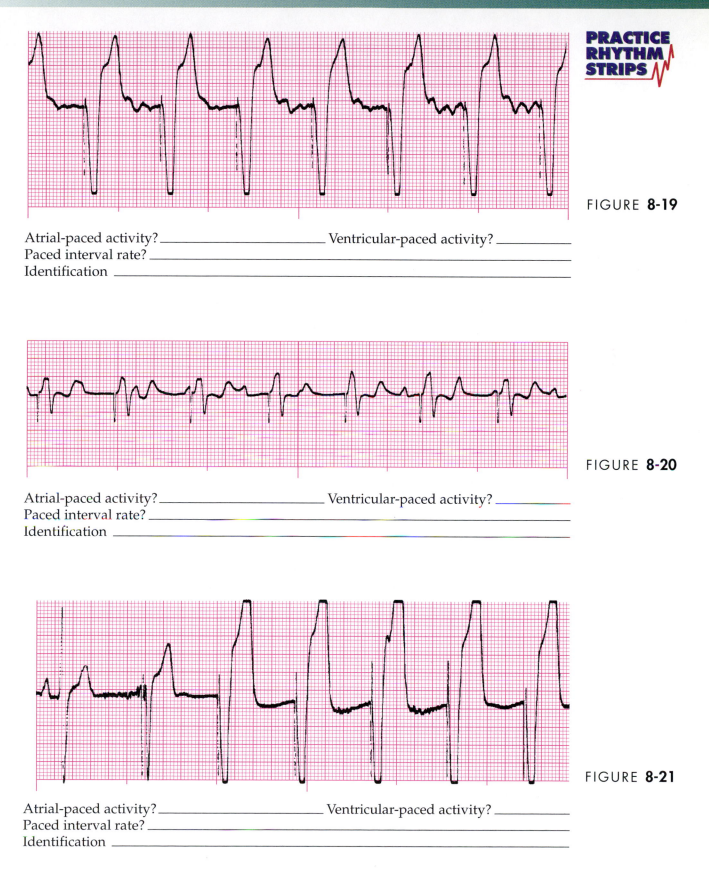

PRACTICE RHYTHM STRIPS

FIGURE **8-19**

Atrial-paced activity? _____ Ventricular-paced activity? _____
Paced interval rate? _____
Identification _____

FIGURE **8-20**

Atrial-paced activity? _____ Ventricular-paced activity? _____
Paced interval rate? _____
Identification _____

FIGURE **8-21**

Atrial-paced activity? _____ Ventricular-paced activity? _____
Paced interval rate? _____
Identification _____

CHAPTER 9

Introduction to the 12-Lead ECG

OBJECTIVES

On completion of this chapter, you will be able to:

1. List the leads that make up the standard 12-lead ECG.
2. Compare bipolar, unipolar, and precordial leads.
3. Describe correct anatomic placement of the precordial leads.
4. Describe the portion of the heart viewed by each lead of the 12-lead ECG.
5. Explain the term *electrical axis* and its significance.
6. Determine electrical axis using leads I and aVF.
7. Describe ECG changes that may reflect evidence of myocardial ischemia and injury.
8. Identify the ECG changes characteristically seen during the evolution of an acute myocardial infarction.
9. Explain the mechanism of a ST-segment elevation (Q wave) and non-ST-segment elevation (non-Q-wave) myocardial infarction.
10. Describe the sequence of normal R-wave progression.
11. Describe a method for recognizing a posterior wall myocardial infarction.
12. Identify the ECG features of right ventricular myocardial infarction.
13. Describe differentiation of right and left bundle branch block using leads V_1 and V_6.
14. Explain what is meant by the terms *dilatation, hypertrophy,* and *enlargement.*
15. Identify the ECG changes characteristically produced by electrolyte imbalances.
16. Describe ECG changes characteristically produced by digitalis toxicity.

INTRODUCTION TO THE 12-LEAD ECG

A standard 12-lead ECG provides views of the heart in both the frontal and horizontal planes and views the surfaces of the left ventricle from 12 different angles. Multiple views of the heart can provide useful information, including recognition of bundle branch blocks; identification of ST segment and T wave changes associated with myocardial ischemia, injury, and infarction; and identification of ECG changes associated with certain medications and electrolyte imbalances.

ANATOMY REVIEW

Right Coronary Artery (RCA)

The right coronary artery (RCA) originates from the right side of the aorta and passes along the atrioventricular sulcus between the right atrium and right ventricle (Figure 9-1). The marginal branch of the RCA supplies the right atrium and right ventricle. In 50% to 60% of individuals, a branch of the RCA supplies the SA node. In 85% to 90% of hearts, the RCA also branches into the AV node artery.[1]

The posterior descending branch supplies blood to the walls of both ventricles. The posterior descending artery has several branches, including the septal branch that supplies the posterior one third of the interventricular septum. Occlusion of the RCA can result in disturbances in AV nodal conduction.

Left Coronary Artery (LCA)

The left coronary artery (LCA) originates from the left side of the aorta and consists of the left main coronary artery that divides into two main branches—the left anterior descending (also called the *anterior interventricular*) artery and the left circumflex artery. The left anterior descending (LAD) branch travels to the anterior interventricular sulcus, and its branches supply blood to the anterior surfaces of both ventricles. Branches of the LAD include the diagonal and septal arteries.

Occlusion of the LAD can result in pump failure and/or intraventricular conduction delays, including right bundle branch block, left anterior hemiblock, or a combination of these (bifascicular block). The left circumflex (LC) branch follows the coronary sulcus between the right and left ventricle and supplies blood to the left atrium and left

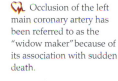 Occlusion of the left main coronary artery has been referred to as the "widow maker" because of its association with sudden death.

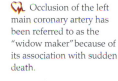 The LC artery supplies the SA node in 40% to 60% of individuals and the AV node in 10% to 15%.

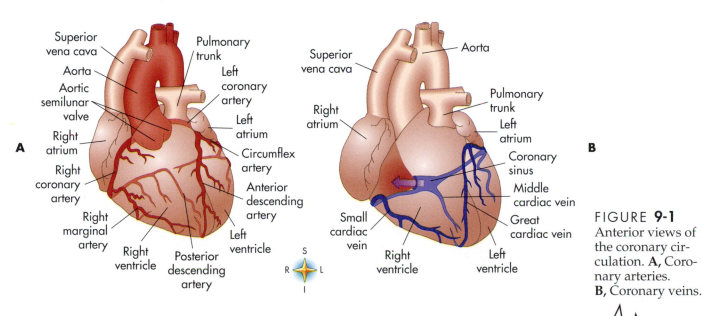

FIGURE 9-1 Anterior views of the coronary circulation. **A,** Coronary arteries. **B,** Coronary veins.

ventricle. Branches of the circumflex include the anterolateral and posterolateral marginal arteries. The left circumflex supplies the lateral wall of the left ventricle. In some patients, the circumflex artery may also supply the inferior portion of the left ventricle.

PLANES

Frontal Plane Leads

Leads allow viewing of the heart's electrical activity in two different planes: frontal (coronal) or horizontal (transverse). Each lead records the *average* current flow at a specific time in a portion of the heart. Frontal plane leads view the heart from the front of the body. Directions in the frontal plane are superior, inferior, right, and left. Leads I, II, and III (bipolar leads) and leads aVR, aVL, and aVF (unipolar leads) view the heart in the frontal plane (Figure 9-2).

Horizontal Plane Leads

Horizontal plane leads view the heart as if the body were sliced in half. Directions in the horizontal plane are anterior, posterior, right, and left. Six precordial (chest or V) leads view the heart in the horizontal plane, allowing a view of the front and left side of the heart (Figure 9-3).

LEADS

A 12-lead ECG is obtained by using electrodes placed on the body in specific locations. Each lead has a negative (−) and positive (+) electrode (pole). Each lead of the standard 12-lead ECG views the left ventricle from the position of its positive electrode.

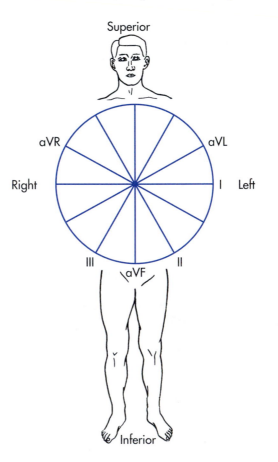

FIGURE **9-2**
Frontal plane
leads.

Standard Limb Leads

Leads I, II, and III make up the standard limb leads. If an electrode is placed on the right arm, left arm, and left leg, three leads are formed. Remember that an imaginary line joining the positive and negative electrodes of a lead is called the *axis* of the lead. The axes of these three limb leads form an equilateral triangle with the heart at the center (Einthoven's triangle) (Figure 9-4).

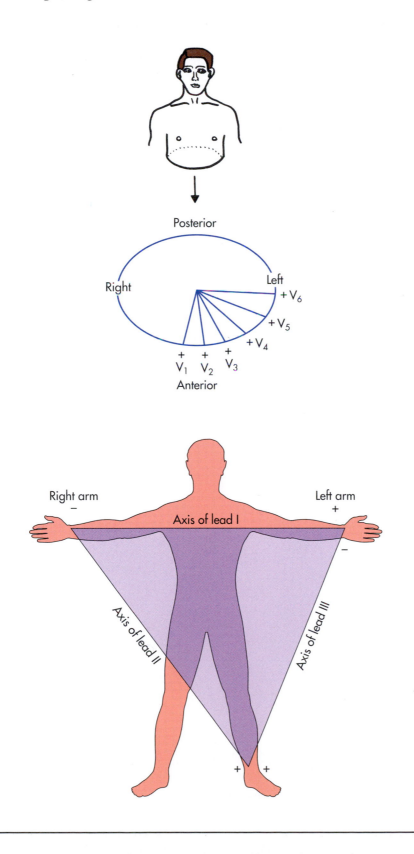

FIGURE **9-3**
Horizontal plane leads.

FIGURE **9-4**
Einthoven's triangle.

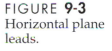

⚕ When viewing leads I, II, and III, if the R wave in lead II does not appear to be the sum of the voltage of the R waves in leads I and III, the leads may have been incorrectly applied.

In the bipolar leads, the right arm electrode is *always* the electrically negative pole and the left leg electrode is always the electrically positive pole. Einthoven expressed the relationship between leads I, II, and III as the sum of any complex in leads I and III equals that of lead II. Thus lead I + III = II. Stated another way, the voltage of a waveform in lead I plus the voltage of the same waveform in lead III equals the voltage of the same waveform in lead II.

Lead I views the lateral surface of the left ventricle. Leads II and III view the inferior surface of the left ventricle.

Augmented Limb Leads

⚕ Together, the three standard limb leads and the three augmented limb leads are often referred to as the *limb leads*.

Leads aVR, aVL, and aVF make up the augmented limb leads. The augmented limb leads are unipolar consisting of only one electrode (a positive electrode) on the body surface (Figure 9-5). The electrical potential produced by the augmented leads is normally relatively small. The ECG machine augments (magnifies) the amplitude of the electrical potentials detected at each extremity by approximately 50% over those recorded at the bipolar leads.

⚕ The six limb leads view the heart in the frontal plane.

Lead aVR views the heart from the right shoulder (the positive electrode) and views the base of the heart (primarily the atria and the great vessels). This lead does not view any wall of the heart. Lead aVL views the heart from the left shoulder (the positive electrode) and is oriented to the lateral wall of the left ventricle. Lead aVF views the heart from the left foot (leg) (positive electrode) and views the inferior surface of the left ventricle.

The relationship between leads aVR, aVL, and aVF can be expressed as aVR + aVL + aVF = 0. When viewing these leads, if the R waves in leads aVR, aVL, and aVF do not appear to equal zero, the leads may have been incorrectly applied.

Precordial Leads

The six precordial leads are unipolar leads that view the heart in the horizontal plane. The precordial leads are identified as V_1, V_2, V_3, V_4, V_5, and V_6. Each electrode placed in

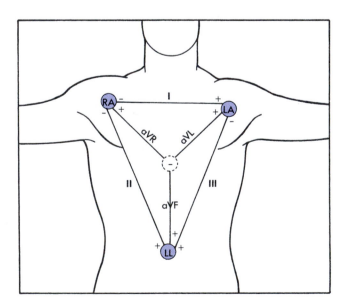

FIGURE 9-5
View of standard limb leads and augmented leads.

a V position is a positive electrode (Figure 9-6). The positive electrode for each of the precordial leads is positioned as follows:

- Lead V_1: Right side of sternum, fourth intercostal space
- Lead V_2: Left side of sternum, fourth intercostal space
- Lead V_3: Midway between V_2 and V_4
- Lead V_4: Left midclavicular line, fifth intercostal space
- Lead V_5: Left anterior axillary line at same level as V_4
- Lead V_6: Left midaxillary line at same level as V_4

Leads V_1 and V_2 view the interventricular septum, V_3 and V_4 view the anterior surface of the left ventricle, and V_5 and V_6 view the lateral surface of the left ventricle.

VECTORS

Leads have a negative (−) and positive (+) electrode pole that senses the magnitude and direction of the electrical force caused by the spread of waves of depolarization and repolarization throughout the myocardium. A **vector (arrow)** is a symbol representing this force. Leads that face the tip or point of a vector record a positive deflection on ECG paper.

A **mean vector** identifies the average of depolarization waves in one portion of the heart. The **mean P vector** represents the average magnitude and direction of both right and left atrial depolarization. The **mean QRS vector** represents the average magnitude

Leads V_1 and V_2 are referred to as right-sided precordial leads. Leads V_3 and V_4 are called midprecordial leads, and leads V_5 and V_6 are called left-sided precordial leads.

Vector: Quantity having direction and magnitude, usually depicted by a straight arrow whose length represents magnitude and whose head represents direction.[2]

A vector points in the direction of depolarization.

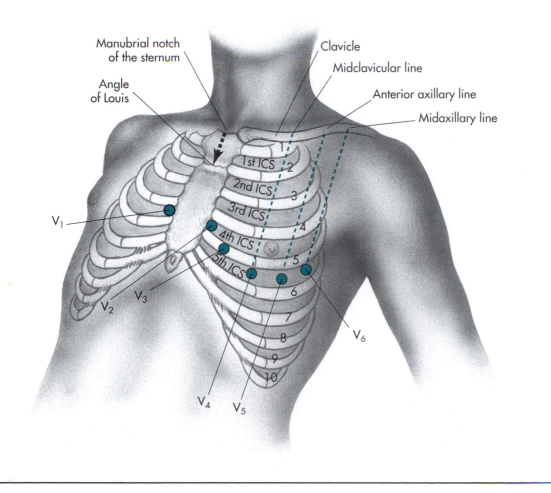

FIGURE **9-6**
Anatomic placement of the precordial leads.

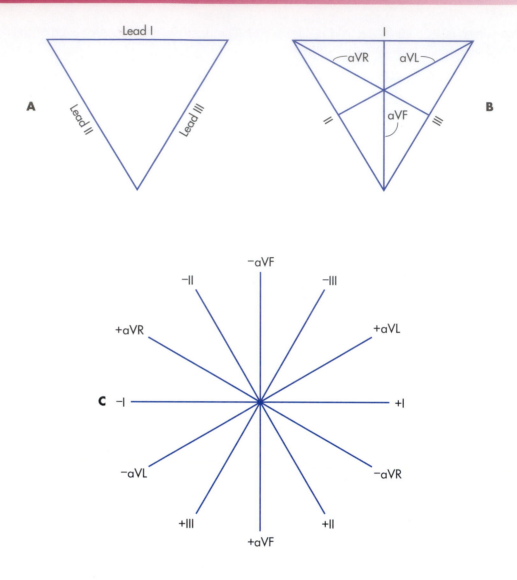

FIGURE 9-7
A, Einthoven's equilateral triangle formed by leads I, II, and III. **B,** Unipolar leads are added to the equilateral triangle. **C,** Hexaxial reference system derived from **B.**

When *axis* is used by itself, it refers to the QRS axis.

and direction of both right and left ventricular depolarization. The average direction of a mean vector is called the **mean axis** and is only identified in the frontal plane. An imaginary line joining the positive and negative electrodes of a lead is called the **axis** of the lead. **Electrical axis** refers to determining the direction (or angle in degrees) in which the main vector of depolarization is pointed.

Axis

During normal ventricular depolarization, the left side of the interventricular septum is stimulated first. The electrical impulse then traverses the septum to stimulate the right side. The left and right ventricles are then depolarized simultaneously. Because the left ventricle is considerably larger than the right, right ventricular depolarization forces are overshadowed on the ECG. As a result, the mean QRS vector points down (inferior) and to the left.

The axes of leads I, II, and III form an equilateral triangle with the heart at the center (Einthoven's triangle). If the augmented limb leads are added to this configuration and the axes of the six leads moved in a way in which they bisect each other, the result is the **hexaxial reference system** (Figure 9-7).

TABLE 9-1 TWO-LEAD METHOD OF AXIS DETERMINATION

Axis	Normal	Left	Right	Indeterminate ("no man's land")
Lead I QRS direction	Positive	Positive	Negative	Negative
Lead aVF QRS direction	Positive	Negative	Positive	Negative

The hexaxial reference system represents all of the frontal plane (limb) leads with the heart in the center and is the means used to express the location of the frontal plane axis. This system forms a 360-degree circle surrounding the heart. The positive end of lead I is designated at 0 degrees. The six frontal plane leads divide the circle into segments, each representing 30 degrees. All degrees in the upper hemisphere are labeled as negative degrees, and all degrees in the lower hemisphere are labeled as positive degrees. The mean QRS vector (normal electrical axis) lies between 0 and +90 degrees.

Current flow to the right of normal is called **right axis deviation** (+90 to +180 degrees). Current flow to the left of normal is called **left axis deviation** (−1 to −90 degrees). Current flow in the direction opposite of normal is called **indeterminate, "no man's land," northwest** or **extreme right axis deviation** (−91 to −179 degrees).

In the hexaxial reference system, the axes of some leads are perpendicular to each other. Lead I is perpendicular to lead aVF. Lead II is perpendicular to aVL, and lead III is perpendicular to aVR. If the electrical force moves toward a positive electrode, a positive (upright) deflection will be recorded. If the electrical force moves away from a positive electrode, a negative (downward) deflection will be recorded. If the electrical force is parallel to a given lead, the largest deflection in that lead will be recorded. Whether the deflection is positive or negative depends on whether the electrical force moves toward or away from the positive electrode. If the electrical force is perpendicular to a lead axis, the resulting ECG complex will be small or biphasic in that lead.

Leads I and aVF divide the heart into four quadrants. These two leads can be used to quickly estimate electrical axis. In leads I and aVF, the QRS complex is normally positive. If the QRS complex in either or both of these leads is negative, axis deviation is present (Table 9-1).

Right axis deviation may be a normal variant, particularly in the young and in thin individuals. Other causes of right axis deviation include mechanical shifts associated with inspiration or emphysema, right ventricular hypertrophy, dextrocardia, and left posterior hemiblock.

Left axis deviation may be a normal variant, particularly in older individuals and obesity. Other causes of left axis deviation include mechanical shifts associated with expiration; a high diaphragm caused by pregnancy, ascites, or abdominal tumors; left anterior hemiblock, hyperkalemia, inspiration or emphysema, right ventricular hypertrophy, and dextrocardia.

ISCHEMIA, INJURY, AND INFARCTION

The sudden occlusion of a coronary artery because of a thrombus may result in ischemia, injury, and/or necrosis of the area of the myocardium supplied by the affected artery. The area supplied by the obstructed artery goes through a characteristic sequence

Some forms of VT are associated with left axis deviation or an axis in "no man's land," but right axis deviation may occur in some.[3]

Axis determination can provide clues in the differential diagnosis of wide QRS tachycardia, hemiblocks, and localization of accessory pathways.

The processes of ischemia, injury, and infarction are called *the three Is* of an acute coronary event.

of events identified as "zones" of ischemia, injury, and infarction. Each zone is associated with characteristic ECG changes (Figure 9-8).

Acute coronary syndromes (ACS) is a term used to refer to patients presenting with ischemic chest pain. Acute coronary syndromes consist of three major syndromes that are related:

- Unstable angina
- Non-ST-segment elevation (non-Q-wave) myocardial infarction
- ST-segment elevation (Q-wave) myocardial infarction

These syndromes represent a continuum of a similar disease process involving a ruptured or eroded atheromatous plaque. Each syndrome is associated with specific strategies in prognosis and management.

Which acute coronary syndrome a patient has is determined by:[4]

- Rapidity of vessel occlusion
- Whether the obstruction is complete or incomplete
- Ability of the infarct-related artery to recruit distal collaterals
- Whether the occlusion is transient, with recurrent cycles of thrombosis and spontaneous lysis that may allow time for myocardial conditioning and development of collateral vessels

Ischemia

Myocardial ischemia results when the heart's demand for oxygen exceeds its supply from the coronary circulation. Myocardial ischemia can occur because of a decrease in myocar-

Acute coronary syndromes consist of: unstable angina, non-ST-elevation MI, ST-elevation MI.

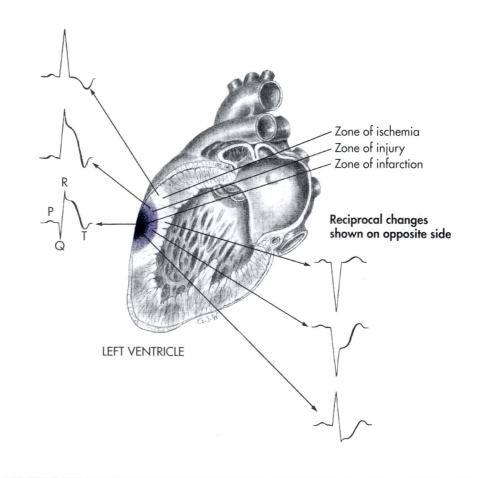

Zone of ischemia
Zone of injury
Zone of infarction

Reciprocal changes shown on opposite side

LEFT VENTRICLE

FIGURE **9-8**
Zones of ischemia, injury, and infarction, showing ECG waveforms and reciprocal waveforms corresponding to each zone.

dial oxygen supply or an increase in myocardial oxygen demand. This imbalance may be caused by decreased coronary artery blood flow because of blood vessel obstruction (atherosclerosis, vasospasm, thrombosis, embolism), decreased filling time (e.g., tachycardia), or decreased filling pressure in the coronary arteries (e.g., severe hypotension, aortic valve disease). Angina pectoris is a symptom of myocardial ischemia. The pain that accompanies angina is typically described as chest heaviness, pressure, squeezing, or constriction.

If the process is not reversed and blood flow restored, severe myocardial ischemia may lead to cellular injury and, eventually, infarction. Ischemia can quickly resolve by either reducing the oxygen needs of the heart (by resting or slowing the heart rate with medications such as beta-blockers) or increasing blood flow by dilating the coronary arteries with medications such as nitroglycerin. Myocardial ischemia delays the process of repolarization; thus, the ECG changes characteristic of ischemia include temporary changes in the ST segment and T wave. ST segment depression is suggestive of myocardial ischemia and is considered significant when the ST segment is more than 1 mm below the baseline at a point 0.04 sec (one small box) to the right of the J point (the point where the QRS ends and the ST segment begins) (Figure 9-9) and is seen in two or more leads facing the same anatomic area of the heart.

If ischemia is present through the full thickness of the myocardium, a negative (inverted) T wave will be present in the leads facing the affected area of the ventricle. In leads opposite the affected area, reciprocal (mirror image) changes may be seen. If ischemia is present only in the subendocardial layer, the T wave is usually positive (upright) because the direction of repolarization is unaffected (repolarization normally occurs from epicardium to endocardium) but may be abnormally tall.[5]

T wave inversion may be seen in conditions other than myocardial ischemia, including pericarditis, bundle branch block, ventricular hypertrophy, shock, electrolyte disorders, and subarachnoid hemorrhage ("cerebral T waves").

Injury

Myocardial injury occurs when the period of ischemia is prolonged more than just a few minutes. This period is a time of severe threat to the myocardium because injured myocardial cells can live or die. If blood flow is restored to the affected area, no tissue death occurs. However, without rapid intervention, the injured area will become necrotic. Methods to restore blood flow may include administration of fibrinolytic agents, coronary angioplasty, or a coronary artery bypass graft (CABG), among others.

Injured myocardium does not function normally, affecting both muscle contraction and the conduction of electrical impulses. The injured area depolarizes incompletely and remains electrically more positive than the uninjured areas surrounding it. Thus ST segment elevation will be present in the leads facing the affected area. ST segment elevation is considered significant when the ST segment is elevated more than 1 mm above the baseline at a point 0.04 sec (one small box) to the right of the J point in the limb leads or more than 2 mm in the precordial leads, and these changes are seen in two or more leads facing the same anatomic area of the heart (Figures 9-9 and 9-10).

Angina is most commonly caused by atherosclerotic disease of the coronary arteries.

In a non-Q wave MI, ST segment and T wave changes are the only ECG changes seen.

Symptoms of coronary artery disease are often not manifested until blood flow to an area of the heart is compromised by at least 60%.[6]

The ST elevation that accompanies an acute MI typically (but not always) bows upward, resembling a firefighter's hat.

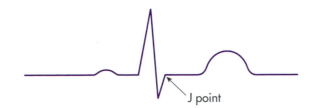
J point

FIGURE 9-9
The point where the QRS complex and the ST segment meet is called the *junction* or *J* point.

FIGURE **9-10**
ST segment.
A, The PR seg-
ment is used as
the baseline from
which to deter-
mine the presence
of ST segment ele-
vation or depres-
sion. **B,** ST seg-
ment elevation.
C, ST segment
depression.

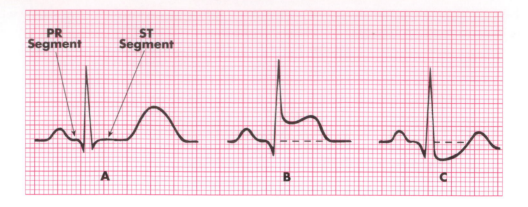

In leads opposite the affected area, ST segment depression (reciprocal changes) may be seen. If injury is present only in the subendocardial layer, the ST segment is usually depressed. A ventricular aneurysm should be suspected if ST segment elevation persists for more than a few months after MI.[7]

Prinzmetal's angina produces ST segment elevation without infarction.

Conditions other than an acute MI may cause ST segment elevation. For example, ST elevation may be present in ventricular hypertrophy, conduction abnormalities, pulmonary embolism, spontaneous pneumothorax, intracranial hemorrhage, hyperkalemia, and pericarditis. In pericarditis, ST segment elevation is usually present in all leads except aVR. In myocardial injury, the ST segment elevation is more localized and accompanied by ST segment depression in the opposite leads.[5]

Infarction

A **myocardial infarction (MI)** is the actual death of injured myocardial cells. MI occurs when there is a sudden decrease or total cessation of blood flow through a coronary artery to an area of the myocardium. This most commonly occurs because of the blockage of a coronary artery by a thrombus. A myocardial infarction often begins in the subendocardial area because this area has a high demand for oxygen and a tenuous blood supply. "The reason for this is explained by following the anatomical pathway of the coronary arteries. The coronary arteries first supply the epicardium and then course deep to supply the endocardium. High intraventricular pressure or a thickened myocardium will tend to decrease blood flow to the subendocardial issue."[7]

Sensitivity refers to a test's ability to identify true disease. Specificity refers to a test that is correctly negative in the absence of disease. A test with high specificity has few false positives.

As myocardial cells die, their cell membranes break and leak substances into the bloodstream. The presence of these substances in the blood can subsequently be measured by means of blood tests to verify the presence of an infarction. These substances (called *cardiac markers* or *serum cardiac markers*) include creatine kinase (CK) MB isoforms, troponin, and myoglobin. Troponin T and troponin I are two tests that may be ordered for a patient with a suspected MI. If the level is elevated (positive test), myocardial necrosis (infarction) has almost certainly occurred. The troponin-I test appears to have better specificity than troponin-T (Table 9-2). Serum cardiac markers are useful for confirming the diagnosis of MI when patients present without ST-segment elevation, when the diagnosis may be unclear, and when physicians must distinguish patients with unstable angina from those with a non-ST-segment elevation (non-Q-wave) MI. They are also useful for confirming the diagnosis of MI for patients with ST-segment elevation.

TABLE 9-2 SERUM CARDIAC MARKERS			
	Rises	Peaks	Duration
Troponin I	4-8 hours	12-16 hours	2 weeks
CK-MB	3-6 hours	12-24 hours	1-3 days
Myoglobin	2-4 hours	9-12 hours	1-2 days

According to the World Health Organization, the diagnosis of myocardial infarction is based on the presence of at least two of the following three criteria:

- Clinical history of ischemic-type chest discomfort
- Changes on serially obtained electrocardiographic tracings
- Rise and fall in serum cardiac markers

The location of a myocardial infarction depends on which coronary artery is obstructed. For many years, a myocardial infarction was classified by its location on the myocardial surface and the muscle layers affected (i.e., nontransmural or transmural MI). A nontransmural infarction was classified as either subendocardial, involving the endocardium and the myocardium, or subepicardial, involving the myocardium and the epicardium.[8] Further, a nontransmural MI was associated with abnormal cardiac enzymes but no pathologic Q waves on the ECG. A transmural MI referred to death of the entire thickness of the myocardium (endocardium, myocardium, and epicardium) in the area supplied by the affected artery. A transmural MI was associated with abnormal cardiac enzymes and pathologic Q waves on the ECG.

Recently, it has been demonstrated that Q waves may not be present in a transmural MI and, conversely, Q waves may be present in a subendocardial MI. "Although non-Q-wave infarction is often referred to as subendocardial infarction and Q-wave infarction as transmural, the implied ECG and anatomic association cannot be verified by autopsy findings in a large number of cases."[5]

Because of these findings, terminology related to myocardial infarctions has changed again. An MI was classified according to its location on the myocardial surface (i.e., anterior, inferior, etc.), and whether it produced Q waves on the ECG (i.e., Q wave vs. non-Q-wave) MI. Today, the World Health Organization recommends classification of infarctions as ST-segment elevation or non-ST-segment elevation infarction rather than Q-wave or non-Q-wave, transmural or subendocardial infarction.

Whether an MI is an ST-segment elevation (Q-wave) or non-ST-segment elevation (non-Q-wave) MI depends on the degree and duration of vessel occlusion and the presence or absence of coronary collateral circulation.

Non-ST-Segment Elevation (Non-Q-Wave) Myocardial Infarction
In the acute phase of a non-ST-segment elevation (non-Q-wave) MI, the ST segment may be depressed in the leads facing the surface of the infarcted area. A non-ST-segment elevation MI can only be diagnosed if the ST segment and T wave changes are accompanied by elevations of serum cardiac markers indicative of myocardial necrosis.[5] Patients with non-ST-segment elevation acute MI are known to be at higher risk for death, reinfarction, and other morbidity than those with unstable angina. Recent data suggest the

incidence of non-ST-segment elevation MI is increasing as the population of older patients with more advanced disease increases.

ST-Segment Elevation (Q-Wave) Myocardial Infarction

Most patients with ST-segment elevation will develop Q-wave MI. Only a minority of patients with ischemic chest discomfort at rest who do not have ST-segment elevation will develop Q-wave MI. A Q-wave MI is diagnosed by the development of abnormal Q waves in serial ECGs. Q-wave MIs tend to be larger than non-Q-wave MIs, reflecting more damage to the left ventricle, and are associated with a more prolonged and complete coronary thrombosis. Q waves may develop quite early in acute coronary syndromes. In one study, 53% of patients presenting within 1 hour of symptom onset already displayed abnormal Q waves.[9] This early development of Q waves appears to predict the size of the infarction.

♥ Q waves are frequently wide and deep in leads III and aVR in normal individuals.

With the exception of leads III and aVR, an abnormal (pathologic) Q wave is more than 0.04 sec in duration and more than 25% of the amplitude of the following R wave in that lead. An abnormal Q wave indicates the presence of dead myocardial tissue and, subsequently, a loss of electrical activity. Although abnormal Q waves can appear within hours after occlusion of a coronary artery, they more commonly appear several hours or days after the onset of signs and symptoms of an acute MI. Q waves do not reflect when an MI occurred. However, when combined with ST segment or T wave changes, their presence suggests a recent (acute) MI. Because the presence of a pathologic Q wave may take hours to develop to confirm the presence of a Q-wave MI, the patient's signs and symptoms, laboratory tests, and the presence of ST segment elevation provides the strongest evidence for the early recognition of MI.

LAYOUT OF THE 12-LEAD ECG

A 12-lead ECG is obtained with a 12-lead monitor that simultaneously records the leads and provides a read-out in a conventional four-column format (Figure 9-11). Each column consists of three rows. The standard limb leads are recorded in the first column, the augmented limb leads in the second column, and the precordial leads in the third and fourth columns (Table 9-3).

12-LEAD CHANGES INDICATING INFARCTION

♥ "Tombstone" T waves are so-called because of their presence in the setting of an acute MI. Because of their size, it is often possible to inscribe "RIP" (rest in peace) in the waveform on the ECG.

During the evolution of an acute Q-wave MI, a typical sequence of ECG events occurs in the leads that face the infarcted area. The earliest changes include an increase in T-wave amplitude. The T waves are tall, may be peaked, and are called "hyperacute" (or "tombstone") T waves. Hyperacute T waves (over 50% of preceding R wave) overlying the affected myocardium may be the first ECG sign of acute MI. They are transient, often seen within minutes or hours after the onset of chest pain, and are believed to be caused by subendocardial ischemia.[5] Hyperacute T waves are followed by ST-segment elevation and then the appearance of pathologic Q waves (in Q-wave infarction) in the leads facing the affected area. The evolution of the MI continues with decreased R-wave amplitude (poor R-wave progression), and T-wave inversion.

In the standard 12-lead ECG, leads II, III, and aVF "look" at tissue supplied by the right coronary artery and eight leads "look" at tissue supplied by the left coronary artery—leads I, aVL, V_1, V_2, V_3, V_4, V_5, and V_6. When evaluating the extent of infarction produced by a left coronary artery occlusion, determine how many of these leads are showing changes consistent with an acute infarction. The more of these eight leads demonstrating acute changes, the larger the infarction is presumed to be.[10]

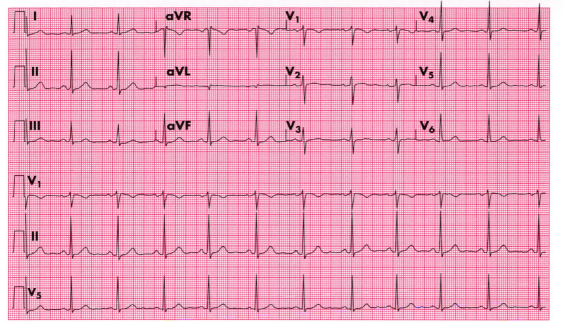

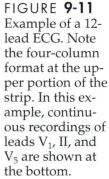

FIGURE **9-11**
Example of a 12-lead ECG. Note the four-column format at the upper portion of the strip. In this example, continuous recordings of leads V_1, II, and V_5 are shown at the bottom.

TABLE **9-3**	**LAYOUT OF THE FOUR-COLUMN 12-LEAD ECG**		
Limb leads		Precordial leads	
Standard leads	Augmented leads	V_1-V_3	V_4-V_6
Column I	Column II	Column III	Column IV
I: lateral	aVR	V_1: septum	V_4: anterior
II: inferior	aVL: lateral	V_2: septum	V_5: lateral
III: inferior	aVF: inferior	V_3: anterior	V_6: lateral

To view the right ventricle, right precordial leads are used (Figure 9-12). Placement of right precordial leads is identical to placement of the standard precordial leads except on the right side of the chest. If time does not permit obtaining all the right precordial leads, the lead of choice is V_4R. A modification of lead V_4R (MC_4R) using a standard 3-lead system may be used to view the right ventricle. The positive electrode is placed in the fifth intercostal space, right mid-clavicular line. The negative electrode is placed on the left arm and the lead selector on the monitor placed in the lead III position.

Because no leads of the standard 12-lead ECG directly view the posterior wall of the left ventricle, changes in the opposite (anterior) wall of the heart can be viewed as reciprocal changes. Alternately, additional precordial leads may be used to view the heart's posterior surface. These leads are placed further left and toward the back. All of the leads are

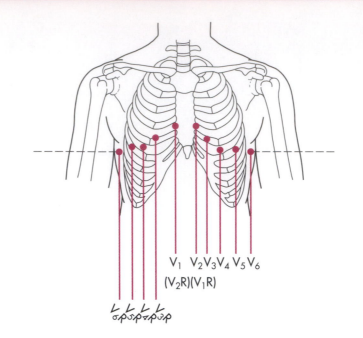

FIGURE **9-12**
Anatomic place-
ment of the left
and right precor-
dial leads.

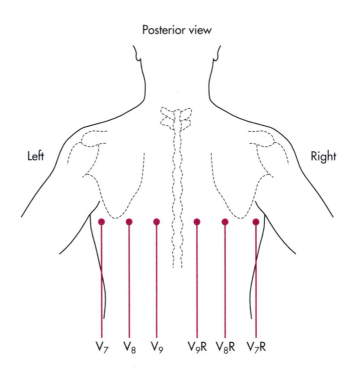

FIGURE **9-13**
Posterior pre-
cordial lead
placement.

placed on the same horizontal line as V_4 to V_6. Lead V_7 is placed at the posterior axillary line. Lead V_8 is placed at the angle of the scapula (posterior scapular line), and Lead V_9 is placed over the left border of spine (Figure 9-13).

R-Wave Progression

Depolarization of the interventricular septum normally occurs from left to right and posteriorly to anteriorly. The wave of ventricular depolarization in the major portions of the ventricles is normally from right to left and in an anterior to posterior direction.

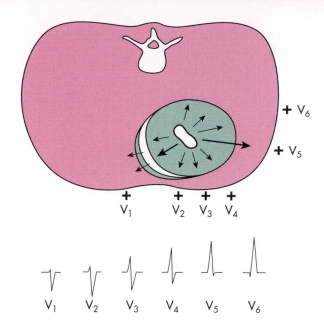

FIGURE **9-14**
Ventricular acti-
vation and
R-wave progres-
sion as viewed in
the precordial
leads.

When viewing the precordial leads in a normal heart, the R wave becomes taller and the S wave becomes smaller as the electrode is moved from right to left. This pattern is called *R-wave progression* (Figure 9-14).

In V_1 and V_2, the QRS deflection is predominantly negative (moving away from the positive precordial electrode), reflecting depolarization of the septum and right ventricle (small R wave) and the left ventricle (large S wave). As the precordial electrode is placed further left, the wave of depolarization is moving toward the positive electrode. V_3 and V_4 normally record an equiphasic (equally positive and negative) RS complex.[11] The area in which this equiphasic complex occurs is called the *transitional zone*. V_5 and V_6 normally record a QR complex in which the Q wave is small, reflecting depolarization of the septum, and the R wave is tall, reflecting ventricular depolarization.

Poor R-wave progression (Figure 9-15) is a phrase used to describe R waves that decrease in size from V_1 to V_4. This is often seen in an anteroseptal infarction but may be a normal variant in young persons, particularly in young women. Other causes of poor R-wave progression include left bundle branch block, left ventricular hypertrophy, severe chronic obstructive pulmonary disease (particularly emphysema), old anteroseptal and anterior infarction.[3]

The R wave in V_6 may actually be smaller than that of V_5 because the V_6 electrode is further from the heart.[11]

LOCALIZATION OF INFARCTIONS

The left ventricle has been divided into four regions where a myocardial infarction may occur—anterior, lateral, inferior, and posterior. Figure 9-16 shows which coronary artery supplies blood to each portion of the heart, the site of infarction if one of these vessels is occluded, and the area of the heart viewed by each of the leads in a standard 12-lead ECG. A myocardial infarction may not be limited to one of the regions previously described. For example, if the precordial leads indicate ECG changes in leads V_3 and V_4, suggestive of an anterior wall MI, and diagnostic changes are also present in V_5 and V_6, the infarction would be called an *anterolateral infarction* or an *anterior infarction with lateral extension*.

It is important to note that the ECG is nondiagnostic in approximately 50% of patients with chest discomfort. A normal ECG does not rule out an acute MI, particularly in the early hours of a coronary artery occlusion.

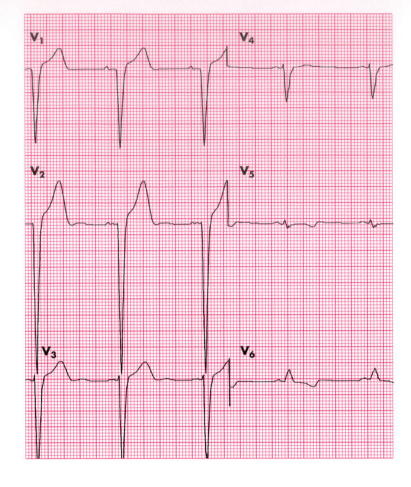

FIGURE **9-15**
Poor R-wave progression in V_1 through V_4; QRS >0.12 sec; left bundle branch block.

Lateral Wall

Leads I, aVL, V_5, and V_6 view the lateral wall of the left ventricle. The lateral wall is usually supplied by the circumflex branch of the left coronary artery. Lateral wall infarctions often occur as extensions of anterior or inferior infarctions. ECG changes suggestive of MI include ST segment elevation in leads I, aVL, V_5, and V_6. Reciprocal ST depression may be seen in V_1. In some patients, the AV node is supplied by a branch of the circumflex artery. In these patients, occlusion of this vessel may result in AV blocks.

Inferior Wall

Because the inferior surface of the heart rests on the diaphragm, the presence of ischemia, injury, or infarction in this area may be called *inferior* or *diaphragmatic*.

Leads II, III, and aVF view the inferior surface of the left ventricle. Reciprocal changes are observed in leads I and aVL. In most individuals, the inferior wall of the left ventricle is supplied by the posterior descending branch of the right coronary artery. ECG changes suggestive of infarction include ST segment elevation in leads II, III, and aVF (Figure 9-17). Early reciprocal changes in leads I and aVL include ST segment depression. Late reciprocal changes include abnormally tall T waves in these leads. Parasympathetic hyperactivity is common with inferior wall MIs, resulting in bradydysrhythmias. Conduction delays such as first-degree AV block and second-degree AV block type I are common and usually transient. Approximately 40% of inferior wall MIs involve the right ventricle.

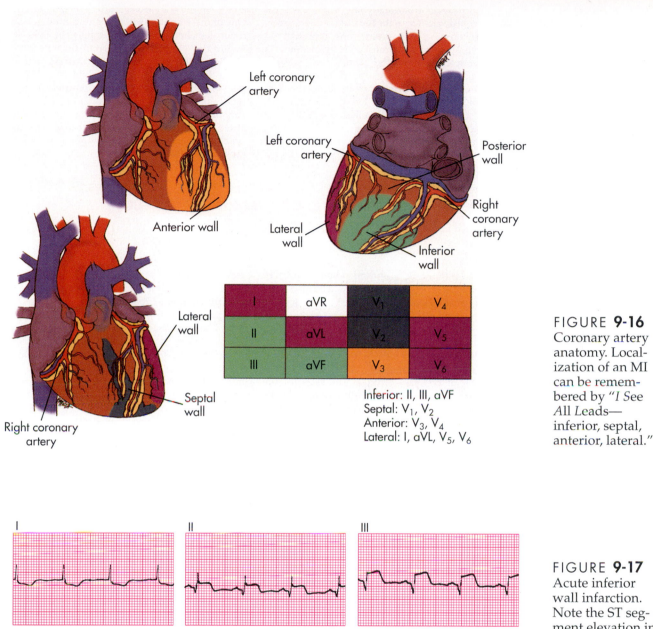

Left coronary
artery

Anterior wall

Left coronary
artery

Posterior
wall

Right
coronary
artery

Lateral
wall

Inferior
wall

Lateral
wall

Septal
wall

Right coronary
artery

I	aVR	V₁	V₄
II	aVL	V₂	V₅
III	aVF	V₃	V₆

Inferior: II, III, aVF
Septal: V₁, V₂
Anterior: V₃, V₄
Lateral: I, aVL, V₅, V₆

FIGURE **9-16**
Coronary artery
anatomy. Local-
ization of an MI
can be remem-
bered by "*I See
All Leads*—
inferior, septal,
anterior, lateral."

I

II

III

aVR

aVL

aVF

FIGURE **9-17**
Acute inferior
wall infarction.
Note the ST seg-
ment elevation in
leads II, III, and
aVF, and the reci-
procal ST depres-
sion in leads I and
aVL. Abnormal Q
waves are also
present in leads
II, III, and aVF.

Septum

Leads V_1 and V_2 face the septal area of the left ventricle. The septum, which contains the bundle of His and bundle branches, is normally supplied by the left anterior descending artery. ECG changes suggestive of infarction include the absence of

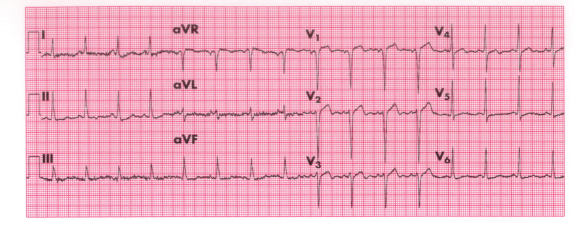

FIGURE **9-18**
Septal infarction.
Poor R-wave
progression.

If the site of infarction is limited to the septum, ECG changes are seen in V_1 and V_2. If the entire anterior wall is involved, ECG changes will be visible in V_1, V_2, V_3, and V_4.

normal "septal" R waves in leads V_1 and V_2 (resulting in QS waves in these leads) (Figure 9-18); absence of normal "septal" Q waves in leads I, II, III, aVF, V_4, V_5, and V_6; and ST segment elevation with tall T waves in leads V_1 and V_2. An occlusion in this area may result in both right and left (more common) bundle branch blocks, second-degree AV block type II, and complete AV block.

Anterior Wall

Patients with an anterior MI gain the most benefit from fibrinolytic therapy.

Leads V_3 and V_4 face the anterior wall of the left ventricle. Reciprocal changes of injury, such as ST depression, appear in leads II, III, and aVF. This area is normally supplied by the diagonal branch of the left anterior descending artery. ECG changes suggestive of infarction include ST segment elevation with tall T waves and taller than normal R waves in leads V_3 and V_4 (Figures 9-19 and 9-20).

Because the left anterior descending artery supplies about 40% of the heart's blood and a critical section of the left ventricle, an occlusion in this area can lead to complications such as left ventricular dysfunction, including congestive heart failure (CHF) and cardiogenic shock. Sympathetic hyperactivity is common with resulting sinus tachycardia and/or hypertension. An anterior wall MI may cause other dysrhythmias, including PVCs, atrial flutter, or atrial fibrillation. Because the bundle branches travel through this area, bundle branch blocks may result from injury in this area.

Posterior Wall

A posterior MI often occurs in conjunction with an inferior wall MI.

The posterior wall of the left ventricle is supplied by the left circumflex coronary artery in most patients; however, in some patients it is supplied by the right coronary artery. On the standard 12-lead ECG, no leads directly view the posterior wall of the left ventricle. Changes in the opposite (anterior) wall of the heart can be viewed as reciprocal changes (Figures 9-21 and 9-22). A posterior wall MI usually produces tall R waves and ST segment depression in leads V_1 through V_4. Complications of a posterior wall MI may include left ventricular dysfunction. If the posterior wall is supplied by the right coronary artery, complications may include dysrhythmias involving the SA node, AV node, and bundle of His.

To assist in the recognition of ECG changes suggesting a posterior wall MI, the "mirror test" is helpful. Flip over the ECG to the blank side and turn it upside down. When held

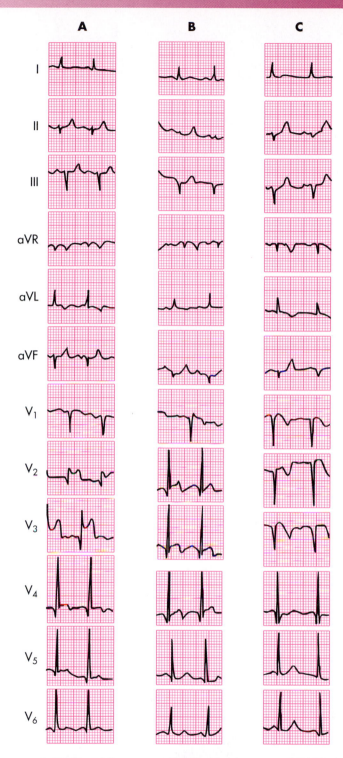

FIGURE **9-19**
Evolutionary changes in anteroseptal myocardial infarction reflected in leads V_2 to V_4. **A,** At admission, hyperacute phase is reflected by ST-segment elevation. **B,** At 24 hours. **C,** At 48 hours, there are abnormal (pathologic) Q waves.

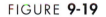

FIGURE **9-20**
Extensive anterior infarction. Reciprocal changes present in leads II, III, and aVF.

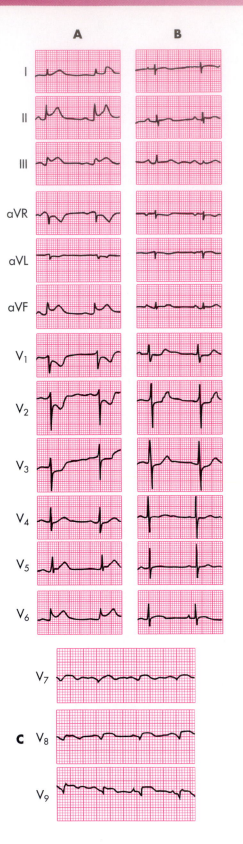

FIGURE 9-21
Evolutionary changes in inferior and posterior myocardial infarction (MI). **A,** Acute inferior and apical injury. **B,** At 24 hours. Note tall R wave in lead V$_1$ not present in **A,** suggesting posterior MI. **C,** Posterior infarction confirmed.

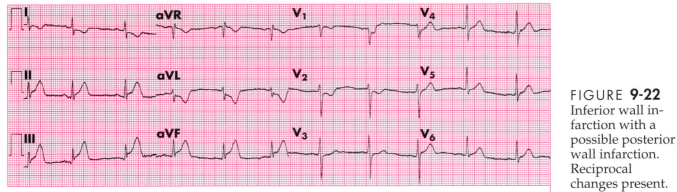

FIGURE **9-22**
Inferior wall infarction with a possible posterior wall infarction. Reciprocal changes present.

up to the light, the tall R waves become deep Q waves and ST depression becomes ST elevation—the "classic" ECG changes associated with MI.

Right Ventricular Infarction

Right ventricular infarction (RVI) should be suspected when ECG changes suggesting an acute inferior wall MI (viewed in leads II, III, and aVF) are observed. When RVI is suspected, right precordial leads are used. ST segment elevation of 1 mm or more in lead V_4R has a sensitivity of 70% to 93% and a specificity of 77% to 100%.[5] Complications associated with RVI include hypotension, cariogenic shock, AV blocks, atrial flutter or fibrillation, and PACs (Figures 9-23 and 9-24).

A right ventricular MI should be suspected in the patient with an inferior left ventricular MI; unexplained, persistent hypotension; clear lung fields; and jugular venous distention. During right ventricular infarction, the right ventricle dilates acutely and does not effectively pump blood to the pulmonary system. Jugular venous distention occurs because of the backup of blood into the systemic venous vessels. Signs of pulmonary edema are absent because the right ventricle is unable to effectively pump blood into the pulmonary vasculature. Filling of the left ventricle is subsequently decreased, resulting in decreased cardiac output and, ultimately, hypotension (Table 9-4).

Although a RVI may occur by itself, it is more commonly associated with an inferior wall MI. RVI has been noted with a frequency approaching 40% of all inferior wall infarctions.[1]

INTRAVENTRICULAR CONDUCTION DELAYS

Intraventricular conduction delays are best identified by using leads MCL_1, MCL_6, V_1, and/or V_6.

Structures of the Intraventricular Conduction System

After passing through the AV node, the electrical impulse enters the bundle of His (also referred to as the *common bundle* or the *atrioventricular bundle*). The bundle of His is normally the only electrical connection between the atria and the ventricles. It is located in the upper portion of the interventricular septum and connects the AV node with the two bundle branches. The bundle of His conducts the electrical impulse to the right and left bundle branches.

The right bundle branch travels down the right side of the interventricular septum to conduct the electrical impulse to the right ventricle. Structurally, the right bundle branch is long, thin, and more fragile than the left. Because of its structure, a relatively small lesion in the right bundle branch can result in delays or interruptions in electrical impulse transmission.

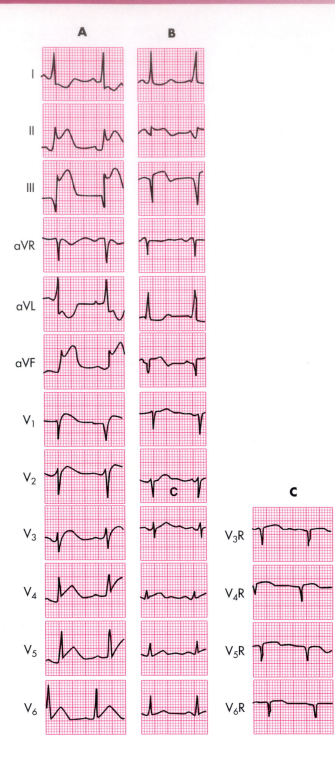

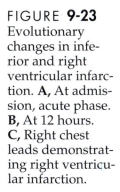

FIGURE **9-23**
Evolutionary changes in inferior and right ventricular infarction. **A,** At admission, acute phase. **B,** At 12 hours. **C,** Right chest leads demonstrating right ventricular infarction.

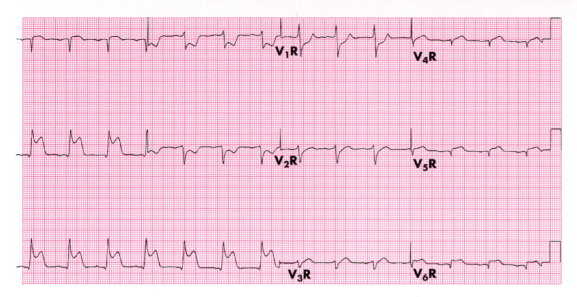

FIGURE **9-24**
12-lead ECG obtained using the right-sided precordial leads. Inferior infarction with evidence of right ventricular injury (V$_4$R).

TABLE **9-4**	LOCALIZATION OF A MYOCARDIAL INFARCTION		
Location of MI	**Indicative changes (leads facing affected area)**	**Reciprocal changes (leads opposite affected area)**	**Affected coronary artery**
Lateral	I, aVL, V$_5$, V$_6$	V$_1$-V$_3$	Left coronary artery—circumflex branch
Inferior	II, III, aVF	I, aVL	Right coronary artery—posterior descending branch
Septum	V$_1$, V$_2$	None	Left coronary artery—left anterior descending artery, septal branch
Anterior	V$_3$, V$_4$	II, III, aVF	Left coronary artery—left anterior descending artery, diagonal branch
Posterior	Not visualized	V$_1$, V$_2$, V$_3$, V$_4$	Right coronary artery or left circumflex artery
Right ventricle	V$_1$R-V$_6$R		Right coronary artery—proximal branches

The left bundle branch begins as a single structure that is short and thick (the left common bundle branch or main stem) and then divides into three divisions (fascicles) called the *anterior fascicle, posterior fascicle,* and the *septal fascicle.*[12] The anterior fascicle spreads the electrical impulse to the anterior and lateral walls of the left ventricle. This fascicle is thin and vulnerable to disruptions in electrical impulse transmission. The posterior fascicle relays the impulse to the posterior (inferior) portions of the left ventricle, and the septal fascicle relays the impulse to the midseptum (Figure 9-25). The posterior fascicle is short, thick, and rarely disrupted because of its structure and dual blood supply from both the left anterior descending artery and the right coronary artery. As a rule, only two divisions of the left bundle branch (the anterior and posterior fascicles) are explained when discussing bundle branch blocks, despite the existence of its three distinct divisions.

The anterior fascicle is also called the *superior fascicle.* The posterior fascicle is also called the *inferior fascicle.*

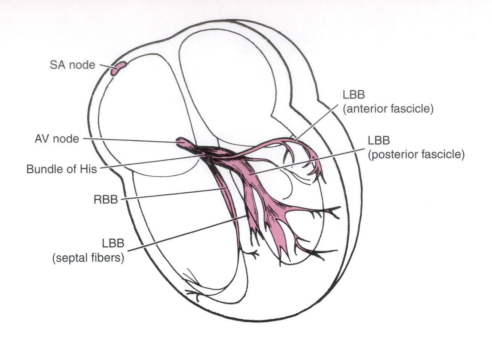

SA node

LBB
(anterior fascicle)

AV node

LBB
(posterior fascicle)

Bundle of His

RBB

LBB
(septal fibers)

FIGURE **9-25**
Conduction
system.

Blood Supply to the Intraventricular Conduction System

The bundle of His receives a dual blood supply from the left anterior and posterior descending coronary arteries making this portion of the conduction system less vulnerable to ischemic damage.[12] The posterior descending artery is the right coronary artery in 90% of individuals.[11] The right bundle branch and the anterior division of the left bundle branch are supplied by the left anterior descending artery.

Bundle Branch Activation

♥ The wave of depolarization moves from endocardium to epicardium.

During normal ventricular depolarization, the left side of the interventricular septum (stimulated by the left posterior fascicle) is stimulated first. The electrical impulse (wave of depolarization) then traverses the septum to stimulate the right side. The left and right ventricles are then depolarized simultaneously.

♥ A left anterior hemiblock is also called *anterior hemiblock* or *anterior fascicular block*. A left posterior hemiblock is also called *posterior hemiblock* or *posterior fascicular block*.

A delay or block can occur in any part of the intraventricular conduction system. A block in only one of the fascicles of the bundle branches is called a **monofascicular block.** A block in any two divisions of the bundle branches is a **bifascicular block.** Although this term may be used to describe a block in both the anterior and posterior branches of the left bundle branch, it is more commonly used to describe a combination of a right bundle branch block and either a left anterior fascicular block (LAFB) or a left posterior fascicular block (LPFB). A **trifascicular block** is a block in the three primary divisions of the bundle branches (i.e., right bundle branch, left anterior fascicle, and left posterior fascicle). A **hemiblock** is a block in either of the fascicles of the left bundle branch (e.g., left anterior hemiblock, left posterior hemiblock). A hemiblock can be complete or intermittent. Because the right bundle branch has only one fascicle, there is no right hemiblock.

ECG Characteristics

If a delay or block occurs in one of the bundle branches, the ventricles will be depolarized asynchronously. The impulse travels first down the unblocked branch and stimulates that ventricle. Because of the block, the impulse must then travel from cell to cell through the myocardium (rather than through the normal conduction pathway) to stimulate the other ventricle. This means of conduction is slower than normal, and the QRS

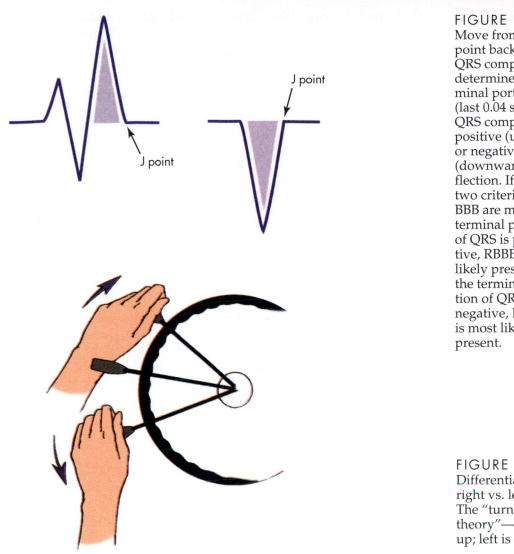

FIGURE **9-26**
Move from J point back into QRS complex and determine if terminal portion (last 0.04 sec) of QRS complex is positive (upright) or negative (downward) deflection. If the two criteria for BBB are met and terminal portion of QRS is positive, RBBB is most likely present. If the terminal portion of QRS is negative, LBBB is most likely present.

FIGURE **9-27**
Differentiating right vs. left BBB. The "turn signal theory"—right is up; left is down.

complex appears widened on the ECG. The ventricle with the blocked bundle branch is the last to be depolarized.

A QRS measuring 0.10 to 0.12 sec is called an **incomplete** right or left bundle branch block. A QRS measuring more than 0.12 sec is called a **complete** right or left bundle branch block. If the QRS is wide but there is no BBB pattern, the term *wide QRS* or *intraventricular conduction delay* is used to describe the QRS.

ECG criteria for identification of a right or left BBB are:

- A QRS duration of more than 0.12 sec (if a complete BBB)
- QRS complexes produced by supraventricular activity (i.e., the QRS complex is not a paced beat nor did it originate in the ventricles)

To determine right vs. left BBB:

- View lead V_1 or MCI_1
- Move from the J point back into the QRS complex and determine if the terminal portion (last 0.04 sec) of the QRS complex is a positive (upright) or negative (downward) deflection (Figures 9-26 and 9-27)

A bundle branch block is abbreviated BBB. A right bundle branch block is RBBB. A left bundle branch block is LBBB. When used alone, LBBB implies a **complete** LBBB.

The width of a QRS complex is most accurately determined when it is viewed and measured in more than one lead. The measurement should be taken from the QRS complex with the longest duration and clearest onset and end.

A delay in conduction in the right bundle branch causes right ventricular activation to occur after left ventricular activation is completed, producing a R' deflection. A delay in the left bundle branch markedly postpones left ventricular activation, resulting in an abnormally prominent S wave.[13]

- If the two criteria for bundle branch block are met and the terminal portion of the QRS is positive, a RBBB is most likely present (Figure 9-28)
- If the terminal portion of the QRS is negative, a LBBB is most likely present (Figure 9-29)

Causes

RBBB can occur in individuals with no underlying heart disease but more commonly occurs in the presence of organic heart disease—coronary artery disease being the most common cause. In patients with acute myocardial infarction, complete RBBB is present in 3% to 7% of the cases. In such cases, it is often accompanied by left anterior hemiblock and is the result of an anterior myocardial infarction.[5] RBBB occurring as the result of acute myocardial infarction may require pacemaker intervention. The progression of RBBB to complete AV block occurs twice as often as that of LBBB, especially when RBBB is associated with a fascicular block.[1]

LBBB may be acute or chronic. Acute LBBB may occur secondary to an anteroseptal (more common) or inferior MI, acute congestive heart failure, or acute pericarditis or myocarditis. The most common causes of chronic LBBB are coronary artery disease, hypertensive heart disease, or a combination of the two, and dilated cardiomyopathy.[5]

Infarction in the Presence of BBB

If RBBB occurs, stimulation of the septum and left ventricle is unaffected because the electrical impulse travels down the left bundle branch into the interventricular septum.

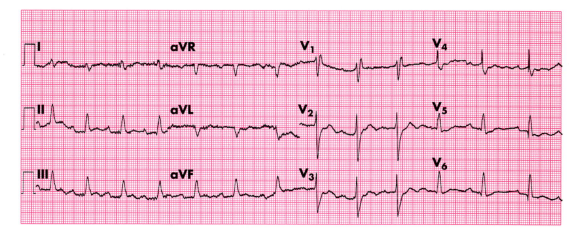

FIGURE 9-28 Right bundle branch block (RBBB).

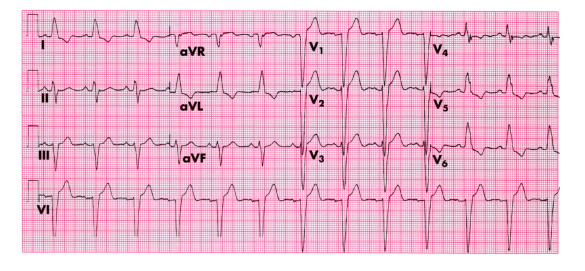

FIGURE 9-29 Left bundle branch block (LBBB).

The septum is activated by the left posterior fascicle and is depolarized from left to right. The left ventricle is then stimulated and depolarizes from right to left. In RBBB, the ECG changes suggestive of an acute MI are normally still visible. Abnormal Q waves are visible, and ST-segment elevation is superimposed on the RBBB ECG pattern.

If LBBB occurs, septal activation is altered and the right ventricle depolarizes before the left. Thus abnormal Q waves originating from the left ventricle may be obscured. Further, ST segment and T wave changes are often present with LBBB, making the diagnosis of acute MI even more difficult. In LBBB, ST segment and T wave are normally of opposite polarity (direction) to the terminal portion of the QRS. If a LBBB pattern is observed in V_5 or V_6 and the ST segment and T wave are of the same polarity as the terminal portion of the QRS, ischemia should be suspected.

CHAMBER ENLARGEMENT

Enlargement of the atrial and/or ventricular chambers of the heart may occur if there is a volume or pressure overload in the heart. **Dilatation** is an increase in the diameter of a chamber of the heart caused by volume overload. Dilatation may be acute or chronic. **Hypertrophy** is an increase in the thickness of a heart chamber because of chronic pressure overload. **Enlargement** is a term that implies the presence of dilatation or hypertrophy or both.

The vertical axis of ECG graph paper represents *voltage* or *amplitude* of the ECG waveforms or deflections. The size or amplitude of a waveform is measured in millivolts (mV) or millimeters (mm). The ECG machine's sensitivity must be calibrated so that a 1-mV electrical signal will produce a deflection measuring exactly 10-mm tall (Figure 9-30). Clinically, the height of a waveform is usually stated in millimeters not millivolts. When evaluating the ECG for the presence of chamber enlargement, it is particularly important to check the standardization marker to ensure it is 10-mm high.

Atrial Enlargement

The first half of the P wave is recorded when the electrical impulse that originated in the SA node stimulates the right atrium and reaches the AV node. The downslope of the P wave reflects stimulation of the left atrium. A normal P wave is smooth and rounded, no more than 2.5 mm in height, and no more than 0.11 sec in duration (width). Normal P waves are positive (upright) in leads I, II, aVF, and V_4 through V_6.

Right Atrium
Enlargement of the right atrium produces an abnormally tall initial part of the P wave. The P wave is tall (2.5 mm or more in height in leads II, III, and aVF), peaked, and of normal duration. This type of P wave is called *P pulmonale* because right atrial enlargement

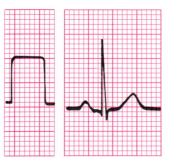

FIGURE **9-30**
When the ECG machine is properly calibrated, a 1-mV electrical signal will produce a deflection measuring exactly 10-mm tall.

The presence of right atrial enlargement (RAE) is suggested by the presence of tall, peaked P waves of normal duration on the ECG. RAE equals increased amplitude.

The presence of left atrial enlargement (LAE) is suggested by the presence of wide, notched P waves on the ECG. LAE equals increased time.

(RAE) is usually caused by conditions that increase the work of the right atrium, such as chronic obstructive pulmonary disease with or without pulmonary hypertension, congenital heart disease, or right ventricular failure of any cause (Figure 9-31). The P wave may be biphasic in lead V_1 with a more prominent positive portion.

Left Atrium

The latter part of the P wave is prominent in left atrial enlargement (LAE). This is because the impulse starts in the right atrium where the SA node is located and chamber size is normal. The electrical impulse then travels to the left to depolarize the left atrium. The waveform inscribed on the ECG is widened (latter part of the P wave) because it takes longer to depolarize an enlarged muscle. The P wave is more than 0.11 sec in duration and often notched in leads I, II, aVL, and V_4, V_5, and V_6 (Figure 9-32). The P wave may be biphasic in lead V_1 with a more prominent negative portion. LAE occurs because of conditions that increase left atrial pressure or volume overload or both. These conditions include mitral regurgitation, mitral stenosis, left ventricular failure, and systemic hypertension. Because of the frequent association of LAE with mitral valve disease, the wide, notched P wave that is usually seen is called *P mitrale*.

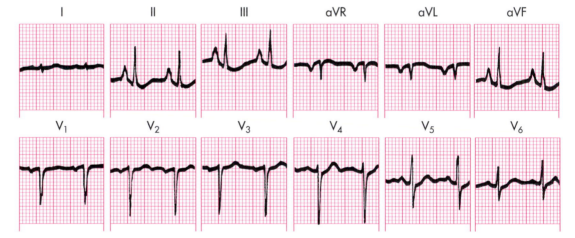

FIGURE 9-31 Right atrial enlargement. P pulmonale pattern in a 44-year-old woman with chronic obstructive pulmonary disease (COPD). Negative P waves are visible in the right precordial leads (V_1, V_2).

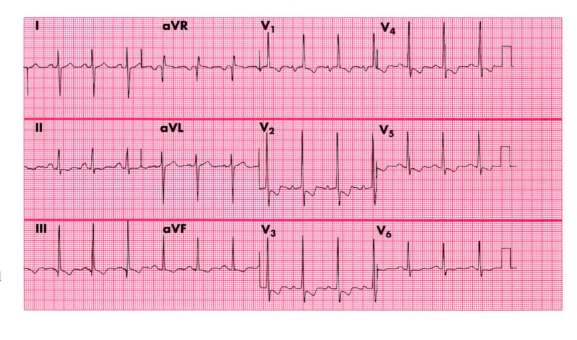

FIGURE 9-32 Left atrial enlargement. Note the wide, notched P waves in leads II, III, and aVF.

Ventricular Enlargement

Ventricular muscle thickens (hypertrophies) when it sustains a persistent pressure over-load. Dilatation occurs because of persistent volume overload. The two often go hand in hand. Hypertrophy increases the QRS amplitude and is often associated with ST-segment depression and asymmetric T-wave inversion. The ST-segment depression and T-wave inversion pattern is called *ventricular strain* or *secondary repolarization changes.*

The amplitude (voltage) of the QRS complex can be affected by various factors, including age, body weight, and lung disease. Increased QRS amplitude may occur normally in thin-chested individuals or young adults because the chest electrodes are closer to the heart in these patients.[7]

Right Ventricle

Because the right ventricle is normally considerably smaller than the left, it must become extremely enlarged before changes are visible on the ECG. Right axis deviation is one of the earliest and most reliable findings of right ventricular hypertrophy (RVH).[7] Further, normal R-wave progression is reversed in the precordial leads, revealing taller than normal R waves and small S waves in V_1 and V_2 and deeper than normal S waves and small R waves in V_5 and V_6. Ventricular activation time (VAT) is delayed in V_1. Causes of RVH include pulmonary hypertension and chronic lung diseases, valvular heart disease, and congenital heart disease (Figure 9-33).

Left Ventricle

Recognition of left ventricular hypertrophy (LVH) on the ECG is not always obvious, and many methods to assist in its recognition have been suggested. ECG signs of LVH include deeper than normal S waves and small R waves in V_1 and V_2 and taller than normal R waves and small S waves in V_5 and V_6. If S-wave amplitude in lead V_1 added to the R-wave amplitude in V_5 is greater than or equal to 35 mV, LVH should be suspected. Other ECG changes suggesting the presence of LVH include an R-wave amplitude in lead aVL greater than or equal to 12 mV. Evidence of delayed ventricular activation time may be visible in V_6, and secondary repolarization changes (strain pattern) are often seen in V_5 and V_6 (Figure 9-34). Causes of LVH include systemic hypertension, hypertrophic cardiomyopathy, aortic stenosis, and aortic insufficiency.

LVH may be accompanied by left axis deviation.

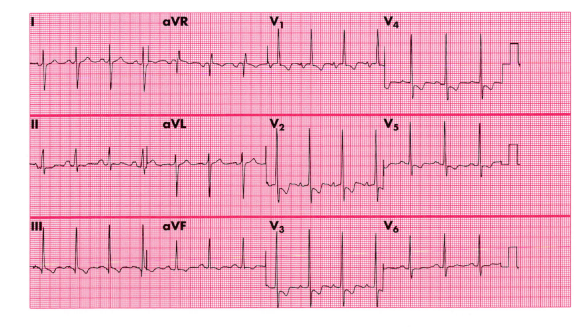

FIGURE **9-33**
Right ventricular hypertrophy. Right axis deviation and secondary repolarization changes are present.

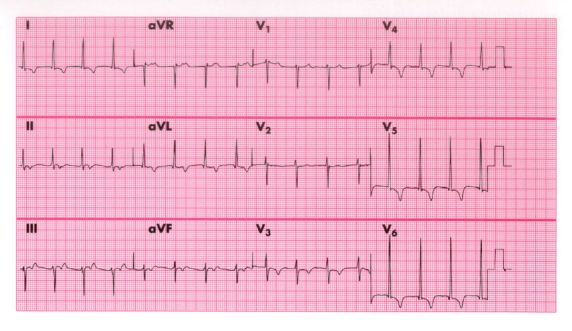

FIGURE 9-34
Left ventricular hypertrophy with first-degree AV block, ST-segment depression, and T-wave inversion.

ECG CHANGES ASSOCIATED WITH ELECTROLYTE DISTURBANCES

The primary ions involved in propagation of impulses from cell to cell in the myocardium are sodium, potassium, and calcium.

There are two types of action potentials in the heart: fast and slow. This classification is based on the rate of voltage change during depolarization of cardiac cells. Fast-response action potentials occur in the cells of the atria, ventricles, and Purkinje fibers. The fast-response action potential occurs because of the presence of many voltage-sensitive sodium channels that allow a rapid influx of sodium when these channels are open and prevent influx when they are closed. Myocardial fibers with a fast-response action potential can conduct impulses at relatively rapid rates.

Slow-response action potentials normally occur in cells such as the SA and AV nodes. These cells do not have fast sodium channels but have slow calcium and slow sodium channels that result in a slower rate of depolarization compared to the depolarization of cardiac cells with fast sodium channels. Slow-response action potentials can occur abnormally anywhere in the heart, usually secondary to ischemia, injury, or an electrolyte imbalance (Table 9-5).[12]

Sodium

Sodium: normal values: 135 to 145 mEq/L.

Causes of hypernatremia (sodium excess) include hypertonic parenteral fluid administration, significantly deficient water intake, excessive salt ingestion, high-protein liquid diets without adequate fluid intake, severe watery diarrhea, or severe insensible water losses (e.g., heat stroke, prolonged high fever). Hypernatremia does not cause any significant changes on the ECG.

Hyponatremia (sodium deficit) may occur because of prolonged diuretic therapy, excessive diaphoresis, and excessive loss of sodium from trauma (e.g., burns); adrenal insufficiency; severe gastrointestinal fluid losses from gastric suctioning or lavage; pro-

TABLE 9-5	ECG Changes Associated With Electrolyte Disturbances						
Medication	P wave	PR interval	QRS complex	ST segment	T wave	QT interval	Heart rate
Hypocalcemia				Long, flattened		Prolonged	
Hypercalcemia		Prolonged		Shortened		Shortened	
Hypokalemia			Widened as level decreases	Depressed	Flattened; U wave present	Prolonged	
Hyperkalemia	Disappear as level increases	Normal or prolonged	Widened as level increases	Disappears as level increases	Tall, peaked/ tented		Slows
Hypomagnesemia	Diminished voltage (amplitude)		Widened as level decreases; diminished voltage	Depressed	Flattened; U wave present	Prolonged	
Hypermagnesemia		Prolonged	Widened		Tall/elevated		

longed vomiting or diarrhea or laxative use; and an insufficient intake of sodium. Hyponatremia does not cause any significant changes on the ECG.

Calcium

Causes of hypercalcemia (calcium excess) include prolonged immobility, excessive vitamin D intake, thyrotoxicosis, metastatic carcinoma, excessive use of calcium-containing antacids, and an excessive intake of calcium supplements. ECG changes include a prolonged PR interval, prolonged QRS complex, and shortened QT interval (because of shortening of the ST segment).

Hypocalcemia (calcium deficit) may occur because of acute or chronic renal failure, vitamin D deficiency, hyperphosphatemia, hypomagnesemia, and inadequate exposure to ultraviolet light. ECG changes include a long, flattened ST segment and prolonged QT interval.

Calcium: normal values: 4.5 to 5.5 mEq/L or 9 to 11 mg/dL.

Magnesium

Causes of hypermagnesemia (magnesium excess) include renal failure, excessive use of parenteral magnesium, and excessive use of magnesium-containing antacids or laxatives. ECG changes include a prolonged PR interval, prolonged QRS complex, and elevated T wave.

Hypomagnesemia (magnesium deficit) may occur because of prolonged or excessive diuretic therapy, excessive calcium or vitamin D intake, administration of intravenous fluids or total parenteral nutrition without magnesium replacement, hypercalcemia, high-dose steroid use, cancer chemotherapy, and sepsis. ECG changes include diminished voltage of P waves and QRS complexes, flattened T waves, slightly widened QRS complexes, and prominent U waves.

Magnesium: normal values: 1.2 to 2.6 mEq/L.

Potassium

Hyperkalemia (potassium excess) may occur because of an excessive administration of potassium supplements, excessive use of salt substitutes, potassium-sparing diuretics (e.g., spironolactone), widespread cell damage (e.g., crush injuries, burns), metabolic or respiratory acidosis, and acute or chronic renal failure. ECG changes include tall, peaked (tented) T waves; widened QRS complexes, prolonged PR intervals, flattened ST segments, and flattened or absent P waves. Hyperkalemia may lead to ventricular dysrhythmias and asystole if not reversed.

FIGURE **9-35**
Serial ECG tracings in patient with marked changes in serum potassium (K+) level. In 11 AM tracing, depressed ST segment and low-amplitude T wave blending into a probable U wave (this cannot be seen with clarity because of superimposed P waves) indicate presence of hypokalemia. After administration of K+, 2 PM tracing becomes relatively normal. Continued K+ administration results in hyperkalemia with disappearance of atrial activity on the ECG and some prolongation of the QRS complex. By 6 PM, QRS complex is more prolonged, and by 9:45 PM, QRS complex is greatly prolonged. Secondary ST-T wave changes are present. Improvement follows administration of bicarbonate, glucose, and insulin at 10:45 PM with reduction in serum K+ level; improvement in ECG results.

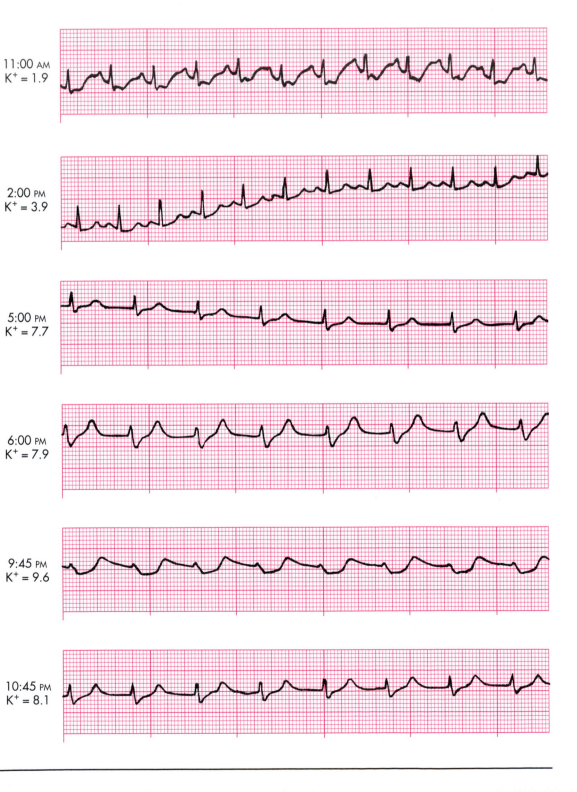

11:00 AM
K+ = 1.9

2:00 PM
K+ = 3.9

5:00 PM
K+ = 7.7

6:00 PM
K+ = 7.9

9:45 PM
K+ = 9.6

10:45 PM
K+ = 8.1

Hypokalemia (potassium deficit) may be the result of prolonged diuretic therapy with thiazide diuretics or furosemide, an inadequate dietary intake of potassium, administration of potassium-deficient parenteral fluids, severe gastrointestinal fluid losses from gastric suctioning or lavage, prolonged vomiting or diarrhea, or laxative use without replacement of potassium. ECG changes include a depressed ST segment, flattened T wave, and prominent U wave (Figure 9-35). Hypokalemia may increase the patient's sensitivity to digitalis toxicity.

A summary of antidysrhythmic medication classifications and the ECG changes associated with the medications can be found in Tables 9-6 and 9-7.

TABLE 9-6 CLASSIFICATION OF ANTIDYSRHYTHMIC MEDICATIONS

Classification	Action	Medication examples
Class I	Fast sodium channel blockers	
Ia	Moderately depress conduction; prolong repolarization time	Disopyramide, procainamide, quinidine
Ib	Modestly slow conduction; shorten repolarization time	Lidocaine, mexiletine, tocainide
Ic	Markedly depress conduction; little effect on repolarization time	Flecainide, propafenone
Class II	Beta-adrenergic blockers; repolarization time unchanged	Esmolol, metoprolol, atenolol
Class III	Potassium channel blockers; markedly prolong repolarization time	Amiodarone, ibutilide, sotalol, bretylium
Class IV		
IVa	AV node calcium channel blocker; repolarization time unchanged	Verapamil, diltiazem
IVb	Calcium channel openers; repolarization time unchanged	ATP, adenosine

TABLE 9-7   ECG Changes Associated With Medications

Medication	Classification	Indications	ECG characteristics				
			Heart rate	PR interval	QRS duration	QT interval	Comments
Adenosine (Adenocard)	Endogenous nucleoside; Class IVb antidysrhythmic	PSVT involving the AV node	Slows	Prolongs			May result in brief period of bradycardia or asystole after IV bolus administration
Amiodarone (Cordarone)	Class III antidysrhythmic	VT, VF, polymorphic VT, SVT, atrial fibrillation, atrial flutter	Slows	Prolongs	May prolong	Prolongs	May cause AV block, hypotension, bradycardia
Atenolol (Tenormin)	Class II antidysrhythmic (beta-blocker)	SVT, angina, hypertension	Slows	Prolongs			Possible AV block
Atropine sulfate	Parasympatholytic	Symptomatic bradycardia, asystole	Increases	Shortens			May result in tachycardia with higher doses
Digoxin (Lanoxin)	Cardiac glycoside	PSVT, uncontrolled atrial fibrillation or flutter, CHF	Slows	Prolongs		Shortens	Downward sloping of ST segment ("dig dip"); T wave inversion or flattening
Diltiazem (Cardizem)	Class IVa antidysrhythmic (calcium channel blocker)	PSVT, uncontrolled atrial fibrillation or flutter, angina	Slows	Prolongs			Possible AV block
Disopyramide (Norpace)	Class Ia antidysrhythmic	Ventricular dysrhythmias, atrial fibrillation or flutter with WPW	Variable	Prolongs	Prolongs	Prolongs	May precipitate torsades de pointes, possible AV block
Epinephrine (Adrenaline)	Sympathomimetic, natural catecholamine	VT, VF, pulseless electrical activity (PEA), asystole (IV bolus); symptomatic bradycardia (IV infusion)	Increases	Decreases			May result in tachycardia
Esmolol (Brevibloc)	Class II antidysrhythmic (beta-blocker)	SVT, angina, hypertension	Slows	Prolongs		May shorten	Possible AV block
Flecainide (Tambocor)	Class Ic antidysrhythmic	Ventricular and supraventricular dysrhythmias	May slow	Prolongs	Prolongs	Prolongs	Possible SA block, AV block, BBB

Drug	Classification	Uses	Heart Rate	PR	QRS	QT	ECG Changes
Ibutilide (Corvert)	Class III antidysrhythmic	For rapid conversion of recent-onset atrial fibrillation or atrial flutter to sinus rhythm	Slows	Prolongs		Prolongs	Can induce or worsen ventricular dysrhythmias, including torsades de pointes
Lidocaine (Xylocaine)	Class Ib antidysrhythmic	VF, VT			May prolong		Possible AV block
Magnesium sulfate	Electrolyte	Torsades de pointes	May increase			May shorten	
Metoprolol (Lopressor)	Class II antidysrhythmic (beta-blocker)	SVT, angina, hypertension	Slows	Prolongs			Possible AV block
Norepinephrine (Levophed)	Sympathomimetic	Significant hypotension not caused by hypovolemia	Increases	Shortens			Increases ventricular irritability
Procainamide (Pronestyl)	Class Ia antidysrhythmic	Ventricular and supraventricular tachydysrhythmias	Variable	Prolongs	Prolongs	Prolongs	May precipitate torsades de pointes, possible AV block
Propafenone (Rythmol)	Class Ic antidysrhythmic	Prevention of recurrence of chronic or paroxysmal atrial fibrillation; WPW (stable patient), life-threatening ventricular rhythms	Slows or no change	Prolongs	Prolongs	Usually not affected	
Propranolol (Inderal)	Class II antidysrhythmic (beta-blocker)	Angina, hypertension, supraventricular and ventricular dysrhythmias	Slows	Prolongs		May shorten	May worsen existing AV block
Quinidine (Duraquin, Quinaglute)	Class Ia antidysrhythmic	Supraventricular and ventricular dysrhythmias	Variable	Prolongs	Prolongs	Prolongs	May precipitate torsades de pointes, BBB sign of toxicity; wide, notched P waves
Sotalol (Betapace)	Class III antidysrhythmic	Supraventricular and serious ventricular dysrhythmias	Slows	Prolongs		Prolongs	Possible AV block
Verapamil (Isoptin, Calan)	Class IVa antidysrhythmic (calcium channel blocker)	PSVT, MAT, angina	Slows	Prolongs			Possible SA and AV block

ANALYZING THE 12-LEAD ECG

When analyzing a 12-lead ECG, it is important to use a systematic method. Findings suggestive of an acute MI are considered significant if viewed in two or more leads looking at the same area of the heart. If these findings are viewed in leads that look directly at the affected area, they are called *indicative changes.* If findings are observed in leads opposite the affected area, they are called *reciprocal changes.*

- Rate: atrial and ventricular
- Rhythm: atrial and ventricular
- Intervals: PR interval, QRS duration, QT interval
- Waveforms: P waves, Q waves, R waves (R-wave progression), T waves, U waves
- ST segment: elevation, depression
- Axis
- Hypertrophy/chamber enlargement
- Myocardial ischemia, injury, infarction
- Effects of medications and electrolyte imbalances

For additional information and review of practice strips regarding the 12-lead ECG, the following texts are recommended:

- Phalen: T: *The 12-lead ECG in acute myocardial infarction,* St Louis, 1996, Mosby.
- Purdie RB, Earnest SL: *Pure practice for 12-lead ECGs: a practice workbook,* St Louis, 1997, Mosby.

REFERENCES

1. Huszar RJ: *Basic dysrhythmias: interpretation and management,* ed 2, St Louis, 1994, Mosby.
2. Anderson KN, Anderson LE, Glanze WD, editors: *Mosby's medical, nursing, and allied health dictionary,* ed 4, St Louis, 1994, Mosby.
3. Kahn MG: *Rapid ECG interpretation,* Philadelphia, 1997, WB Saunders.
4. Murphy JG: *Mayo clinical cardiology review,* ed 2, Philadelphia, 2000, Lippincott, Williams & Wilkins.
5. Chou T, Knilans TK: *Electrocardiography in clinical practice: adult and pediatric,* Philadelphia, 1996, WB Saunders.
6. Kinney MR, editor: *Andreoli's comprehensive cardiac care,* ed 8, St Louis, 1996, Mosby.
7. Johnson R, Swartz MH: *A simplified approach to electrocardiography,* Philadelphia, 1986, WB Saunders.
8. Thelan LA, Davie JK, Urden LD, Lough ME: *Critical care nursing: diagnosis and management,* ed 2, St Louis, 1994, Mosby.
9. Bar FW, Volders PG, Hoppener P, et al: Development of ST-segment elevation and Q- and R-wave changes in acute myocardial infarction and the influence of thrombolytic therapy, *Am J Cardiol* 77:337-343, 1996.
10. Phalen T: *The 12-lead ECG in acute myocardial infarction,* St Louis, 1996, Mosby.
11. Conover MB: *Understanding electrocardiography,* ed 7, St Louis, 1996, Mosby.
12. Marriott HJL, Conover MB: *Advanced concepts in arrhythmias,* ed 3, St Louis, 1998, Mosby.
13. Wagner GS: *Marriott's practical electrocardiography,* ed 9, Baltimore, 1994, Williams & Wilkins.

BIBLIOGRAPHY

Chou T, Knilans TK: *Electrocardiography in clinical practice: adult and pediatric,* Philadelphia, 1996, WB Saunders.
Clochesy JM, Breu C, Cardin S, et al: *Critical care nursing,* ed 2, Philadelphia, 1996, WB Saunders.
Conover MB: *Understanding electrocardiography,* ed 7, St Louis, 1996, Mosby.
Crawford MV, Spence MI: *Common sense approach to coronary care,* ed 6, St Louis, 1995, Mosby.

Gibler WB: *Emergency cardiac care,* St Louis, 1994, Mosby.

Goldberger AL: *Clinical electrocardiography: a simplified approach,* ed 6, St Louis, 1999, Mosby.

Goldman L, Braunwald E: *Primary cardiology,* Philadelphia, 1998, WB Saunders.

Huszar RJ: *Basic dysrhythmias: interpretation and management,* ed 2, St Louis, 1994, Mosby.

Johnson R, Swartz MH: *A simplified approach to electrocardiography,* Philadelphia, 1986, WB Saunders.

Kahn MG: *Rapid ECG interpretation,* Philadelphia, 1997, WB Saunders.

Kinney MR, Packa DR, editors: *Andreoli's comprehensive cardiac care,* ed 8, St Louis, 1996, Mosby.

Marriott HJL, Conover MB: *Advanced concepts in arrhythmias,* ed 3, St Louis, 1998, Mosby.

Murphy JG: *Mayo clinical cardiology review,* ed 2, Philadelphia, 2000, Lippincott, Williams & Wilkins.

Padrid PJ, Kowey PR, editors: *Cardiac arrhythmia: mechanisms, diagnosis, and management,* Baltimore, 1995, Williams & Wilkins.

Paradis NA, Halperin HR, Nowak RM, editors: *Cardiac arrest: the science and practice of resuscitation medicine,* Baltimore, 1996, Williams & Wilkins.

Phalen T: *The 12-Lead ECG in acute myocardial infarction,* St Louis, 1996, Mosby.

Thelan LA, Davie JK, Urden LD, Lough ME: *Critical care nursing: diagnosis and management,* ed 2, St Louis, 1994, Mosby.

Weil MH, Tang W: *CPR: Resuscitation of the arrested heart,* Philadelphia, 1999, WB Saunders.

Woods SL, Sivarajan Froelicher ES, Motzer SA: *Cardiac nursing,* ed 4, Philadelphia, 2000, Lippincott, Williams & Wilkins.

S T O P & R E V I EW

MATCHING

___ 1. Leads that view the inferior wall of the heart

___ 2. Occlusion of the right coronary artery may result in a(n) ___ myocardial infarction

___ 3. Indicator of the magnitude and direction of current flow

___ 4. Lead I is perpendicular to lead ___

___ 5. Lead I + lead III = ___

___ 6. Lead located at the fourth intercostal space, right sternal border

___ 7. Common ECG finding in hyperkalemia

___ 8. Leads that view the heart in the frontal plane

___ 9. The zone of ___ is typically characterized by ST-segment elevation

___ 10. Leads used to view the right ventricle

___ 11. Lead located at the fifth intercostal space, left midclavicular line

___ 12. Leads that view the septum

___ 13. Lead III is perpendicular to lead ___

___ 14. Leads that view the heart in the horizontal plane

___ 15. Occlusion of the left anterior descending coronary artery may result in a(n) ___ myocardial infarction

___ 16. Leads that view the lateral wall of the heart

___ 17. Direction of the mean QRS vector

___ 18. The zone of ___ is typically characterized by Q waves

___ 19. Lead located at the fourth intercostal space, left sternal border

___ 20. Lead II is perpendicular to lead ___

A. aVL
B. V_1
C. V_1, V_2
D. II, III, aVF
E. Anterior
F. Precordial
G. aVR
H. V_2
I. I, aVL, V_5, V_6
J. Electrical axis
K. Infarction
L. Limb
M. Inferior
N. Vector
O. V_1R-V_6R
P. Tall, tented T waves
Q. V_4
R. Lead II
S. Injury
T. aVF

IDENTIFICATION AND MEASUREMENTS—PRACTICE RHYTHM STRIPS

The 12-lead ECG below is from a 48-year-old female complaining of substernal chest pain radiating to her back. Her symptoms began while driving to work. She has a history of hypertension and asthma. She takes a blood pressure medication but cannot recall the name. BP 132/84, RR 16.

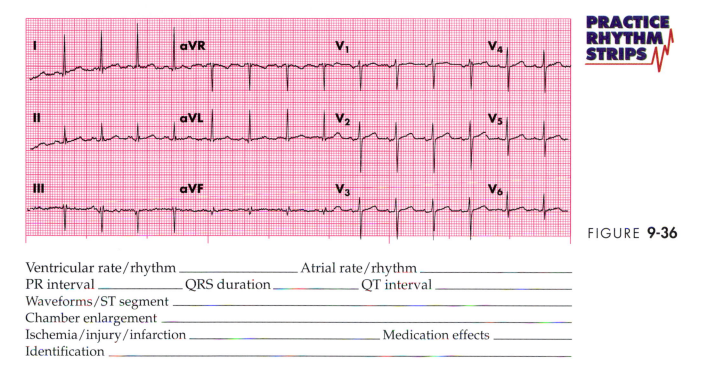

PRACTICE RHYTHM STRIPS

FIGURE **9-36**

Ventricular rate/rhythm _____ Atrial rate/rhythm _____
PR interval _____ QRS duration _____ QT interval _____
Waveforms/ST segment _____
Chamber enlargement _____
Ischemia/injury/infarction _____ Medication effects _____
Identification _____

The 12-lead ECG below is from an 83-year-old female complaining of substernal chest pain that has been present for the past 6 hours. She had a myocardial infarction 5 years ago and has a history of emphysema. The patient is on home oxygen. She has taken one nitroglycerin tablet with no relief of pain. BP 162/108. RR 18.

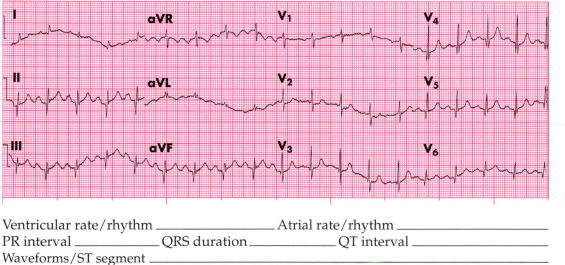

FIGURE **9-37**

Ventricular rate/rhythm _____ Atrial rate/rhythm _____
PR interval _____ QRS duration _____ QT interval _____
Waveforms/ST segment _____
Chamber enlargement _____
Ischemia/injury/infarction _____ Medication effects _____
Identification _____

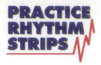

The 12-lead ECG below is from a 72-year-old male complaining of chest pain. BP 138/72, RR 28. The patient has a history of angina, two prior myocardial infarctions, coronary artery bypass surgery 3 years ago, abdominal aortic aneurysm repair 5 years ago, atrial fibrillation, and emphysema. Medications include aspirin, lorazepam, nitroglycerin, and dexamethasone.

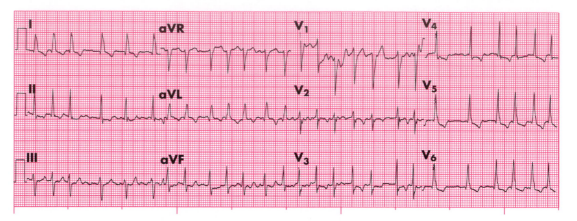

FIGURE **9-38**

Ventricular rate/rhythm _____ Atrial rate/rhythm _____
PR interval _____ QRS duration _____ QT interval _____
Waveforms/ST segment _____
Chamber enlargement _____
Ischemia/injury/infarction _____ Medication effects _____
Identification _____

The 12-lead ECG below is from a 58-year-old male complaining of a headache, nausea, and a burning sensation in his chest. He states the pain radiates to his jaw and tongue. BP 140/90, RR 16. Skin warm and dry.

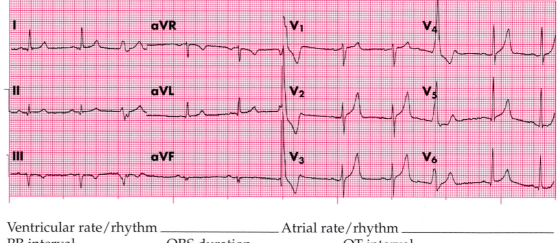

FIGURE **9-39**

Ventricular rate/rhythm _____ Atrial rate/rhythm _____
PR interval _____ QRS duration _____ QT interval _____
Waveforms/ST segment _____
Chamber enlargement _____
Ischemia/injury/infarction _____ Medication effects _____
Identification _____

CHAPTER 10

Post-Test

MULTIPLE CHOICE AND TRUE/FALSE

1. The basic contractile unit of a myofibril is the:
   a. Sinoatrial (SA) node
   b. Sarcomere
   c. Intercalated disk
   d. Action potential
2. *True or False.* The augmented leads are the only unipolar leads in the standard 12-lead ECG.
3. The QRS complex represents:
   a. Atrial contraction
   b. Atrial depolarization
   c. Ventricular depolarization
   d. Ventricular repolarization
4. The primary pacemaker of the heart is the:
   a. Bundle of His
   b. Purkinje fibers
   c. Sinoatrial (SA) node
   d. Atrioventricular (AV) node
5. Automaticity refers to the ability of cardiac cells to:
   a. Reach threshold and respond to a stimulus
   b. Spontaneously initiate an electrical impulse without being stimulated from another source
   c. Receive an electrical stimulus and conduct that impulse to an adjacent cardiac cell
   d. Shorten, causing contraction of cardiac muscle in response to an electrical stimulus
6. Atrial repolarization is obscured by the _____ on the ECG.
7. *True or False.* The electrocardiogram (ECG) represents mechanical activity of the heart.
8. Each small box on ECG paper represents _____ second.

9. Which of the following reflects the correct electrode position for lead V$_4$?
   a. Left midclavicular line, fifth intercostal space
   b. Left side of sternum, fourth intercostal space
   c. Left anterior axillary line, fifth intercostal space
   d. Left midaxillary line, fourth intercostal space

10. The _____ is used as the baseline from which to evaluate the degree of displacement (elevation or depression) of the ST segment from the isoelectric line.

11. In the majority of the population, the SA and AV nodes are supplied by the _____ coronary artery.

12. The external layer of the heart wall is the:
   a. Epicardium
   b. Myocardium
   c. Endocardium
   d. Fibrous pericardium

13. Which of the following are atrioventricular (AV) valves?
   a. Aortic and tricuspid
   b. Tricuspid and mitral
   c. Mitral and pulmonary
   d. Pulmonary and aortic

14. The right atrium receives deoxygenated blood from three vessels. Can you name them? _____ , _____ and, the _____

15. The anterior surface of the heart consists primarily of the:
   a. Left atrium
   b. Right atrium
   c. Left ventricle
   d. Right ventricle

16. Cardiac output may be defined as:
   a. The amount of blood flowing into the right atrium each minute from the systemic circulation.
   b. The amount of blood ejected by either ventricle during one contraction.
   c. The force exerted by the blood on the walls of the ventricles at the end of diastole.
   d. The amount of blood pumped into the aorta each minute by the heart.

17. The heart is enclosed in a fibrous sac called the:
   a. Endocardium
   b. Myocardium
   c. Pericardium
   d. Subendocardium

18. The left atrium receives blood from the:
   a. Aorta
   b. Pulmonary veins
   c. Pulmonary arteries
   d. Inferior vena cava

19. Thin strands of fibrous connective tissue extend from the AV valves to the papillary muscles and prevent the AV valves from bulging back into the atria during ventricular systole. These strands are called:
   a. Cardiac cilia
   b. Chordae tendineae
   c. Purkinje fibers
   d. Medullary fibers

20. The coronary arteries originate:
    a. At the base of the pulmonary artery, immediately above the leaflets of the pulmonic valve.
    b. At the base of the aorta, immediately above the leaflets of the aortic valve.
    c. At the base of the superior vena cava, immediately above the sinoatrial node.
    d. At the base of the pulmonary artery, immediately above the leaflets of the tricuspid valve.
21. *True or False.* The right atrium and ventricle make up a high-pressure pump whose purpose is to pump blood to the systemic circulation.
22. The primary neurotransmitter of the sympathetic division of the autonomic nervous system is:
    a. Norepinephrine
    b. Dopamine
    c. Acetylcholine
    d. Monoamine oxidase
23. Sympathetic stimulation of the heart typically results in:
    a. Slowing of the rate of discharge of the SA node.
    b. An increase in the force of myocardial contraction.
    c. A decrease in the rate of conduction through the AV node.
    d. A decrease in myocardial oxygen demand.
24. The two primary branches of the left coronary artery are the:
    a. Circumflex and anterior descending
    b. Marginal and posterior descending
    c. Marginal and circumflex
    d. Anterior and posterior descending
25. Beginning with the right atrium, trace the normal pathway of blood flow through the heart and pulmonary circulation.

_1_ Right atrium	___ Left ventricle
___ Mitral valve	___ Pulmonary arteries
___ Aorta	___ Tricuspid valve
___ Right ventricle	___ Pulmonary veins
___ Pulmonic valve	___ Aortic valve
___ Left atrium	___ Systemic circulation

26. Which of the following medications may decrease myocardial contractility?
    a. Propranolol
    b. Digitalis
    c. Calcium chloride
    d. Epinephrine
27. *True or False.* If the systolic blood pressure decreases, the body's normal compensatory response to increase blood pressure is peripheral vasodilation, decreased heart rate, and decreased myocardial contractility.
28. Stroke volume is influenced by:
    a. Contractility, heart rate, afterload
    b. Blood pressure, afterload, heart rate
    c. Preload, blood pressure, contractility
    d. Preload, afterload, contractility
29. *True or False.* Stimulation of alpha-receptor sites results in constriction of blood vessels in the skin, cerebral, and splanchnic circulation.
30. *True or False.* A response by the sympathetic division of the autonomic nervous system is also called a *cholinergic response.*
31. The S wave is the:
    a. First negative deflection after the R wave
    b. First negative deflection before the R wave
    c. First positive waveform of the cardiac cycle
    d. Second positive waveform of the cardiac cycle

32. Ventricular rate and rhythm are determined by measuring from:
    a. P wave to P wave
    b. P wave to R wave
    c. R wave to R wave
    d. Q wave to T wave

33. A segment:
    a. Is a line between waveforms
    b. Is a waveform and a segment
    c. Consists of several waveforms
    d. Is movement away from the baseline in either a positive or negative direction

34. A delta wave is an ECG characteristic associated with which of the following dysrhythmias?
    a. Sinus arrest
    b. Sinus dysrhythmia
    c. Junctional escape rhythm
    d. Wolff-Parkinson-White (WPW) syndrome

35. An accelerated junctional rhythm is characterized by a regular ventricular response occurring at a rate of:
    a. 20 to 40 beats/min
    b. 40 to 60 beats/min
    c. 60 to 100 beats/min
    d. 100 to 180 beats/min

36. Atrial fibrillation is characterized by:
    a. An erratic, wavy baseline and irregular ventricular rhythm
    b. "Saw-tooth" or "picket-fence" waves preceding each QRS
    c. P waves occurring before, during, or after the QRS complex; when seen they are inverted
    d. One P wave before each QRS and a regular ventricular rate of 60 to 100 beats/min

37. Torsades de pointes is a type of polymorphic VT associated with:
    a. A long QT interval
    b. Complete AV block
    c. ST segment elevation
    d. A prolonged PR interval

38. The first letter of the pacemaker identification code represents:
    a. The chamber paced
    b. The chamber sensed
    c. The mode of response
    d. Programmable functions

39. In second-degree AV block with 2:1 conduction, the PR interval:
    a. Shortens
    b. Lengthens
    c. Remains constant
    d. Is completely variable

40. *True or False.* The QRS complex associated with a complete AV block is always wide.

41. An interpolated PVC is described as a:
    a. Series of PVCs that look different from one another
    b. Ventricular complex that occurs after the next expected sinus beat
    c. Type of PVC in which the R wave of the PVC falls on the T wave of the preceding beat
    d. PVC that is "squeezed" between two regular complexes and does not disturb the underlying rhythm

42. *True or False.* Failure to pace is the inability of the pacemaker stimulus to depolarize the myocardium and is recognized on the ECG by pacemaker spikes not followed by P waves (if the electrode is located in the atrium) or by QRS complexes (if the electrode is located in the right ventricle).

43. In second-degree and complete AV block:
    a. P waves occur regularly
    b. Every other P wave is dropped
    c. P waves are periodically dropped
    d. There are more QRS complexes than P waves

44. Explain the difference between a PVC and a ventricular escape beat:

    _____
    _____
    _____
    _____
    _____

45. An 83-year-old male is complaining of weakness and fatigue. The cardiac monitor (lead II) reveals a regular rhythm at a rate of 180 beats/min with absent P waves. The QRS measures 0.16 sec. This rhythm is most likely:
    a. Ventricular tachycardia
    b. An idioventricular rhythm
    c. Supraventricular tachycardia
    d. An accelerated junctional rhythm

TEST RHYTHM STRIPS

For each of the following rhythm strips, determine the atrial and ventricular rates, measure the PR interval, QRS duration, and QT interval, and then identify the rhythm. All strips lead II unless otherwise noted.

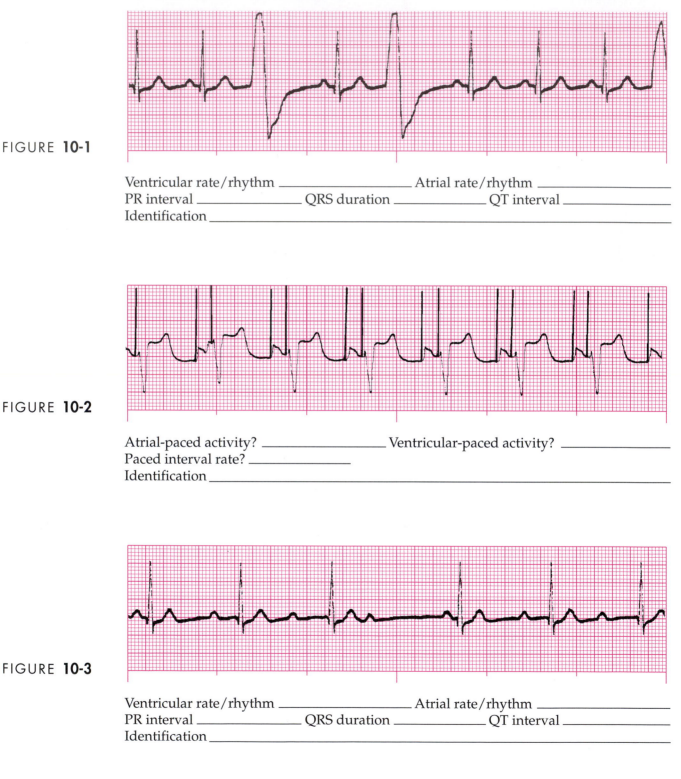

FIGURE **10-1**

Ventricular rate/rhythm _____ Atrial rate/rhythm _____
PR interval _____ QRS duration _____ QT interval _____
Identification _____

FIGURE **10-2**

Atrial-paced activity? _____ Ventricular-paced activity? _____
Paced interval rate? _____
Identification _____

FIGURE **10-3**

Ventricular rate/rhythm _____ Atrial rate/rhythm _____
PR interval _____ QRS duration _____ QT interval _____
Identification _____

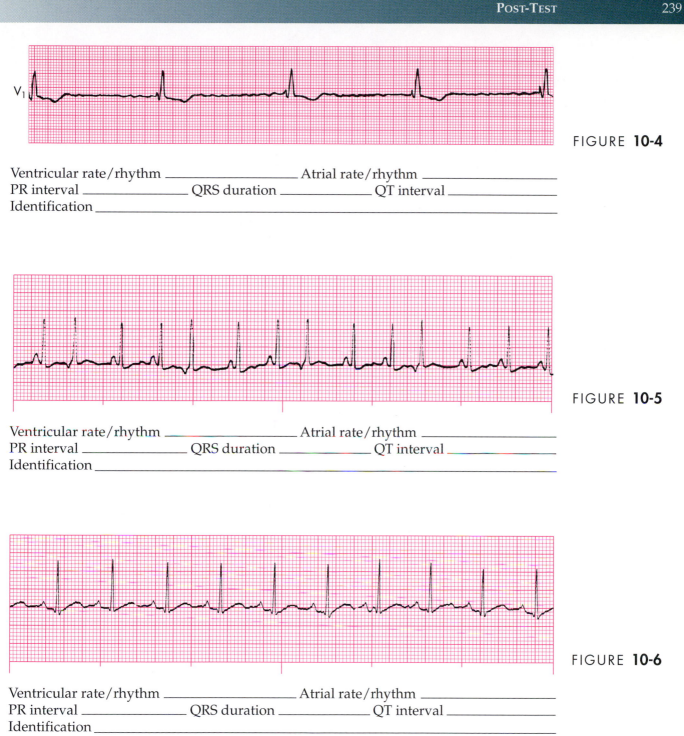

FIGURE **10-4**

Ventricular rate/rhythm _____ Atrial rate/rhythm _____
PR interval _____ QRS duration _____ QT interval _____
Identification _____

FIGURE **10-5**

Ventricular rate/rhythm _____ Atrial rate/rhythm _____
PR interval _____ QRS duration _____ QT interval _____
Identification _____

FIGURE **10-6**

Ventricular rate/rhythm _____ Atrial rate/rhythm _____
PR interval _____ QRS duration _____ QT interval _____
Identification _____

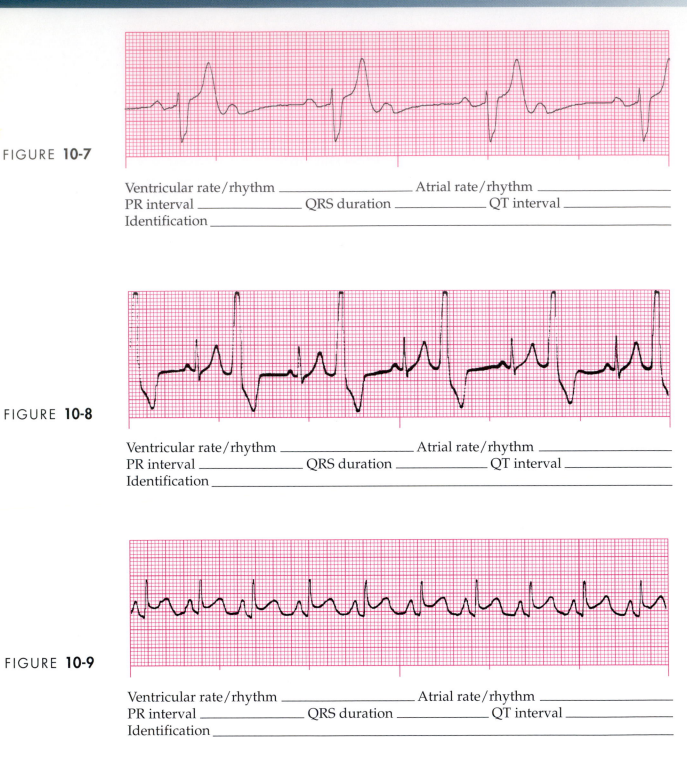

FIGURE **10-7**

Ventricular rate/rhythm _____ Atrial rate/rhythm _____
PR interval _____ QRS duration _____ QT interval _____
Identification _____

FIGURE **10-8**

Ventricular rate/rhythm _____ Atrial rate/rhythm _____
PR interval _____ QRS duration _____ QT interval _____
Identification _____

FIGURE **10-9**

Ventricular rate/rhythm _____ Atrial rate/rhythm _____
PR interval _____ QRS duration _____ QT interval _____
Identification _____

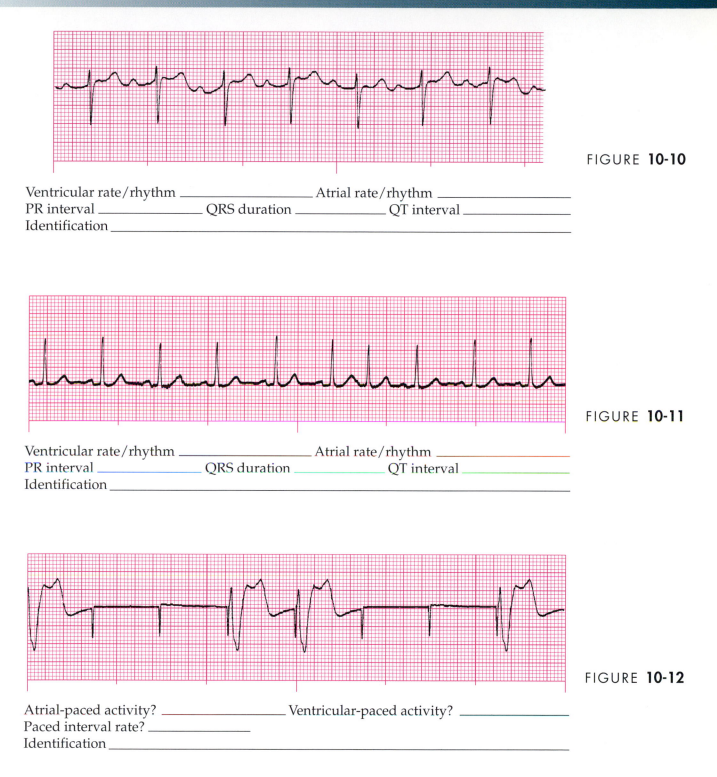

FIGURE **10-10**

Ventricular rate/rhythm _____ Atrial rate/rhythm _____
PR interval _____ QRS duration _____ QT interval _____
Identification _____

FIGURE **10-11**

Ventricular rate/rhythm _____ Atrial rate/rhythm _____
PR interval _____ QRS duration _____ QT interval _____
Identification _____

FIGURE **10-12**

Atrial-paced activity? _____ Ventricular-paced activity? _____
Paced interval rate? _____
Identification _____

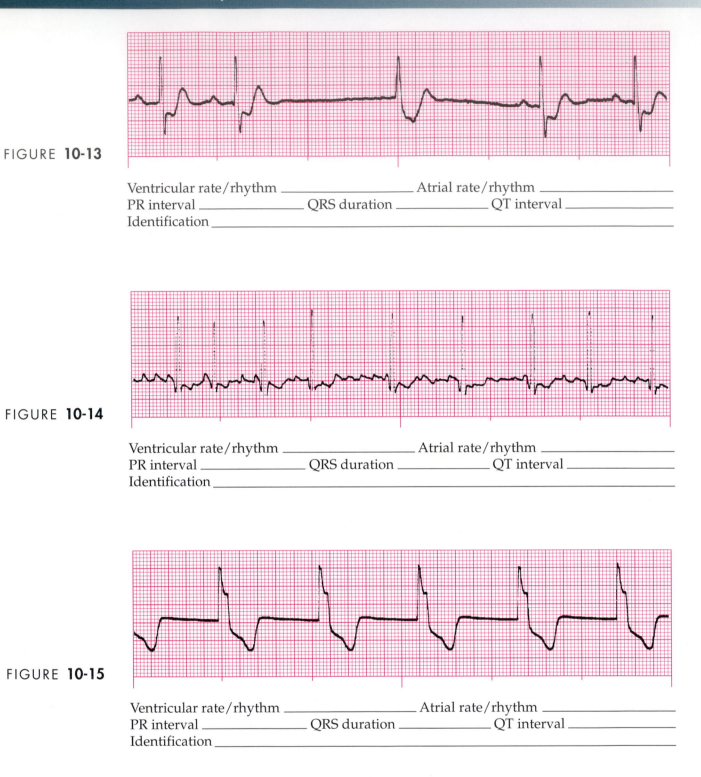

FIGURE **10-13**

FIGURE **10-14**

FIGURE **10-15**

Ventricular rate/rhythm _____ Atrial rate/rhythm _____
PR interval _____ QRS duration _____ QT interval _____
Identification _____

Ventricular rate/rhythm _____ Atrial rate/rhythm _____
PR interval _____ QRS duration _____ QT interval _____
Identification _____

Ventricular rate/rhythm _____ Atrial rate/rhythm _____
PR interval _____ QRS duration _____ QT interval _____
Identification _____

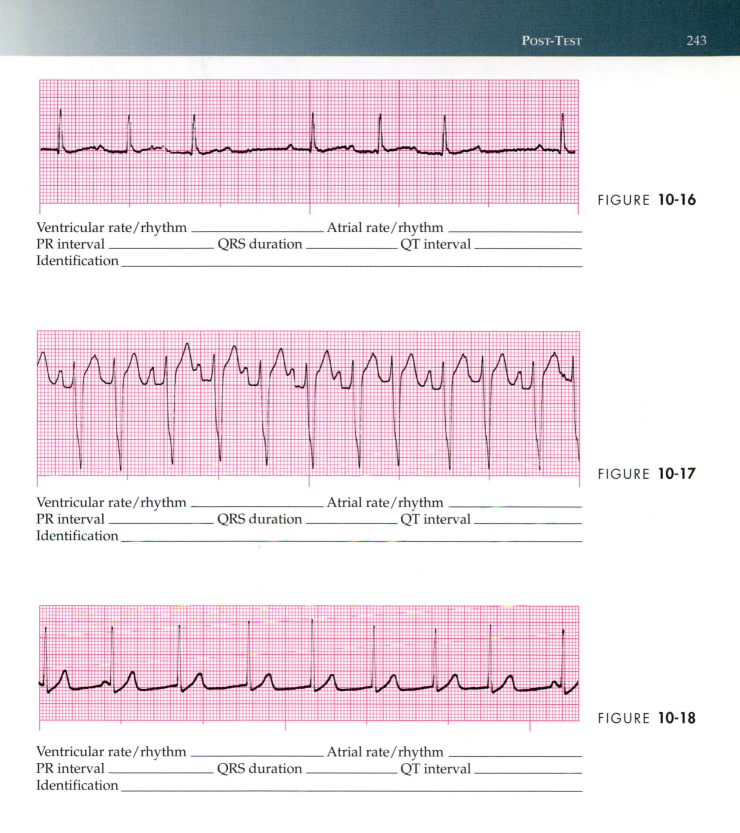

FIGURE **10-16**

Ventricular rate/rhythm _____ Atrial rate/rhythm _____
PR interval _____ QRS duration _____ QT interval _____
Identification _____

FIGURE **10-17**

Ventricular rate/rhythm _____ Atrial rate/rhythm _____
PR interval _____ QRS duration _____ QT interval _____
Identification _____

FIGURE **10-18**

Ventricular rate/rhythm _____ Atrial rate/rhythm _____
PR interval _____ QRS duration _____ QT interval _____
Identification _____

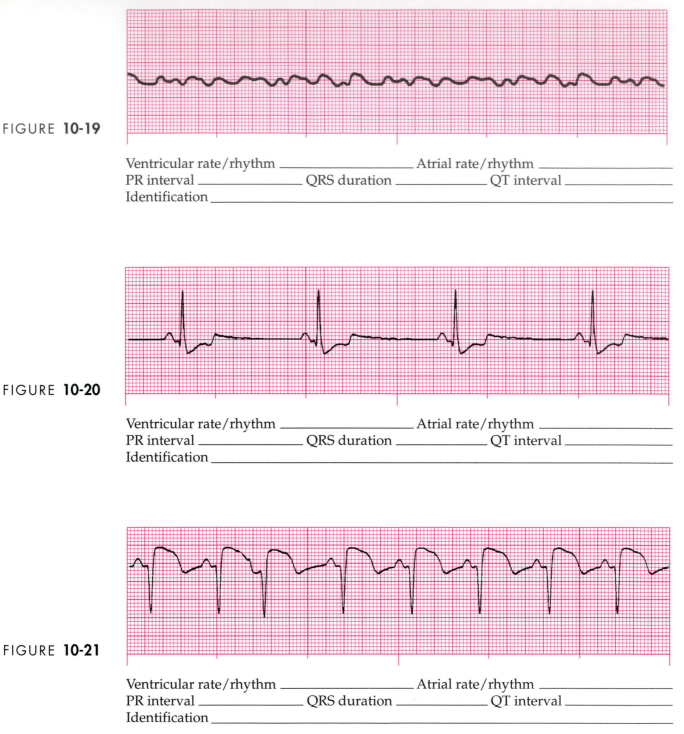

FIGURE **10-19**

Ventricular rate/rhythm _____ Atrial rate/rhythm _____
PR interval _____ QRS duration _____ QT interval _____
Identification _____

FIGURE **10-20**

Ventricular rate/rhythm _____ Atrial rate/rhythm _____
PR interval _____ QRS duration _____ QT interval _____
Identification _____

FIGURE **10-21**

Ventricular rate/rhythm _____ Atrial rate/rhythm _____
PR interval _____ QRS duration _____ QT interval _____
Identification _____

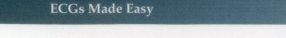

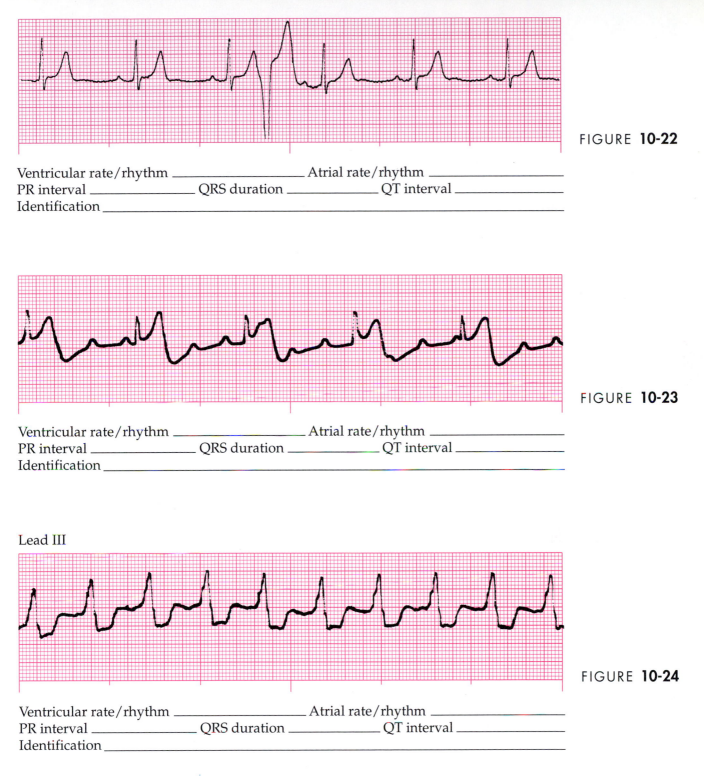

FIGURE **10-22**

Ventricular rate/rhythm _____ Atrial rate/rhythm _____
PR interval _____ QRS duration _____ QT interval _____
Identification _____

FIGURE **10-23**

Ventricular rate/rhythm _____ Atrial rate/rhythm _____
PR interval _____ QRS duration _____ QT interval _____
Identification _____

Lead III

FIGURE **10-24**

Ventricular rate/rhythm _____ Atrial rate/rhythm _____
PR interval _____ QRS duration _____ QT interval _____
Identification _____

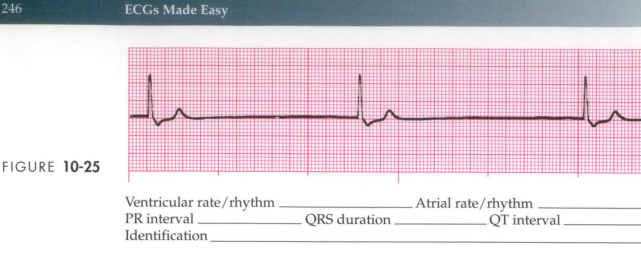

FIGURE **10-25**

Ventricular rate/rhythm _____ Atrial rate/rhythm _____
PR interval _____ QRS duration _____ QT interval _____
Identification _____

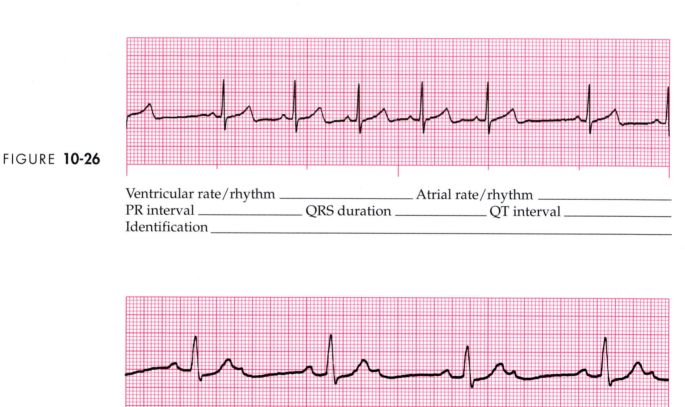

FIGURE **10-26**

Ventricular rate/rhythm _____ Atrial rate/rhythm _____
PR interval _____ QRS duration _____ QT interval _____
Identification _____

FIGURE **10-27**

Ventricular rate/rhythm _____ Atrial rate/rhythm _____
PR interval _____ QRS duration _____ QT interval _____
Identification _____

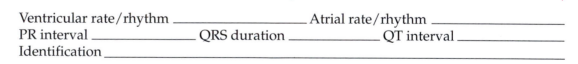

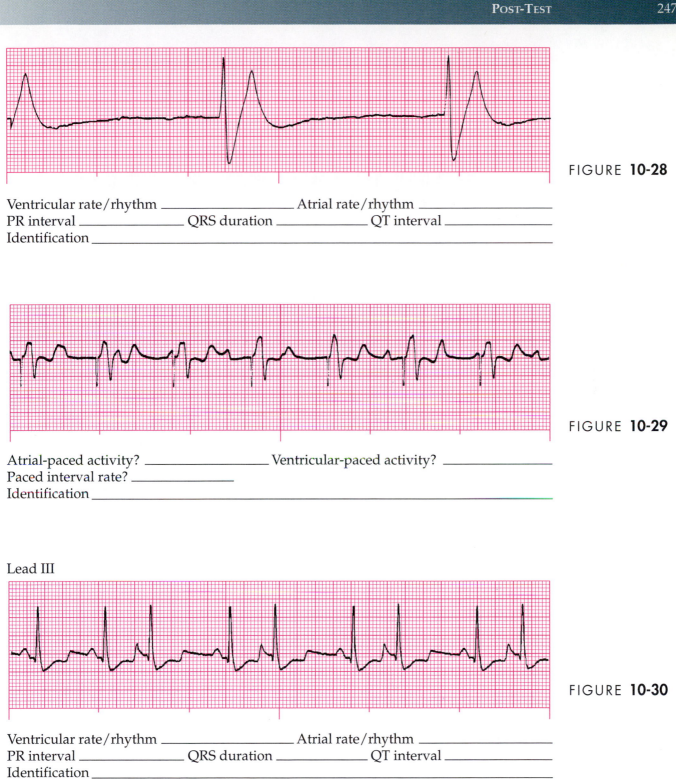

FIGURE **10-28**

Ventricular rate/rhythm _____ Atrial rate/rhythm _____
PR interval _____ QRS duration _____ QT interval _____
Identification _____

FIGURE **10-29**

Atrial-paced activity? _____ Ventricular-paced activity? _____
Paced interval rate? _____
Identification _____

Lead III

FIGURE **10-30**

Ventricular rate/rhythm _____ Atrial rate/rhythm _____
PR interval _____ QRS duration _____ QT interval _____
Identification _____

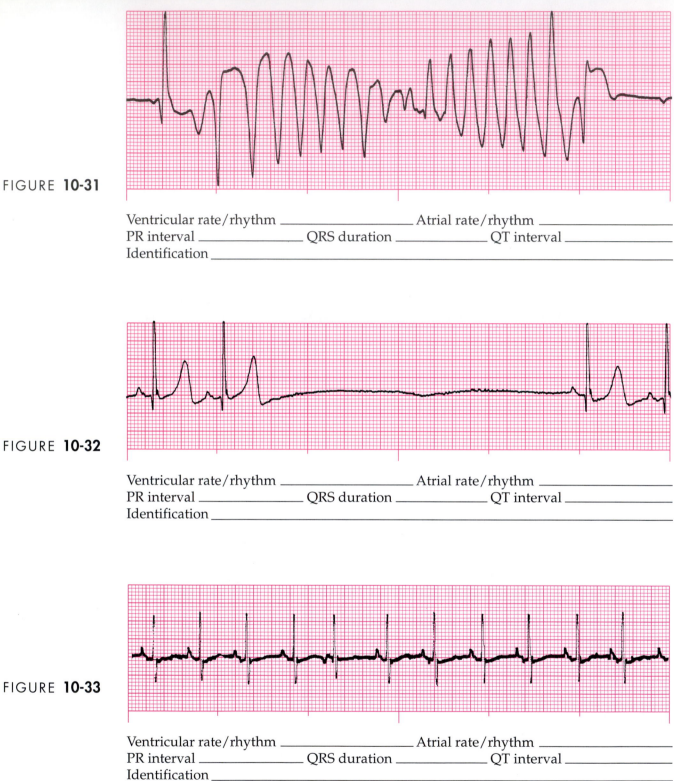

FIGURE 10-31

Ventricular rate/rhythm _____ Atrial rate/rhythm _____
PR interval _____ QRS duration _____ QT interval _____
Identification _____

FIGURE 10-32

Ventricular rate/rhythm _____ Atrial rate/rhythm _____
PR interval _____ QRS duration _____ QT interval _____
Identification _____

FIGURE 10-33

Ventricular rate/rhythm _____ Atrial rate/rhythm _____
PR interval _____ QRS duration _____ QT interval _____
Identification _____

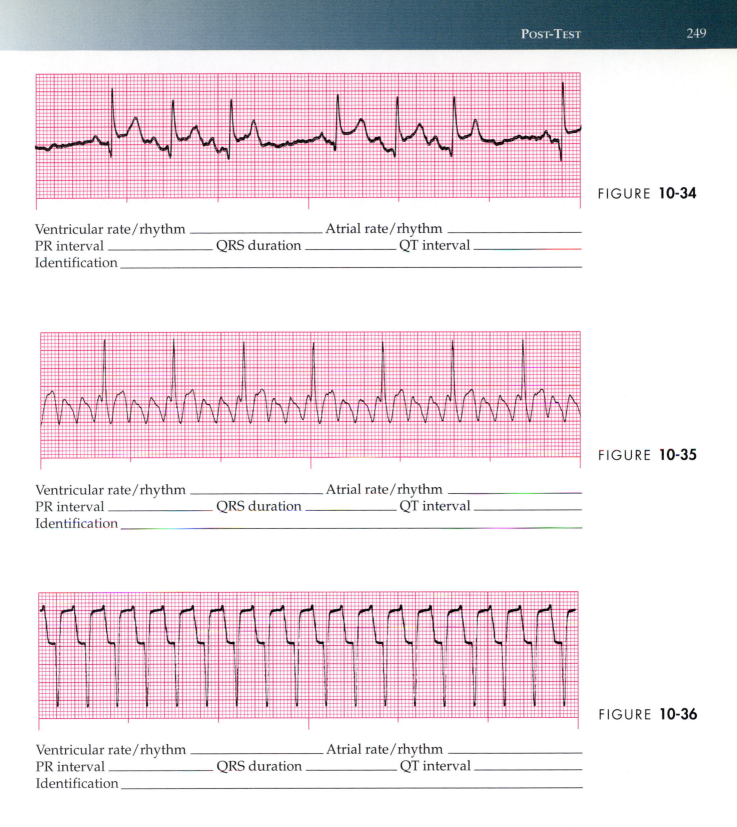

FIGURE **10-34**

Ventricular rate/rhythm _____ Atrial rate/rhythm _____
PR interval _____ QRS duration _____ QT interval _____
Identification _____

FIGURE **10-35**

Ventricular rate/rhythm _____ Atrial rate/rhythm _____
PR interval _____ QRS duration _____ QT interval _____
Identification _____

FIGURE **10-36**

Ventricular rate/rhythm _____ Atrial rate/rhythm _____
PR interval _____ QRS duration _____ QT interval _____
Identification _____

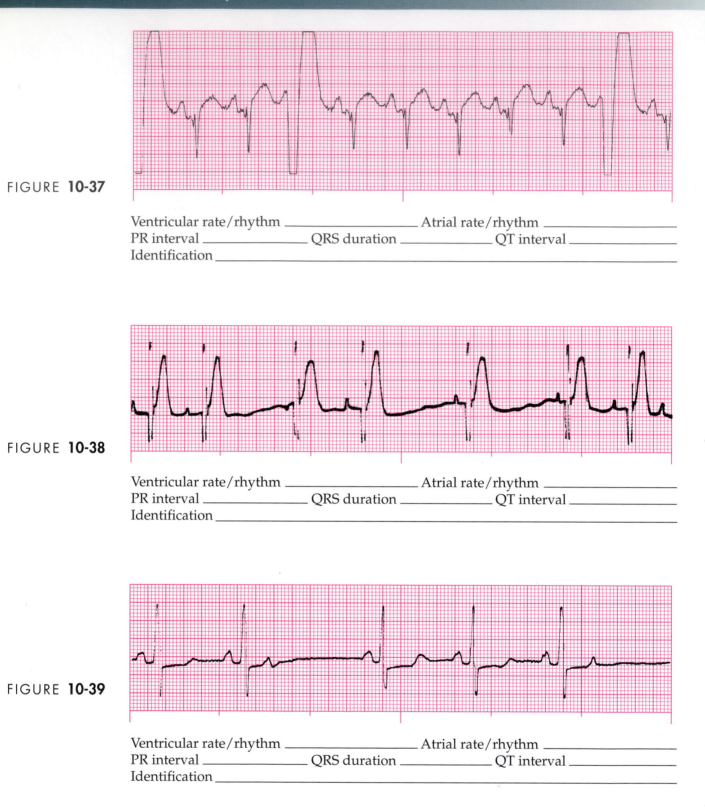

FIGURE **10-37**

Ventricular rate/rhythm _____ Atrial rate/rhythm _____
PR interval _____ QRS duration _____ QT interval _____
Identification _____

FIGURE **10-38**

Ventricular rate/rhythm _____ Atrial rate/rhythm _____
PR interval _____ QRS duration _____ QT interval _____
Identification _____

FIGURE **10-39**

Ventricular rate/rhythm _____ Atrial rate/rhythm _____
PR interval _____ QRS duration _____ QT interval _____
Identification _____

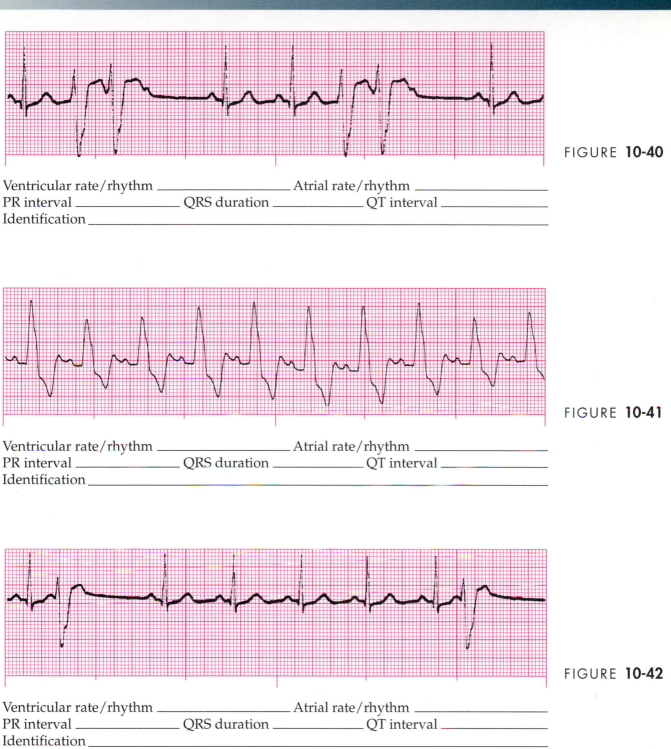

FIGURE **10-40**

Ventricular rate/rhythm _____ Atrial rate/rhythm _____
PR interval _____ QRS duration _____ QT interval _____
Identification _____

FIGURE **10-41**

Ventricular rate/rhythm _____ Atrial rate/rhythm _____
PR interval _____ QRS duration _____ QT interval _____
Identification _____

FIGURE **10-42**

Ventricular rate/rhythm _____ Atrial rate/rhythm _____
PR interval _____ QRS duration _____ QT interval _____
Identification _____

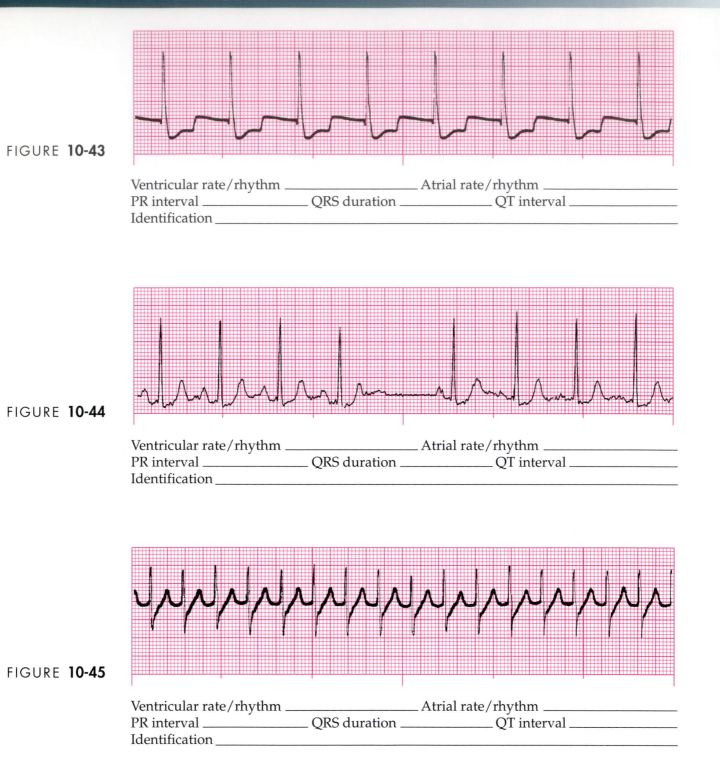

FIGURE **10-43**

Ventricular rate/rhythm _____ Atrial rate/rhythm _____
PR interval _____ QRS duration _____ QT interval _____
Identification _____

FIGURE **10-44**

Ventricular rate/rhythm _____ Atrial rate/rhythm _____
PR interval _____ QRS duration _____ QT interval _____
Identification _____

FIGURE **10-45**

Ventricular rate/rhythm _____ Atrial rate/rhythm _____
PR interval _____ QRS duration _____ QT interval _____
Identification _____

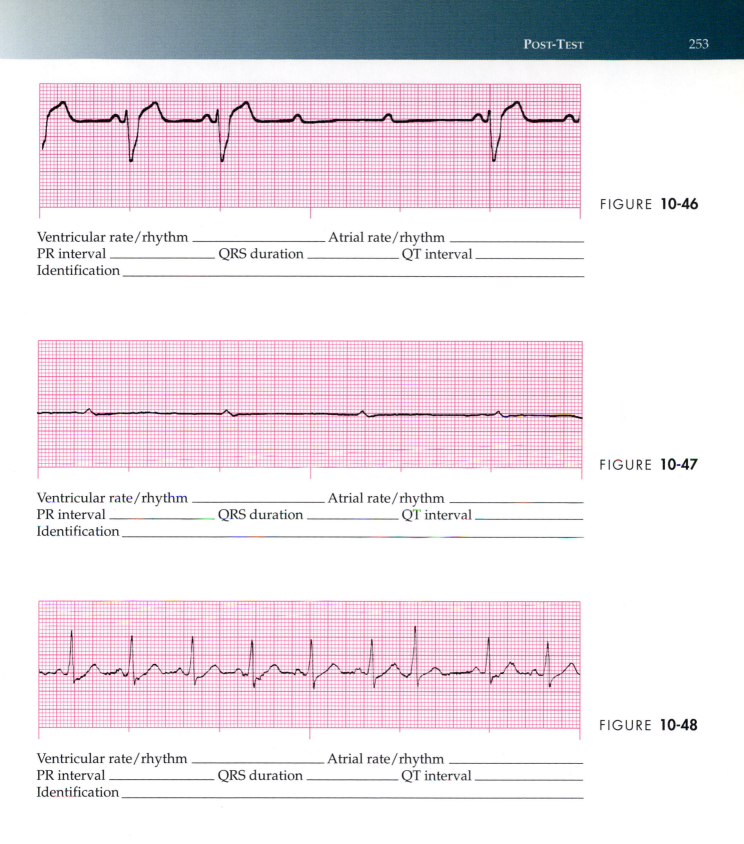

FIGURE **10-46**

Ventricular rate/rhythm _____ Atrial rate/rhythm _____
PR interval _____ QRS duration _____ QT interval _____
Identification _____

FIGURE **10-47**

Ventricular rate/rhythm _____ Atrial rate/rhythm _____
PR interval _____ QRS duration _____ QT interval _____
Identification _____

FIGURE **10-48**

Ventricular rate/rhythm _____ Atrial rate/rhythm _____
PR interval _____ QRS duration _____ QT interval _____
Identification _____

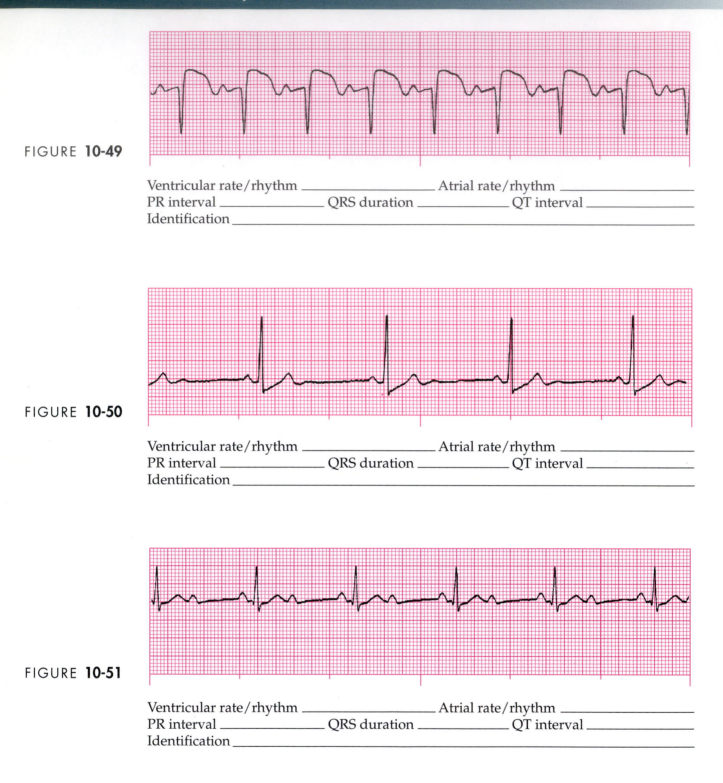

FIGURE **10-49**

Ventricular rate/rhythm _____ Atrial rate/rhythm _____
PR interval _____ QRS duration _____ QT interval _____
Identification _____

FIGURE **10-50**

Ventricular rate/rhythm _____ Atrial rate/rhythm _____
PR interval _____ QRS duration _____ QT interval _____
Identification _____

FIGURE **10-51**

Ventricular rate/rhythm _____ Atrial rate/rhythm _____
PR interval _____ QRS duration _____ QT interval _____
Identification _____

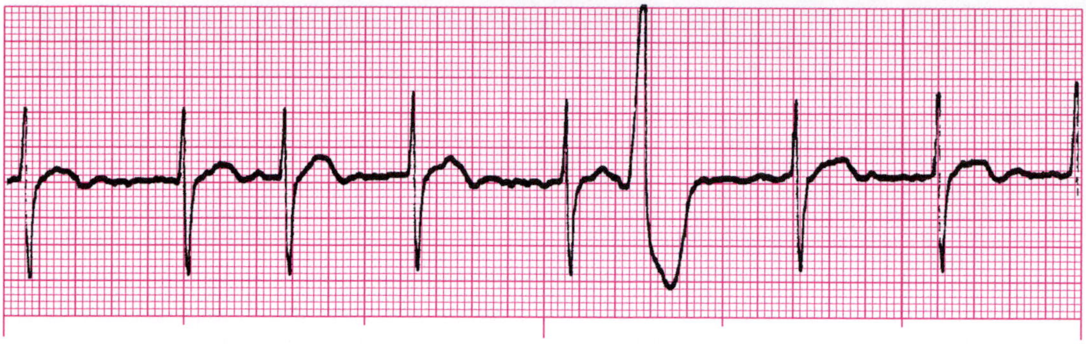

FIGURE **10-52**

Ventricular rate/rhythm _____ Atrial rate/rhythm _____
PR interval _____ QRS duration _____ QT interval _____
Identification _____

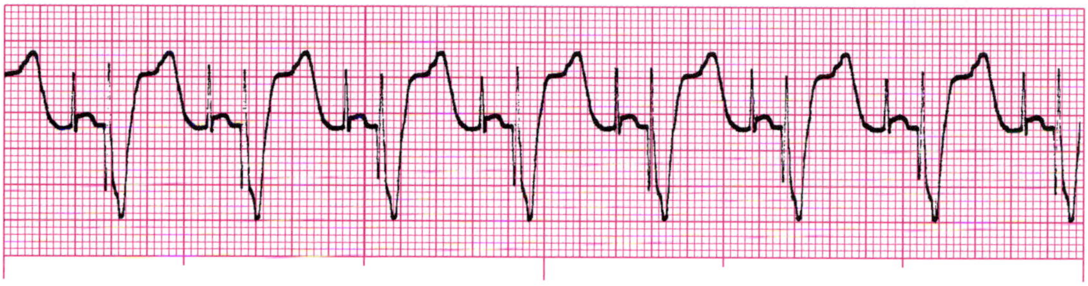

FIGURE **10-53**

Atrial-paced activity? _____ Ventricular-paced activity? _____
Paced interval rate? _____
Identification _____

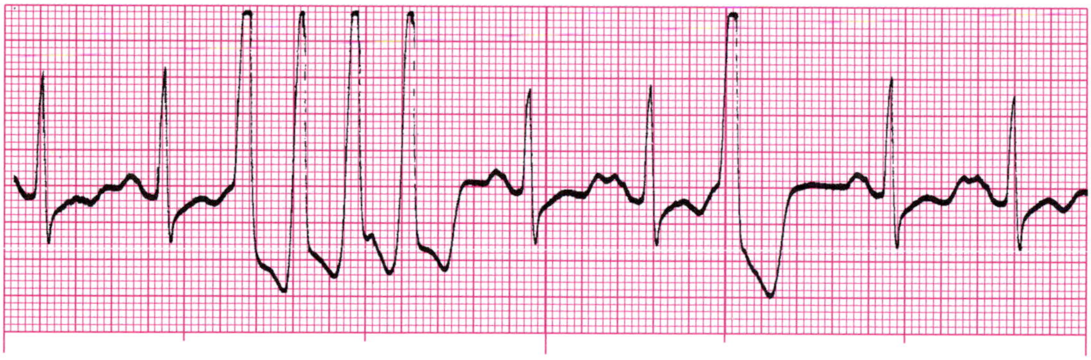

FIGURE **10-54**

Ventricular rate/rhythm _____ Atrial rate/rhythm _____
PR interval _____ QRS duration _____ QT interval _____
Identification _____

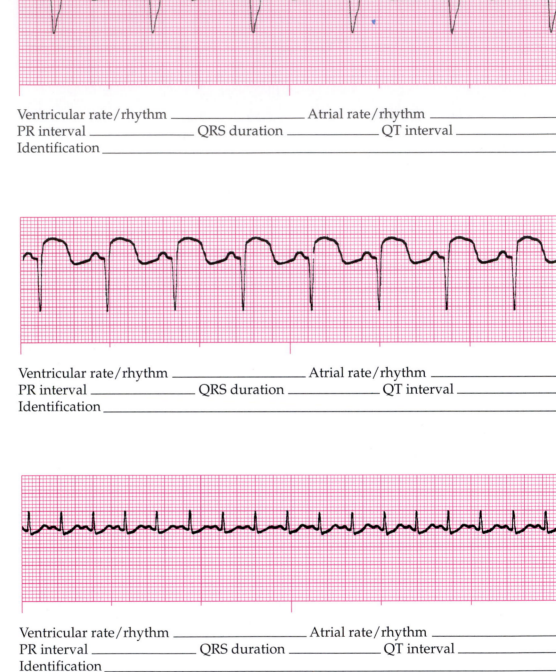

FIGURE **10-55**

Ventricular rate/rhythm _____ Atrial rate/rhythm _____
PR interval _____ QRS duration _____ QT interval _____
Identification _____

FIGURE **10-56**

Ventricular rate/rhythm _____ Atrial rate/rhythm _____
PR interval _____ QRS duration _____ QT interval _____
Identification _____

FIGURE **10-57**

Ventricular rate/rhythm _____ Atrial rate/rhythm _____
PR interval _____ QRS duration _____ QT interval _____
Identification _____

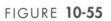

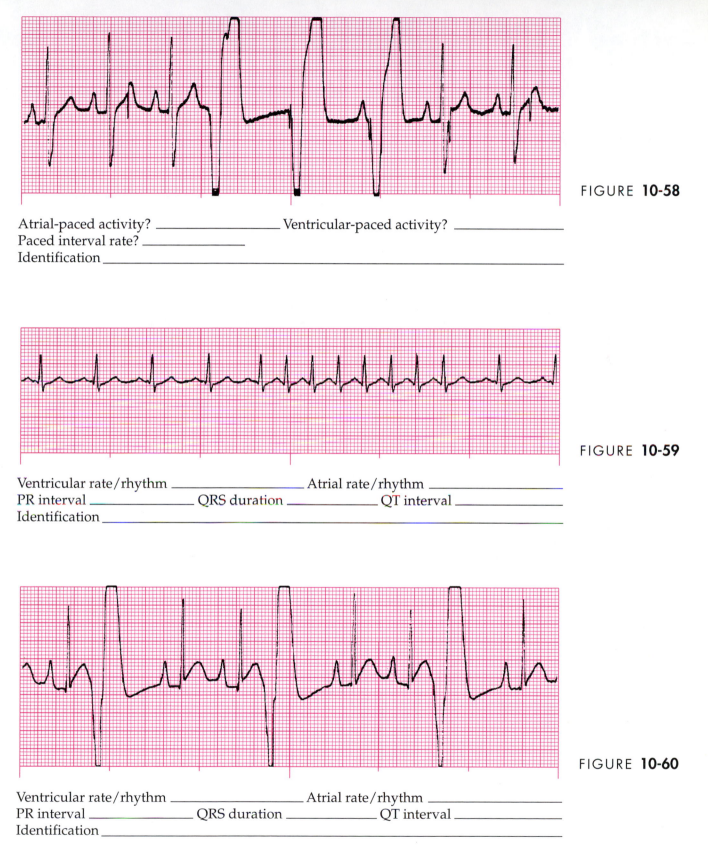

FIGURE **10-58**

Atrial-paced activity? _____ Ventricular-paced activity? _____
Paced interval rate? _____
Identification _____

FIGURE **10-59**

Ventricular rate/rhythm _____ Atrial rate/rhythm _____
PR interval _____ QRS duration _____ QT interval _____
Identification _____

FIGURE **10-60**

Ventricular rate/rhythm _____ Atrial rate/rhythm _____
PR interval _____ QRS duration _____ QT interval _____
Identification _____

Chapter 1 Stop and Review Answers

MATCHING

M	1.	The pressure or resistance against which the ventricles must pump to eject blood
K	2.	Occlusion of this vessel has been referred to as the "widow maker" because of its association with sudden death
L	3.	A repetitive pumping process that includes all of the events associated with the flow of blood through the heart
J	4.	Blood flows from the right atrium through the ___ valve into the right ventricle
A	5.	The amount of blood pumped into the aorta each minute by the heart
G	6.	A double-walled sac that encloses the heart and helps protect it from trauma and infection
O	7.	A positive ___ effect results in an increase in myocardial contractility
F	8.	Blood flows from the left atrium through the ___ valve into the left ventricle
N	9.	Specialized nerve tissue located in the internal carotid arteries and the aortic arch that detects changes in blood pressure
D	10.	The largest vein that drains the heart
E	11.	Coronary artery that supplies the SA node and AV node in most of the population
I	12.	This results when the heart's demand for oxygen exceeds its supply from the coronary circulation
H	13.	A negative ___ effect refers to a decrease in heart rate
B	14.	Sensors in the internal carotid arteries and aortic arch that detect changes in the concentration of hydrogen ions (pH), oxygen, and carbon dioxide in the blood
C	15.	The amount of blood flowing into the right atrium each minute from the systemic circulation

A. Cardiac output
B. Chemoreceptors
C. Venous return
D. Coronary sinus
E. Right coronary artery
F. Mitral (bicuspid)
G. Pericardium
H. Chronotropic
I. Myocardial ischemia
J. Tricuspid
K. Left main coronary artery
L. Cardiac cycle
M. Afterload
N. Baroreceptors
O. Inotropic

Chapter 2 Stop and Review Answers

MATCHING

O	1.	QT interval
G	2.	Intrinsic rate of AV junction
J	3.	Excitability
H	4.	Refractoriness
Q	5.	Repolarization
R	6.	Intrinsic rate of ventricles
E	7.	Myocardial cells
K	8.	Absolute refractory period
C	9.	Depolarization
I	10.	Pacemaker cells
A	11.	Intrinsic rate of SA node
D	12.	Inferior
L	13.	Bipolar limb leads
B	14.	Relative refractory period
P	15.	Lateral
M	16.	Time
N	17.	Unipolar limb leads
F	18.	Amplitude/voltage

A. 60 to 100 beats/min
B. Corresponds with the downslope of the T wave
C. Movement of ions across a cell membrane, causing the inside of the cell to become more positive
D. Surface of the left ventricle viewed by leads II, III, and aVF
E. Working cells of the myocardium that contain contractile filaments
F. Measured on the vertical axis of ECG paper
G. 40 to 60 beats/min
H. Extent to which a cell is able to respond to a stimulus
I. Specialized cells of the heart's electrical conduction system capable of spontaneously generating and conducting electrical impulses
J. Ability of cardiac muscle cells to respond to an external stimulus
K. Corresponds with the onset of the QRS complex to the peak of the T wave
L. I, II, III
M. Measured on the horizontal axis of ECG paper
N. aVR, aVL, aVF
O. Represents total ventricular activity—the time from ventricular depolarization to repolarization
P. Surface of the left ventricle viewed by leads I, aVL, V_5, and V_6
Q. Movement of ions across a cell membrane in which the inside of the cell is restored to its negative charge
R. 20 to 40 beats/min

Practice Rhythm Strips

Note: WNL, within normal limits; *UTD,* unable to determine. (Strips shown for labeling.)

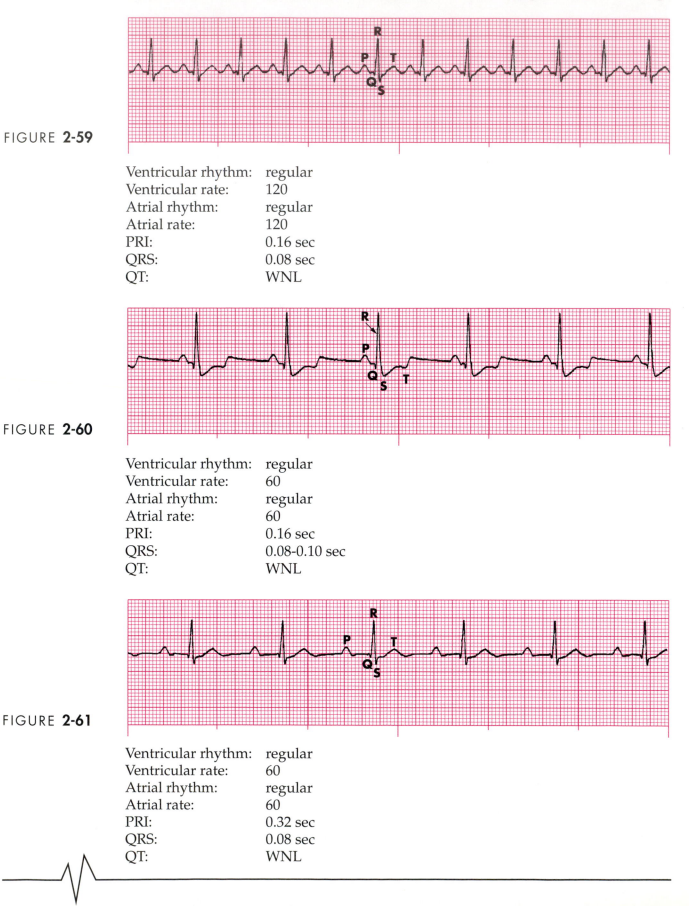

FIGURE **2-59**

Ventricular rhythm:	regular
Ventricular rate:	120
Atrial rhythm:	regular
Atrial rate:	120
PRI:	0.16 sec
QRS:	0.08 sec
QT:	WNL

FIGURE **2-60**

Ventricular rhythm:	regular
Ventricular rate:	60
Atrial rhythm:	regular
Atrial rate:	60
PRI:	0.16 sec
QRS:	0.08-0.10 sec
QT:	WNL

FIGURE **2-61**

Ventricular rhythm:	regular
Ventricular rate:	60
Atrial rhythm:	regular
Atrial rate:	60
PRI:	0.32 sec
QRS:	0.08 sec
QT:	WNL

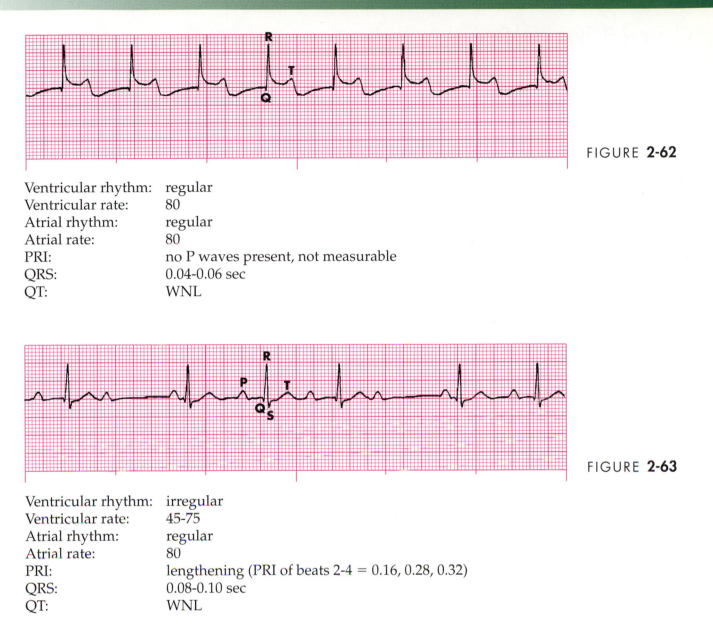

FIGURE **2-62**

Ventricular rhythm:	regular
Ventricular rate:	80
Atrial rhythm:	regular
Atrial rate:	80
PRI:	no P waves present, not measurable
QRS:	0.04-0.06 sec
QT:	WNL

FIGURE **2-63**

Ventricular rhythm:	irregular
Ventricular rate:	45-75
Atrial rhythm:	regular
Atrial rate:	80
PRI:	lengthening (PRI of beats 2-4 = 0.16, 0.28, 0.32)
QRS:	0.08-0.10 sec
QT:	WNL

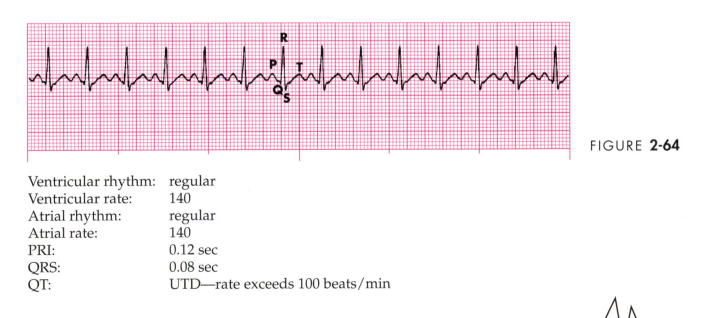

FIGURE **2-64**

Ventricular rhythm:	regular
Ventricular rate:	140
Atrial rhythm:	regular
Atrial rate:	140
PRI:	0.12 sec
QRS:	0.08 sec
QT:	UTD—rate exceeds 100 beats/min

Chapter 3 Stop and Review Answers

MATCHING

H	1.	Common dysrhythmia associated with respiratory rate
J	2.	Appearance of P waves that originate from the SA node
F	3.	Rate associated with sinus bradycardia
G	4.	If the SA node fails to generate an impulse, the next (escape) pacemaker that should generate an impulse
I	5.	Dysrhythmia with a pause that is the same as (or an exact multiple of) the distance between two other P-P intervals
B	6.	Normal rate for a sinus rhythm
D	7.	Pacemaker with an intrinsic rate of 20 to 40 beats/min
C	8.	Dysrhythmia that originates from the SA node and has a ventricular rate of 101 to 180 beats/min
A	9.	Dysrhythmia with a pause of undetermined length that is not the same distance as other P-P intervals
E	10.	Normal QRS duration in an adult

A. Sinus arrest
B. 60 to 100 beats/min
C. Sinus tachycardia
D. Ventricles
E. Less than 0.10 sec
F. Less than 60 beats/min
G. AV junction
H. Sinus arrhythmia
I. Sinoatrial (SA) block
J. Positive (upright) in lead II, one precedes each QRS

Practice Rhythm Strips

Note: WNL, within normal limits; *UTD,* unable to determine; *bpm,* beats/min

Figure 3-7

Ventricular rhythm: regular
Ventricular rate: 65
Atrial rhythm: regular
Atrial rate: 65
PRI: 0.16 sec
QRS: 0.08-0.10 sec
QT: WNL

Identification: Sinus rhythm at 65 bpm, ST segment elevation

Figure 3-8

Ventricular rhythm: regular
Ventricular rate: 40
Atrial rhythm: regular
Atrial rate: 40
PRI: 0.16 sec
QRS: 0.08 sec
QT: WNL

Identification: Sinus bradycardia at 40 bpm; ST segment depression, inverted T waves

Figure 3-9

Ventricular rhythm: regular
Ventricular rate: 100
Atrial rhythm: regular
Atrial rate: 100
PRI: 0.16 sec
QRS: 0.14 sec
QT: WNL

Identification: Sinus rhythm with a wide QRS at 100 bpm; ST segment depression, inverted T waves

Figure 3-10

Ventricular rhythm: irregular
Ventricular rate: 0-75
Atrial rhythm: irregular
Atrial rate: 0-75
PRI: 0.16 sec
QRS: 0.08 sec
QT: UTD

Identification: Sinus rhythm at approximately 75 bpm with a 4.0-sec sinus arrest, elevated T waves

Figure 3-11

Ventricular rhythm: regular
Ventricular rate: 85
Atrial rhythm: regular
Atrial rate: 85
PRI: 0.16 sec
QRS: 0.08 sec
QT: WNL

Identification: Sinus rhythm at 85 bpm

Figure 3-12

Ventricular rhythm: regular
Ventricular rate: 140
Atrial rhythm: regular
Atrial rate: 140
PRI: 0.12 sec
QRS: 0.08 sec
QT: UTD, rate exceeds 100 bpm

Identification: Sinus tachycardia at 140 bpm

Figure 3-13

Ventricular rhythm: regular
Ventricular rate: 60
Atrial rhythm: regular
Atrial rate: 60
PRI: 0.12 sec
QRS: 0.08 sec
QT: UTD

Identification: Sinus rhythm at 60 bpm

Figure 3-14

Ventricular rhythm: regular
Ventricular rate: 60
Atrial rhythm: regular
Atrial rate: 60
PRI: 0.16 sec
QRS: 0.08 sec
QT: WNL

Identification: Sinus rhythm at 60 bpm; ST segment depression, inverted T waves

Figure 3-15

Ventricular rhythm:	regular
Ventricular rate:	95
Atrial rhythm:	regular
Atrial rate:	95
PRI:	0.16 sec
QRS:	0.08 sec
QT:	WNL

Identification: Sinus rhythm at 95 bpm

Figure 3-16

Ventricular rhythm:	regular
Ventricular rate:	44
Atrial rhythm:	regular
Atrial rate:	44
PRI:	0.16 sec
QRS:	0.06 sec
QT:	WNL

Identification: Sinus bradycardia at 44 bpm, ST segment depression; note the upright U waves following each T wave

Figure 3-17

Ventricular rhythm:	irregular
Ventricular rate:	71-100
Atrial rhythm:	irregular
Atrial rate:	71-100
PRI:	0.16 sec
QRS:	0.04 sec
QT:	WNL

Identification: Sinus arrhythmia at 71-100 bpm

Figure 3-18

Ventricular rhythm:	regular
Ventricular rate:	83
Atrial rhythm:	regular
Atrial rate:	83
PRI:	0.18 sec
QRS:	0.12 sec
QT:	WNL

Identification: Sinus rhythm with a wide QRS at 83 bpm

Figure 3-19

Ventricular rhythm:	regular
Ventricular rate:	58
Atrial rhythm:	regular
Atrial rate:	58
PRI:	0.16 sec
QRS:	0.08 sec
QT:	WNL

Identification: Sinus bradycardia at 58 bpm

Figure 3-20

Ventricular rhythm:	irregular
Ventricular rate:	54-88
Atrial rhythm:	irregular
Atrial rate:	54-88
PRI:	0.12 sec
QRS:	0.08 sec
QT:	WNL

Identification: Sinus arrhythmia at 54-88 bpm

Chapter 4 Stop and Review Answers

MATCHING

F	1.	Updated term for wandering atrial pacemaker	A.	400 to 600 beats/min
N	2.	The most common preexcitation syndrome	B.	Decreased stroke volume
I	3.	Atrial rate associated with type I atrial flutter	C.	Atrial fibrillation
B	4.	Consequence of decreased ventricular filling time	D.	An early P wave with no QRS following it
O	5.	Verapamil, diltiazem	E.	Beta-blocker
H	6.	Digoxin	F.	Multiformed atrial rhythm
D	7.	ECG characteristic of a nonconducted PAC	G.	Paroxysmal
M	8.	Adenosine	H.	Cardiac glycoside
A	9.	Atrial rate associated with atrial fibrillation	I.	250 to 350 beats/min
E	10.	Esmolol, atenolol, metoprolol, propranolol	J.	Atrial flutter
G	11.	Term referring to the sudden onset or cessation of a dysrhythmia	K.	Anticoagulants
			L.	Premature atrial complex
J	12.	Ventricular rhythm may be regular or irregular, waveforms resembling teeth of a saw or picket fence before QRS	M.	First-line medication used for most types of PSVT
L	13.	Early beat initiated by an irritable atrial site	N.	Wolff-Parkinson-White syndrome
C	14.	Irregularly irregular ventricular rhythm, no identifiable P waves	O.	Calcium channel blocker
K	15.	Before elective cardioversion, prophylactic treatment with ___ is recommended for the patient in atrial fibrillation		

Practice Rhythm Strips

Note: WNL, within normal limits; *UTD*, unable to determine; *bpm*, beats/min

Figure 4-17

Ventricular rhythm: regular except for the event
Ventricular rate: 78
Atrial rhythm: regular except for the event
Atrial rate: 78
PRI: 0.16 sec
QRS: 0.06 sec
QT: UTD

Identification: Sinus rhythm at 78 bpm with a PAC, ST segment elevation (PAC is the third complex from left)

Figure 4-18

Ventricular rhythm: regular
Ventricular rate: 170
Atrial rhythm: regular
Atrial rate: 170
PRI: 0.08 sec
QRS: 0.06 sec
QT: UTD, rate >100 bpm

Identification: Atrial tachycardia (SVT) at 170 bpm

Figure 4-19

Ventricular rhythm: irregular
Ventricular rate: 115-214
Atrial rhythm: irregular
Atrial rate: UTD
PRI: not measurable
QRS: 0.06 sec
QT: UTD, rate >100 bpm

Identification: Uncontrolled AF at 115-224 bpm, ST segment depression

Figure 4-20

Ventricular rhythm: regular except for the event
Ventricular rate: 93
Atrial rhythm: regular except for the event
Atrial rate: 93
PRI: 0.16 sec
QRS: 0.04 sec
QT: WNL

Identification: Sinus rhythm at 93 bpm with a PAC (PAC is the seventh complex from the left)

Figure 4-21

Ventricular rhythm: irregular
Ventricular rate: 54-115
Atrial rhythm: irregular
Atrial rate: UTD
PRI: UTD
QRS: 0.08 sec
QT: UTD

Identification: Atrial fibrillation at 54-115 bpm

Figure 4-22

Ventricular rhythm: regular except for events
Ventricular rate: 117
Atrial rhythm: regular except for events
Atrial rate: 117
PRI: 0.16 sec
QRS: 0.12 sec
QT: UTD, rate >100 bpm

Identification: Sinus tachycardia at 117 bpm with 3 PACs (beats 2, 8 and 10 from the left are PACs) and a wide QRS, ST segment elevation

Figure 4-23

Ventricular rhythm:	regular except for events
Ventricular rate:	60 (sinus beats)
Atrial rhythm:	regular except for events
Atrial rate:	60 (sinus beats)
PRI:	0.16-0.18 sec
QRS:	0.08 sec
QT:	0.56 sec

Identification: Sinus rhythm at 60 bpm with two nonconducted (blocked) PACs, ST segment depression (the nonconducted PACS can be seen after second and fifth QRS complexes)

Figure 4-24

Ventricular rhythm:	regular
Ventricular rate:	168
Atrial rhythm:	UTD
Atrial rate:	UTD
PRI:	not measurable
QRS:	0.08 sec
QT:	UTD, rate >100 bpm

Identification: SVT at 168 bpm, ST segment depression

Figure 4-25

Ventricular rhythm:	regular
Ventricular rate:	150
Atrial rhythm:	UTD
Atrial rate:	UTD
PRI:	not measurable
QRS:	0.04-0.06 sec
QT:	UTD, rate >100 bpm

Identification: SVT vs. atrial flutter with 2:1 conduction at 150 bpm

Figure 4-26

Ventricular rhythm:	irregular
Ventricular rate:	68-115
Atrial rhythm:	irregular
Atrial rate:	UTD
PRI:	not measurable
QRS:	0.06 sec
QT:	not measurable

Identification: Atrial fibrillation at 68-115 bpm

Figure 4-27

Ventricular rhythm:	regular except for events
Ventricular rate:	83 (sinus beats)
Atrial rhythm:	regular except for events
Atrial rate:	83 (sinus beats)
PRI:	0.16 sec
QRS:	0.04-0.08 sec
QT:	WNL

Identification: Sinus rhythm at 83 bpm with frequent PACs (atrial bigeminy), ST segment depression, inverted T waves (beats 3, 5, 7, and 9 are PACs)

Figure 4-28

Ventricular rhythm:	regular
Ventricular rate:	70
Atrial rhythm:	UTD
Atrial rate:	70 (sinus beats)
PRI:	varies
QRS:	varies
QT:	WNL

Identification: Underlying rhythm is sinus but pacemaker site varies; ventricular rate approximately 70 bpm; patient with known WPW; note delta waves

Figure 4-29

Ventricular rhythm:	irregular
Ventricular rate:	79-164
Atrial rhythm:	irregular
Atrial rate:	UTD
PRI:	not measurable
QRS:	0.08 sec
QT:	not measurable

Identification: Atrial fibrillation at 79-164 bpm (lead MCL$_1$)

Figure 4-30

Ventricular rhythm:	regular
Ventricular rate:	85
Atrial rhythm:	regular
Atrial rate:	375
PRI:	not measurable
QRS:	0.08 sec
QT:	not measurable

Identification: Atrial flutter at 85 bpm (lead III), ST segment depression, inverted T waves

Chapter 5 Stop and Review Answers

MATCHING

M	1.	Impulse(s) originating from a source other than the sinoatrial node
K	2.	Name given to a dysrhythmia that originates in the AV junction with a ventricular rate between 61 to 100 beats/min
H	3.	___ toxicity/excess is a common cause of junctional dysrhythmias
N	4.	A beat originating from the AV junction that appears later than the next expected beat
J	5.	Location of the P wave on the ECG if atrial and ventricular depolarization occur simultaneously
L	6.	Medication that increases heart rate (positive chronotropic effect) by accelerating the SA node discharge rate and blocking the vagus nerve
E	7.	Normal duration of a QRS complex in a junctional dysrhythmia
B	8.	Characteristic of specialized cardiac cells to spontaneously initiate an electrical impulse without being stimulated from another source
G	9.	In a junctional rhythm, location of the P wave on the ECG if ventricular depolarization precedes atrial depolarization
A	10.	Normal duration of a PR interval
D	11.	A beat originating from the AV junction that appears earlier than the next expected sinus beat
I	12.	The ability of a cardiac cell to receive an electrical stimulus and propagate that impulse to an adjacent cardiac cell
O	13.	Primary waveform used to differentiate PJCs from PACs
F	14.	Normal (intrinsic) rate for the AV junction
C	15.	In a junctional rhythm, location of the P wave on the ECG if atrial depolarization precedes ventricular depolarization

A. 0.12 to 0.20 sec
B. Automaticity
C. Inverted P wave precedes the QRS complex in leads II, III, and aVF
D. Premature junctional complex (PJC)
E. 0.10 sec or less
F. 40 to 60 beats/min
G. Inverted P wave occurs after the QRS complex in leads II, III, and aVF
H. Digitalis
I. Conductivity
J. Hidden within the QRS complex (not visible)
K. Accelerated junctional rhythm
L. Atropine
M. Ectopic
N. Junctional escape beat
O. P wave

Practice Rhythm Strips

Note: WNL, within normal limits; *UTD*, unable to determine; *bpm*, beats/min

Figure 5-7

Ventricular rhythm:	regular except for the event(s)
Ventricular rate:	136 (sinus beats)
Atrial rhythm:	regular except for the event(s)
Atrial rate:	136 (sinus beats)
PRI:	0.10 sec
QRS:	0.06 sec
QT:	UTD, rate >100 bpm

Identification: Sinus tachycardia at 136 bpm with frequent PJCs (the PJCs are beats 2, 5, 8, and 11 from the left)

Figure 5-8

Ventricular rhythm:	regular
Ventricular rate:	75
Atrial rhythm:	regular
Atrial rate:	75
PRI:	0.16 sec
QRS:	0.08 sec
QT:	WNL

Identification: Accelerated junctional rhythm at 75 bpm

Figure 5-9

Ventricular rhythm:	regular (junctional beats)
Ventricular rate:	115-214
Atrial rhythm:	UTD (junctional beats)
Atrial rate:	UTD (junctional beats)
PRI:	not measurable in junctional beats
QRS:	0.06 sec
QT:	WNL

Identification: Sinus rhythm changing to an accelerated junctional rhythm at 79 bpm, back to a sinus rhythm

Figure 5-10

Ventricular rhythm:	irregular
Ventricular rate:	19-26
Atrial rhythm:	UTD
Atrial rate:	UTD
PRI:	UTD
QRS:	0.04 sec
QT:	0.44 sec

Identification: Junctional escape rhythm (junctional bradycardia) with a ventricular response of 19-26 bpm, ST segment depression

Figure 5-11

Ventricular rhythm:	regular except for event(s)
Ventricular rate:	94 (sinus beats)
Atrial rhythm:	regular except for event(s)
Atrial rate:	94 (sinus beats)
PRI:	0.12 sec
QRS:	0.06 sec
QT:	WNL

Identification: Sinus rhythm at 94 bpm with a PAC (second beat from left) and a junctional escape beat (third beat from left)

Figure 5-12

Ventricular rhythm:	regular except for the event
Ventricular rate:	115 (sinus beats)
Atrial rhythm:	regular except for the event
Atrial rate:	115 (sinus beats)
PRI:	0.16 sec
QRS:	0.06 sec
QT:	UTD, rate >100 bpm

Identification: Sinus tachycardia at 115 bpm with a PJC (fifth beat is the PJC)

Figure 5-13

Ventricular rhythm:	regular
Ventricular rate:	52
Atrial rhythm:	regular
Atrial rate:	52
PRI:	0.16 sec
QRS:	0.08 sec
QT:	WNL

Identification: Junctional escape rhythm at 52 bpm with elevated T waves

Figure 5-14

Ventricular rhythm:	essentially regular
Ventricular rate:	37
Atrial rhythm:	UTD
Atrial rate:	UTD
PRI:	not measurable
QRS:	0.10 sec
QT:	WNL

Identification: Junctional rhythm at 37 bpm, converting to a sinus rhythm, ST segment elevation in junctional beats

Figure 5-15

Ventricular rhythm:	regular
Ventricular rate:	83
Atrial rhythm:	regular
Atrial rate:	83
PRI:	0.12 sec
QRS:	0.06 sec
QT:	WNL

Identification: Accelerated junctional rhythm at 83 bpm

Figure 5-16

Ventricular rhythm:	irregular
Ventricular rate:	107 (sinus beats)
Atrial rhythm:	irregular
Atrial rate:	107 (sinus beats)
PRI:	0.16 sec
QRS:	0.08 sec
QT:	UTD, rate >100 bpm

Identification: Sinus tachycardia at 107 bpm with a junctional escape beat (third beat from the left) and a nonconducted PAC (buried in the T wave of the fourth beat from the left), elevated T waves

Figure 5-17

Ventricular rhythm:	regular
Ventricular rate:	125
Atrial rhythm:	regular
Atrial rate:	125
PRI:	0.16 sec
QRS:	0.08 sec
QT:	UTD, rate >100 bpm

Identification: Sinus tachycardia at 125 bpm, changing to a junctional tachycardia at 125 bpm

Figure 5-18

Ventricular rhythm:	regular
Ventricular rate:	70
Atrial rhythm:	regular
Atrial rate:	70
PRI:	0.16 sec
QRS:	0.08 sec
QT:	WNL

Identification: Sinus rhythm at 70 bpm with a nonconducted PAC (note distortion of the T wave of the beat preceding the pause) and a junctional escape beat

Figure 5-19

Ventricular rhythm:	regular
Ventricular rate:	138
Atrial rhythm:	UTD
Atrial rate:	UTD
PRI:	not measurable
QRS:	0.10 sec
QT:	UTD, rate >100 bpm

Identification: SVT (probably junctional tachycardia) at 138 bpm

Figure 5-20

Ventricular rhythm:	regular except for the event
Ventricular rate:	90
Atrial rhythm:	regular except for the event
Atrial rate:	90
PRI:	0.16 sec
QRS:	0.10 sec
QT:	WNL

Identification Sinus rhythm at 90 bpm with a PAC (sixth beat from the left is the PAC)

Chapter 6 Stop and Review Answers

Matching

N	1.	Two sequential PVCs	A. R-on-T phenomenon
K	2.	Medication that should be avoided in the management of IVR or AIVR	B. Asystole
			C. Trigeminy
G	3.	Pattern in which every other beat is an ectopic beat	D. Ventricular tachycardia
I	4.	Clinical situation in which organized electrical activity (other than VT) is observed on the cardiac monitor, but the patient is pulseless	E. Ventricular escape beat
			F. Uniform
			G. Bigeminy
J	5.	Essentially regular ventricular rhythm with a ventricular rate of 40 beats/min or less	H. Accelerated idioventricular rhythm
O	6.	Type of PVC that occurs between two normal beats and does not interrupt the underlying rhythm	I. Pulseless electrical activity
			J. Ventricular escape rhythm
B	7.	Absence of electrical activity on the cardiac monitor	K. Lidocaine
L	8.	Medication used in the management of torsades de pointes	L. Magnesium sulfate
			M. Quinidine, procainamide
H	9.	Essentially regular ventricular rhythm with a ventricular rate of 41 to 100 beats/min	N. Couplet
			O. Interpolated
A	10.	Name given a PVC falling on the T wave of the preceding beat	
F	11.	PVCs of similar configuration in the same lead	
C	12.	Pattern in which every third beat is an ectopic beat	
E	13.	Ventricular beat that occurs later than the next expected sinus beat; protective mechanism	
M	14.	Medications associated with prolongation of the QT interval and precipitation of torsades de pointes	
D	15.	Essentially regular ventricular rhythm with a ventricular rate of more than 100 beats/min	

Practice Rhythm Strips

Note: WNL, within normal limits; *UTD,* unable to determine; *bpm,* beats/min

Figure 6-16

Ventricular rhythm:	regular (sinus beats)
Ventricular rate:	54
Atrial rhythm:	regular (sinus beats)
Atrial rate:	54
PRI:	0.12 sec (sinus beats)
QRS:	0.06-0.08 sec (sinus beats)
QT:	WNL

Identification: Sinus bradycardia at 54 bpm with ventricular bigeminy; ventricular rate approximately 100 bpm if PVCs counted in the rate

Figure 6-17

Ventricular rhythm:	UTD
Ventricular rate:	UTD
Atrial rhythm:	UTD
Atrial rate:	UTD
PRI:	UTD
QRS:	UTD
QT:	UTD

Identification: Coarse ventricular fibrillation

Figure 6-18

Ventricular rhythm:	regular
Ventricular rate:	60
Atrial rhythm:	regular
Atrial rate:	60
PRI:	0.20 sec (sinus beats)
QRS:	0.08 sec (sinus beats)
QT:	0.36 sec (sinus beats)

Identification: Sinus rhythm at 60 bpm with an R-on-T interpolated PVC, elevated T waves

Figure 6-19

Ventricular rhythm:	regular
Ventricular rate:	150
Atrial rhythm:	UTD
Atrial rate:	UTD
PRI:	UTD
QRS:	0.16 sec
QT:	UTD

Identification: Ventricular tachycardia at 150 bpm

Figure 6-20

Ventricular rhythm:	regular except for event (PVCs)
Ventricular rate:	102
Atrial rhythm:	regular except for event (PVCs)
Atrial rate:	102
PRI:	0.16 sec (sinus beats)
QRS:	0.06-0.08 sec (sinus beats)
QT:	UTD, rate >100 bpm

Identification: Sinus tachycardia at 102 bpm with uniform PVCs; ST segment elevation

Figure 6-21

Ventricular rhythm:	essentially regular
Ventricular rate:	94
Atrial rhythm:	UTD
Atrial rate:	UTD
PRI:	UTD
QRS:	0.12 sec
QT:	UTD

Identification: Accelerated idioventricular rhythm (AIVR) at 94 bpm (lead III)

Figure 6-22

Ventricular rhythm:	regular
Ventricular rate:	<25
Atrial rhythm:	UTD
Atrial rate:	UTD
PRI:	UTD
QRS:	0.16 sec
QT:	UTD

Identification: Idioventricular rhythm at <25 bpm (called an *agonal rhythm* when ventricular rate is <20 bpm)

Figure 6-23

Ventricular rhythm:	essentially regular
Ventricular rate:	62
Atrial rhythm:	essentially regular
Atrial rate:	62
PRI:	0.20 sec
QRS:	0.10 sec
QT:	WNL

Identification: Sinus rhythm at 62 bpm with an interpolated PVC; inverted T waves

Figure 6-24

Ventricular rhythm:	irregular
Ventricular rate:	230-300
Atrial rhythm:	UTD
Atrial rate:	UTD
PRI:	UTD
QRS:	variable
QT:	UTD

Identification: Torsades de pointes (TdP)

Figure 6-25

Ventricular rhythm:	irregular
Ventricular rate:	94 (sinus beats)
Atrial rhythm:	irregular
Atrial rate:	94 (sinus beats)
PRI:	0.16 sec (sinus beats)
QRS:	0.08 sec (sinus beats)
QT:	WNL

Identification: Sinus rhythm at 94 bpm with an episode of couplets and a run of VT

Figure 6-26

Ventricular rhythm:	regular except for the events
Ventricular rate:	88 (sinus beats)
Atrial rhythm:	regular except for the events
Atrial rate:	88 (sinus beats)
PRI:	0.20 sec (sinus beats)
QRS:	0.08 sec (sinus beats)
QT:	0.40 sec (sinus beats)

Identification: Sinus rhythm at 88 bpm with a PVC and run of VT, ST segment depression, inverted T waves

Figure 6-27

Ventricular rhythm:	regular except for events (PVCs)
Ventricular rate:	83 (sinus beats)
Atrial rhythm:	regular except for events (PVCs)
Atrial rate:	83 (sinus beats)
PRI:	0.16 sec
QRS:	0.08 sec
QT:	WNL

Identification: Sinus rhythm at 83 bpm with ventricular trigeminy, ST segment depression, inverted T waves

Figure 6-28

Ventricular rhythm:	irregular
Ventricular rate:	150-250
Atrial rhythm:	UTD
Atrial rate:	UTD
PRI:	not measurable
QRS:	0.06 sec
QT:	UTD, rate >100 bpm

Identification: Atrial fib with a rapid ventricular response of 150-250 bpm and a run of VT

Figure 6-29

Ventricular rhythm:	regular except for the event
Ventricular rate:	30 (sinus beats)
Atrial rhythm:	regular except for the event
Atrial rate:	30 (sinus beats)
PRI:	0.12-0.16 sec (sinus beats)
QRS:	0.06 sec (sinus beats)
QT:	UTD

Identification: Sinus bradycardia at 30 bpm with ventricular bigeminy (ventricular rate approximately 60 if PVCs counted), inverted T waves, horizontal ST segments

Chapter 7 Stop and Review Answers

MATCHING

E	1.	PR interval pattern in second-degree AV block, type I
I	2.	A ___ escape rhythm with a complete AV block, usually has a ventricular rate of 40 beats/min or less
H	3.	AV block that often progresses to a complete AV block without warning
K	4.	Location of the block in a second-degree AV block, type II
G	5.	Second-degree AV block type I is most commonly associated with an ___ myocardial infarction
M	6.	Normal duration of the PR interval
C	7.	AV block characterized by regular P-P intervals, regular R-R intervals, and a PR interval with no consistent value or pattern
N	8.	Common location of the block in a second-degree AV block, type I
A	9.	PR interval pattern in second-degree AV block, type II
D	10.	Location of the block in a complete AV block
F	11.	Ventricular rhythm pattern in second-degree AV block, types I and II
B	12.	AV block characterized by a PR interval greater than 0.20 sec and one P wave for each QRS complex
O	13.	Ventricular rhythm pattern in second-degree AV block 2:1 conduction and complete AV block
L	14.	A ___ escape rhythm with a complete AV block, usually has a narrow QRS and a ventricular rate of 40 to 60 beats/min
J	15.	Second-degree AV block type II is most commonly associated with an ___ myocardial infarction

A. Constant
B. First-degree AV block
C. Complete AV block
D. AV node, bundle of His, or bundle branches
E. Progressive lengthening
F. Irregular
G. Inferior wall
H. Second-degree AV block, type II
I. Ventricular
J. Anterior wall
K. Bundle of His or bundle branches
L. Junctional
M. 0.12 to 0.20 sec
N. AV node
O. Regular

Practice Rhythm Strips

Note: WNL, within normal limits; *UTD,* unable to determine; *bpm,* beats/min

Figure 7-9

Ventricular rhythm:	regular
Ventricular rate:	88
Atrial rhythm:	regular
Atrial rate:	88
PRI:	0.28 sec
QRS:	0.08 sec
QT:	WNL

Identification: Sinus rhythm at 88 bpm with first-degree AV block

Figure 7-10

Ventricular rhythm:	regular
Ventricular rate:	30
Atrial rhythm:	regular
Atrial rate:	68
PRI:	0.28 sec
QRS:	0.16 sec
QT:	UTD

Identification: Second-degree AV block, 2:1 conduction, probably type II; ST segment elevation

Figure 7-11

Ventricular rhythm:	regular
Ventricular rate:	50
Atrial rhythm:	regular
Atrial rate:	167
PRI:	variable
QRS:	0.06 sec
QT:	WNL

Identification: Complete AV block at 50 bpm, ST segment elevation

Figure 7-12

Ventricular rhythm:	regular
Ventricular rate:	40
Atrial rhythm:	regular
Atrial rate:	83
PRI:	0.24 sec
QRS:	0.10 sec
QT:	WNL

Identification: Second-degree AV block, 2:1 conduction, probably type I at 40 bpm, ST segment depression

Figure 7-13

Ventricular rhythm:	irregular
Ventricular rate:	50-94
Atrial rhythm:	regular
Atrial rate:	94
PRI:	lengthening
QRS:	0.10 sec
QT:	WNL

Identification: Second-degree AV block type I at 50-94 bpm, ST segment elevation

Figure 7-14

Ventricular rhythm:	irregular
Ventricular rate:	<20-60
Atrial rhythm:	regular
Atrial rate:	60
PRI:	0.16 sec
QRS:	0.12 sec
QT:	WNL

Identification: Second-degree AV block type II at <20-60 bpm, ST segment depression

Figure 7-15

Ventricular rhythm: irregular
Ventricular rate: <20-94
Atrial rhythm: regular
Atrial rate: 94
PRI: lengthening
QRS: 0.08 sec
QT: UTD

Identification: Second-degree AV block type I at <20-94 bpm (leads II and III)

Figure 7-16

Ventricular rhythm: irregular
Ventricular rate: 47-88
Atrial rhythm: regular
Atrial rate: 88
PRI: lengthening
QRS: 0.06 sec
QT: UTD

Identification: Second-degree AV block at 47-88 bpm, ST segment elevation; the fourth beat from the left is a fusion beat

Figure 7-17

Ventricular rhythm: regular
Ventricular rate: 33
Atrial rhythm: regular
Atrial rate: 71
PRI: variable
QRS: 0.06 sec
QT: UTD

Identification: Complete AV block at 33 bpm, ST segment elevation

Chapter 8 Stop and Review Answers

MATCHING

J	1.	Pacemaker that discharges only when the patient's heart rate drops below the preset rate for the pacemaker
H	2.	The time measured between a sensed cardiac event and the next pacemaker output
G	3.	The ECG waveform that results when an intrinsic depolarization and a pacing stimulus occur simultaneously and both contribute to depolarization of that cardiac chamber
L	4.	Rate at which the pulse generator of a pacemaker paces when no intrinsic activity is detected; expressed in pulses/min
M	5.	Pacemaker response in which the output pulse is suppressed when an intrinsic event is sensed
K	6.	In dual-chamber pacing, the interval between a sensed or ventricular-paced event and the next atrial-paced event
E	7.	Ability of a pacing stimulus to successfully depolarize the cardiac chamber that is being paced
C	8.	Ability of a pacemaker to increase the pacing rate in response to physical activity or metabolic demand
B	9.	A vertical line on the ECG that indicates the pacemaker has discharged
A	10.	A pacing system with a lead attached to the right atrium, designed to correct abnormalities in the SA node (sick sinus syndrome)
N	11.	The power source that houses the battery and controls for regulating a pacemaker
O	12.	Period, expressed in milliseconds, between two consecutively paced events in the same cardiac chamber without an intervening sensed event
D	13.	In dual-chamber pacing, the length of time between an atrial-sensed or atrial-paced event and the delivery of a ventricular pacing stimulus; analogous to the P-R interval of intrinsic waveforms
I	14.	Electrical stimulus delivered by a pacemaker's pulse generator
F	15.	Pacemaker that stimulates the atrium and ventricle

A. Atrial pacing
B. Pacemaker spike
C. Rate modulation
D. A-V interval
E. Capture
F. Dual-chamber pacemaker
G. Fusion beat
H. Escape interval
I. Output
J. Demand pacemaker
K. V-A interval
L. Base rate
M. Inhibition
N. Pulse generator
O. Pacing interval

Practice Rhythm Strips

Note: WNL, within normal limits; *UTD*, unable to determine; *bpm*, beats/min

Figure 8-10
Atrial pacing?   No
Ventricular pacing?   Yes
Paced interval: 79 bpm

Identification: 100% ventricular-paced rhythm

Figure 8-11
Atrial pacing?   No
Ventricular pacing?   Yes
Paced interval: 86

Identification: Normal functioning ventricular-demand pacer; underlying rhythm is a sinus rhythm with two uniform PVCs

Figure 8-12
Atrial pacing?   No
Ventricular pacing?   Yes
Paced interval: 76

Identification: 100% ventricular-paced rhythm

Figure 8-13
Atrial pacing?   No
Ventricular pacing?   Yes
Paced interval: 80

Identification: Ventricular-paced rhythm with pacemaker malfunction (loss of capture)

Figure 8-14
Atrial pacing?   No
Ventricular pacing?   Yes
Paced interval: 72

Identification: Malfunctioning ventricular-demand pacemaker (failure to capture); underlying rhythm appears to be atrial flutter

Figure 8-15
Atrial pacing?   Yes
Ventricular pacing?   Yes
Paced interval: 80

Identification: Normal functioning AV sequential pacemaker at 80 bpm

Figure 8-16
Atrial pacing?   No
Ventricular pacing?   Yes
Paced interval: 74

Identification: 100% ventricular-paced rhythm

Figure 8-17
Atrial pacing?   Yes
Ventricular pacing?   No
Paced interval: 80

Identification: Normal atrial pacemaker function; ST segment elevation

Figure 8-18
Atrial pacing?   No
Ventricular pacing?   Yes
Paced interval: 71

Identification: Pacemaker malfunction (failure to sense); underlying rhythm is a sinus rhythm at 88 bpm with a PVC; note the pacer spikes in the T waves of the second and eighth beats from the left

Figure 8-19
Atrial pacing?   No
Ventricular pacing?   Yes
Paced interval: 71

Identification: 100% ventricular-paced rhythm; underlying rhythm is atrial flutter

Figure 8-20

Atrial pacing?	No
Ventricular pacing?	Yes
Paced interval:	71

Identification: 100% ventricular-paced rhythm; underlying rhythm is a complete AV block

Figure 8-21

Atrial pacing?	No
Ventricular pacing?	Yes
Paced interval:	71

Identification: Normal pacemaker function—ventricular-demand pacer

Chapter 9 Stop and Review Answers

MATCHING

D	1.	Leads that view the inferior wall of the heart	A. aVL
M	2.	Occlusion of the right coronary artery may result in a(n) ___ myocardial infarction	B. V_1
N	3.	Indicator of the magnitude and direction of current flow	C. V_1, V_2
T	4.	Lead I is perpendicular to lead	D. II, III, aVF
R	5.	Lead I + lead III = ___	E. Anterior
B	6.	Lead located at the fourth intercostal space, right sternal border	F. Precordial
P	7.	Common ECG finding in hyperkalemia	G. aVR
L	8.	Leads that view the heart in the frontal plane	H. V_2
S	9.	The zone of ___ is typically characterized by ST segment elevation	I. I, aVL, V_5, V_6
O	10.	Leads used to view the right ventricle	J. Electrical axis
Q	11.	Lead located at the fifth intercostal space, left midclavicular line	K. Infarction
C	12.	Leads that view the septum	L. Limb
G	13.	Lead III is perpendicular to lead ___	M. Inferior
F	14.	Leads that view the heart in the horizontal plane	N. Vector
E	15.	Occlusion of the left anterior descending coronary artery may result in a(n) ___ myocardial infarction	O. V_1R-V_6R
I	16.	Leads that view the lateral wall of the heart	P. Tall, tented T waves
J	17.	Direction of the mean QRS vector	Q. V_4
K	18.	The zone of ___ is typically characterized by Q waves	R. Lead II
H	19.	Lead located at the fourth intercostal space, left sternal border	S. Injury
A	20.	Lead II is perpendicular to lead ___	T. aVF

Practice Rhythm Strips

Note: WNL, within normal limits; *UTD,* unable to determine; *bpm,* beats/min

Figure 9-36
Heart rate: 99
PRI: 0.15 sec
QRS: 0.08 sec
QT: 0.36 sec

Interpretation: Sinus rhythm; minimal voltage criteria for LVH, may be normal variant; borderline ECG

Figure 9-37
Heart rate: 110
PRI: 0.19 sec
QRS: 0.08 sec
QT: 0.31 sec

Interpretation: Sinus tachycardia; possible right atrial enlargement; cannot rule out lateral infarct, age undetermined; inferior infarct, age undetermined with posterior extension; abnormal ECG

Figure 9-38
Heart rate: 153
PRI: 0 sec
QRS: 0.96 sec
QT: 0.31 sec

Interpretation: Atrial fibrillation with rapid ventricular response; ST and T wave abnormality, possible anterolateral ischemia or digitalis effect; abnormal ECG

Figure 9-39
Heart rate: 63
PRI: 0.18 sec
QRS: 0.96 sec
QT: 0.39 sec

Interpretation: Sinus rhythm with frequent PVCs; tall T waves, possible hyperkalemia; abnormal ECG

Chapter 10 Post-Test Answers

MULTIPLE CHOICE AND TRUE/FALSE

1. B   The *sarcomere* is the basic contractile unit of a myofibril.
2. False A 12-lead ECG consists of 3 bipolar and 9 unipolar leads. The bipolar leads are the standard limb leads (I, II, III). The unipolar leads include the three augmented leads (aVR, aVL, aVF) and the six precordial (chest or "V") leads (V_1, V_2, V_3, V_4, V_5, and V_6).
3. C   The QRS complex represents ventricular depolarization. The P wave represents atrial depolarization.
4. C   The primary pacemaker of the heart is the sinoatrial (SA) node.
5. B   Automaticity is the ability of cardiac pacemaker cells to spontaneously initiate an electrical impulse without being stimulated from another source (such as a nerve). The SA node, AV junction, and Purkinje fibers normally possess this characteristic. "A" refers to excitability. "C" refers to conductivity. "D" refers to contractility.
6.   Repolarization of the atria is obscured by the *QRS complex* on the ECG.
7. False The ECG can provide information about the orientation of the heart in the chest, conduction disturbances, electrical effects of medications and electrolytes, the mass of cardiac muscle, and the presence of ischemic damage. The ECG does *not* provide information about the mechanical (contractile) condition of the myocardium. The effectiveness of the heart's mechanical activity is evaluated by assessment of the patient's pulse and blood pressure.
8.   Each small box on ECG paper represents 0.04 sec.
9. A   The correct electrode position for lead V_4 is the left midclavicular line, fifth intercostal space.
10.   The PR segment is used as the baseline from which to evaluate the degree of displacement of the ST segment from the isoelectric line (elevation or depression).
11.   In the majority of the population, the SA and AV nodes are supplied by the *right* coronary artery.
12. A   The epicardium, also known as the visceral pericardium, is the external layer of the heart wall.
13. B   The tricuspid and mitral valves are atrioventricular (AV) valves. The aortic and pulmonary valves are semilunar valves.
14.   The right atrium receives deoxygenated blood from the *superior vena cava*, the *inferior vena cava*, and the *coronary sinus*.
15. D   The anterior surface of the heart consists primarily of the right ventricle.
16. D   Cardiac output is the amount of blood pumped into the aorta each minute by the heart.
17. C   The heart is enclosed in a fibrous sac called the *pericardium*.
18. B   The left atrium receives oxygenated blood from the lungs via the right and left pulmonary veins.
19. B   The chordae tendineae are thin strands of fibrous connective tissue that extend from the AV valves to the papillary muscles that prevent the AV valves from bulging back into the atria during ventricular systole (contraction).
20. B   The coronary arteries originate at the base of the aorta, immediately above the leaflets of the aortic valve.
21. F   The right atrium and right ventricle make up a *low-pressure* pump whose purpose is to pump blood to the pulmonary circulation.
22. A   Norepinephrine is the primary neurotransmitter of the sympathetic division of the autonomic nervous system. Acetylcholine is the primary neurotransmitter for the parasympathetic division.

23. B   Sympathetic stimulation accelerates firing of the SA node, enhances conduction through the AV node, and increases the force of contraction (stroke volume).

24. A   The two primary branches of the left coronary artery are the left anterior descending and the circumflex. Two primary branches of the right coronary artery are the posterior descending and right marginal arteries.

25.   The normal pathway of blood flow through the heart and pulmonary circulation:

1	right atrium	9	left ventricle
8	mitral valve	5	pulmonary arteries
11	aorta	2	tricuspid valve
3	right ventricle	6	pulmonary veins
4	pulmonic valve	10	aortic valve
7	left atrium	12	systemic circulation

26. A   A decrease in myocardial contractility may result from severe hypoxia, decreased pH, hypercapnea (elevated carbon dioxide levels), and medications such as propranolol (Inderal).

27. False   If the systolic blood pressure decreases, the body's normal compensatory response to increase blood pressure is peripheral vasoconstriction, increased heart rate (chronotropy), and increased myocardial contractility (inotropy). These compensatory responses occur because of a reflex sympathetic response.

28. D   Stroke volume is influenced by preload, afterload, and contractility.

29. True   Stimulation of alpha-receptor sites results in constriction of blood vessels in the skin, cerebral, and splanchnic circulation.

30. False   A response by the sympathetic division of the autonomic nervous system is also called an *adrenergic* response. A response by the *parasympathetic* division of the autonomic nervous system is also called a *cholinergic* response.

31. A   The S wave is the first negative deflection after the R wave. The first positive waveform of the cardiac cycle is the P wave. The Q wave is the first negative deflection after the P wave. The R wave is the positive deflection after the Q wave.

32. C   Ventricular rate and rhythm are determined by measuring from R wave to R wave.

33. A   A segment is a line between waveforms. A waveform is recorded as movement away from the baseline in either a positive or negative direction. An interval is a waveform and a segment. A complex consists of several waveforms.

34. D   A delta wave is an ECG characteristic associated with Wolff-Parkinson-White (WPW) syndrome.

35. C   An accelerated junctional rhythm is characterized by a regular ventricular response between 61 to 100 beats/min.

36. A   ECG characteristics of atrial fibrillation:

Rate: Atrial rate usually greater than 400 to 600 beats/min; ventricular rate variable
Rhythm: Ventricular rhythm usually irregularly irregular
P waves: No identifiable P waves; fibrillatory waves present; erratic, wavy baseline
PRI: Not measurable
QRS: Usually less than 0.10 sec but may be widened if an intraventricular conduction defect exists

37. A   Torsades de pointes (TdP) is a type of polymorphic VT associated with a long QT interval. Torsades may be precipitated by slow heart rates and is often associated with drugs or electrolyte disturbances that lengthen the QT interval. A lengthening of the QT interval may be the only warning sign suggesting impending torsades.

38. A   The *first letter* of the code identifies which chamber of the heart is being paced. The *second letter* identifies the chamber of the heart being sensed by the pacemaker. The *third letter* indicates how the pacemaker responds to the sensed event. The *fourth letter* identifies the number of reprogrammable functions available, and the *fifth letter* indicates how the pacemaker will respond to tachydysrhythmias.

39. C   In second-degree AV block, 2:1 conduction, the PR interval remains constant.
40. False   In complete AV block, a secondary pacemaker (either junctional or ventricular) stimulates the ventricles; therefore, the QRS may be narrow or wide depending on the location of the escape pacemaker and the condition of the intraventricular conduction system (narrow QRS = junctional pacemaker, wide QRS = ventricular pacemaker).
41. D   An interpolated PVC is "squeezed" between two regular complexes and does not disturb the underlying rhythm (it does not have a compensatory pause).
42. False   The definition given is that for failure to *capture*. Failure to *pace* is a pacemaker malfunction that occurs when the pacemaker fails to deliver an electrical stimulus or when it fails to deliver the correct number of electrical stimulations per minute. Failure to pace is recognized on the ECG as a absence of pacemaker spikes even though the patient's intrinsic rate is less than that of the pacemaker and there is a return of the underlying rhythm for which the pacemaker was implanted.
43. A   In all types of second-degree AV block (type I, type II, 2:1 conduction) and complete AV block there are more P waves than QRS complexes. Despite the type of block, the P waves occur regularly because the SA node is unaffected by the block; the problem lies in AV conduction.
44.   A PVC is *premature* and occurs before the next expected sinus beat. A ventricular escape beat is *late,* occurring after the next expected sinus beat.
45. A   Ventricular tachycardia is characterized by an essentially regular ventricular rhythm at a rate between 100 to 250 beats/min. P waves may be present or absent; if present they have no set relationship to the QRS complexes, appearing between the QRSs at a rate different from that of the VT. The QRS measures greater than 0.12 sec.

Rhythm Strips

Note: WNL, within normal limits; *UTD,* unable to determine; *bpm,* beats/min

Figure 10-1

Ventricular rhythm:	irregular
Ventricular rate:	75
Atrial rhythm:	irregular
Atrial rate:	75
PRI:	0.16 sec (sinus beats)
QRS:	0.08 sec (sinus beats)
QT:	0.36 sec (sinus beats)

Identification: Sinus rhythm at 75 bpm with frequent uniform PVCs

Figure 10-2

Atrial pacing?	Yes
Ventricular pacing?	Yes
Paced interval:	71

Identification: Normal functioning AV sequential pacemaker

Figure 10-3

Ventricular rhythm:	irregular
Ventricular rate:	43-60
Atrial rhythm:	regular
Atrial rate:	68
PRI:	lengthening
QRS:	0.06 sec
QT:	0.32 sec

Identification: Second-degree AV block type I at 43-60 bpm

Figure 10-4

Ventricular rhythm:	regular
Ventricular rate:	33
Atrial rhythm:	UTD
Atrial rate:	UTD
PRI:	not measurable
QRS:	0.12 sec
QT:	UTD

Identification: Atrial fibrillation with complete AV block; notice the right bundle branch morphology of the QRS complexes

Figure 10-5

Ventricular rhythm:	regular except for the event(s)
Ventricular rate:	136 (sinus beats)
Atrial rhythm:	regular except for the event(s)
Atrial rate:	136 (sinus beats)
PRI:	0.10 sec
QRS:	0.06 sec
QT:	UTD, rate >100 bpm

Identification: Sinus tachycardia at 136 bpm with frequent PJCs (the PJCs are beats 2, 5, 8, and 11 from the left)

Figure 10-6

Ventricular rhythm:	regular
Ventricular rate:	95
Atrial rhythm:	regular
Atrial rate:	95
PRI:	0.16 sec
QRS:	0.08 sec
QT:	WNL

Identification: Sinus rhythm at 95 bpm

Figure 10-7

Ventricular rhythm:	regular
Ventricular rate:	30
Atrial rhythm:	regular
Atrial rate:	68
PRI:	0.28 sec
QRS:	0.16 sec
QT:	UTD

Identification: Second-degree AV block, 2:1 conduction, probably type II; ST segment elevation, hyperacute T waves

Figure 10-8

Ventricular rhythm:	regular (sinus beats)
Ventricular rate:	54
Atrial rhythm:	regular (sinus beats)
Atrial rate:	54
PRI:	0.12 sec (sinus beats)
QRS:	0.06-0.08 sec (sinus beats)
QT:	WNL

Identification: Sinus bradycardia at 54 bpm with ventricular bigeminy; ventricular rate approximately 100 bpm if PVCs counted in the rate

Figure 10-9

Ventricular rhythm:	regular
Ventricular rate:	98
Atrial rhythm:	regular
Atrial rate:	98
PRI:	0.16 sec
QRS:	0.04-0.06 sec
QT:	0.32 sec

Identification: Sinus rhythm at 98 bpm; ST segment elevation

Figure 10-10

Ventricular rhythm:	regular
Ventricular rate:	41
Atrial rhythm:	regular
Atrial rate:	41
PRI:	0.36 sec
QRS:	0.08 sec
QT:	WNL

Identification: Sinus bradycardia at 41 bpm with first-degree AV block

Figure 10-11

Ventricular rhythm:	regular except for event
Ventricular rate:	93
Atrial rhythm:	regular except for event
Atrial rate:	93
PRI:	0.16 sec
QRS:	0.04 sec
QT:	WNL

Identification: Sinus rhythm at 93 bpm with a PAC (seventh beat from the left is the PAC)

Figure 10-12

Atrial pacing?	No
Ventricular pacing?	Yes
Paced interval:	80

Identification: Ventricular-paced rhythm with pacemaker malfunction (loss of capture)

Figure 10-13

Ventricular rhythm:	regular except for the event
Ventricular rate:	71 (sinus beats)
Atrial rhythm:	regular except for the event
Atrial rate:	71
PRI:	0.24 sec
QRS:	0.08 sec
QT:	WNL

Identification: Sinus rhythm at 71 bpm with a first-degree AV block, 3.36 period of sinus arrest and a junctional escape beat; ST segment depression

Figure 10-14

Ventricular rhythm:	irregular
Ventricular rate:	68-150
Atrial rhythm:	irregular
Atrial rate:	UTD
PRI:	UTD
QRS:	0.08 sec
QT:	UTD

Identification: Atrial flutter (atrial fib/flutter) with a ventricular response of 68-150 bpm

Figure 10-15

Ventricular rhythm:	regular
Ventricular rate:	56
Atrial rhythm:	UTD
Atrial rate:	UTD
PRI:	UTD
QRS:	0.12 sec
QT:	0.44 sec

Identification: Accelerated idioventricular rhythm (AIVR) at 56 bpm; ST segment depression

Figure 10-16

Ventricular rhythm:	irregular
Ventricular rate:	47-79
Atrial rhythm:	regular
Atrial rate:	88
PRI:	lengthening
QRS:	0.06 sec
QT:	UTD

Identification: Second-degree AV block type I with a ventricular response of 47-79 bpm

Figure 10-17

Ventricular rhythm:	regular except for events
Ventricular rate:	117
Atrial rhythm:	regular except for events
Atrial rate:	117
PRI:	0.16 sec
QRS:	0.12 sec
QT:	UTD, rate >100 bpm

Identification: Sinus tachycardia at 117 bpm with 3 PACs (beats 2, 8 and 10 from the left are PACs) and a wide QRS, ST segment elevation

Figure 10-18

Ventricular rhythm:	regular (junctional beats)
Ventricular rate:	115-214
Atrial rhythm:	UTD (junctional beats)
Atrial rate:	UTD
PRI:	not measurable in junctional beats
QRS:	0.06 sec
QT:	WNL

Identification: Sinus rhythm, changing to an accelerated junction rhythm at 79 bpm, back to a sinus rhythm

Figure 10-19

Ventricular rhythm:	UTD
Ventricular rate:	UTD
Atrial rhythm:	UTD
Atrial rate:	UTD
PRI:	UTD
QRS:	UTD
QT:	UTD

Identification: Ventricular fibrillation

Figure 10-20

Ventricular rhythm:	regular
Ventricular rate:	40
Atrial rhythm:	regular
Atrial rate:	40
PRI:	0.16 sec
QRS:	0.08 sec
QT:	WNL

Identification: Sinus bradycardia at 40 bpm; ST segment depression, inverted T waves

Figure 10-21

Ventricular rhythm:	regular except for the event
Ventricular rate:	93
Atrial rhythm:	regular except for the event
Atrial rate:	93
PRI:	0.16 sec
QRS:	0.04 sec
QT:	UTD

Identification: Sinus rhythm at 93 bpm with a PAC (third beat from left), ST segment elevation

Figure 10-22

Ventricular rhythm:	regular
Ventricular rate:	60
Atrial rhythm:	regular
Atrial rate:	60
PRI:	0.20 sec (sinus beats)
QRS:	0.08 sec (sinus beats)
QT:	0.36 sec (sinus beats)

Identification: Sinus rhythm at 60 bpm with an R-on-T interpolated PVC

Figure 10-23

Ventricular rhythm:	regular
Ventricular rate:	50
Atrial rhythm:	regular
Atrial rate:	167
PRI:	variable
QRS:	0.06 sec
QT:	WNL

Identification: Complete AV block at 50 bpm, ST segment elevation

Figure 10-24

Ventricular rhythm:	essentially regular
Ventricular rate:	94
Atrial rhythm:	UTD
Atrial rate:	UTD
PRI:	UTD
QRS:	0.12 sec
QT:	UTD

Identification: Accelerated idioventricular rhythm (AIVR) at 94 bpm, ST segment depression (lead III)

Figure 10-25

Ventricular rhythm:	irregular
Ventricular rate:	19-26
Atrial rhythm:	UTD
Atrial rate:	UTD
PRI:	UTD
QRS:	0.04 sec
QT:	0.44 sec

Identification: Junctional escape rhythm (junctional bradycardia) at 19-26 bpm

Figure 10-26

Ventricular rhythm:	irregular
Ventricular rate:	54-88
Atrial rhythm:	irregular
Atrial rate:	54-88
PRI:	0.12 sec
QRS:	0.08 sec
QT:	WNL

Identification: Sinus arrhythmia at 54-88 bpm

Figure 10-27

Ventricular rhythm:	regular
Ventricular rate:	40
Atrial rhythm:	regular
Atrial rate:	83
PRI:	0.24 sec
QRS:	0.10 sec
QT:	WNL

Identification: Second-degree AV block, 2:1 conduction, probably type I at 40 bpm, ST segment depression

Figure 10-28

Ventricular rhythm:	regular
Ventricular rate:	<25
Atrial rhythm:	UTD
Atrial rate:	UTD
PRI:	UTD
QRS:	0.16 sec
QT:	UTD

Identification: Idioventricular rhythm at <25 bpm (may also be called an *agonal rhythm* when ventricular rate is <20 bpm)

Figure 10-29

Atrial pacing?	No
Ventricular pacing?	Yes
Paced interval:	71

Identification: 100% ventricular-paced rhythm; underlying rhythm is a complete AV block

Figure 10-30

Ventricular rhythm:	regular except for events
Ventricular rate:	83 (sinus beats)
Atrial rhythm:	regular except for events
Atrial rate:	83 (sinus beats)
PRI:	0.16 sec
QRS:	0.04-0.08 sec
QT:	WNL

Identification: Sinus rhythm at 83 bpm with frequent PACs (atrial bigeminy), ST segment depression, inverted T waves (beats 3, 5, 7, and 9 are PACs)

Figure 10-31

Ventricular rhythm:	irregular
Ventricular rate:	230-300
Atrial rhythm:	UTD
Atrial rate:	UTD
PRI:	UTD
QRS:	variable
QT:	TD

Identification: Sinus (?) beat with an R-on-T PVC, followed by torsades de pointes (TdP)

Figure 10-32

Ventricular rhythm:	irregular
Ventricular rate:	0-75
Atrial rhythm:	irregular
Atrial rate:	0-75
PRI:	0.16 sec
QRS:	0.08 sec
QT:	UTD

Identification: Sinus rhythm at approximately 75 bpm with a 4.0-sec period of sinus arrest

Figure 10-33

Ventricular rhythm:	regular except for the event
Ventricular rate:	115 (sinus beats)
Atrial rhythm:	regular except for the event
Atrial rate:	115 (sinus beats)
PRI:	0.16 sec
QRS:	0.06 sec
QT:	UTD, rate >100 bpm

Identification: Sinus tachycardia at 115 bpm with a PJC (fifth beat is the PJC)

Figure 10-34

Ventricular rhythm:	irregular
Ventricular rate:	50-94
Atrial rhythm:	regular
Atrial rate:	94
PRI:	lengthening
QRS:	0.10 sec
QT:	WNL

Identification: Second-degree AV block type I at 50-94 bpm, ST segment elevation

Figure 10-35

Ventricular rhythm:	regular
Ventricular rate:	76
Atrial rhythm:	regular
Atrial rate:	300
PRI:	UTD
QRS:	0.04 sec
QT:	UTD

Identification: Atrial flutter at 76 bpm

Figure 10-36

Ventricular rhythm:	regular
Ventricular rate:	180
Atrial rhythm:	UTD
Atrial rate:	UTD
PRI: UTD	
QRS:	0.04 sec
QT:	UTD, rate >100 bpm

Identification: Supraventricular tachycardia at 180 bpm; ST segment elevation

Figure 10-37

Ventricular rhythm:	regular except for event(s)
Ventricular rate:	102
Atrial rhythm:	regular except for event(s)
Atrial rate:	102
PRI:	0.16 sec (sinus beats)
QRS:	0.06-0.08 sec (sinus beats)
QT:	UTD, rate >100 bpm

Identification: Sinus tachycardia at 102 bpm with frequent uniform PVCs; ST segment elevation

Figure 10-38

Ventricular rhythm:	irregular
Ventricular rate:	107 (sinus beats)
Atrial rhythm:	irregular
Atrial rate:	107 (sinus beats)
PRI:	0.16 sec
QRS:	0.08 sec
QT:	UTD, rate >100 bpm

Identification: Sinus tachycardia at 107 bpm with a junctional escape beat (third beat from the left) and a nonconducted PAC (buried in the T wave of the fourth beat from the left); hyperacute T waves

Figure 10-39

Ventricular rhythm:	regular except for events
Ventricular rate:	60 (sinus beats)
Atrial rhythm:	regular except for events
Atrial rate:	60 (sinus beats)
PRI:	0.16-0.18 sec
QRS:	0.08 sec
QT:	0.56 sec

Identification: Sinus rhythm at 60 bpm with two nonconducted (blocked) PACs, ST segment depression (the nonconducted PACS can be seen after second and fifth QRS complexes)

Figure 10-40

Ventricular rhythm:	irregular
Ventricular rate:	27-80
Atrial rhythm:	irregular
Atrial rate:	27-80
PRI:	0.16 sec (sinus beats)
QRS:	0.04-0.06 sec (sinus beats)
QT:	WNL (sinus beats)

Identification: Sinus rhythm at 80 bpm with frequent episodes of paired PVCs (couplets)

Figure 10-41

Ventricular rhythm:	regular
Ventricular rate:	100
Atrial rhythm:	regular
Atrial rate:	100
PRI:	0.16 sec
QRS:	0.14 sec
QT:	0.40 sec

Identification: Sinus rhythm with a wide QRS at 100 bpm; ST segment depression, inverted T waves

Figure 10-42

Ventricular rhythm:	regular except for the event(s)
Ventricular rate:	75
Atrial rhythm:	regular except for the event(s)
Atrial rate:	75
PRI:	0.16 sec
QRS:	0.08 sec
QT:	WNL

Identification: Sinus rhythm at 75 bpm with two R-on-T PVCs

Figure 10-43

Ventricular rhythm:	regular
Ventricular rate:	79
Atrial rhythm:	UTD
Atrial rate:	UTD
PRI:	UTD
QRS:	0.08 sec
QT:	WNL

Identification: Accelerated junctional rhythm at 79 bpm; ST segment depression; inverted T waves

Figure 10-44

Ventricular rhythm:	regular except for the event
Ventricular rate:	90
Atrial rhythm:	regular except for the event
Atrial rate:	90
PRI:	0.20 sec
QRS:	0.06 sec
QT:	WNL

Identification: Sinus rhythm at 90 bpm with an episode of sinoatrial (SA) block

Figure 10-45

Ventricular rhythm:	regular
Ventricular rate:	168
Atrial rhythm:	UTD
Atrial rate:	UTD
PRI:	not measurable
QRS:	0.08 sec
QT:	UTD, rate >100 bpm

Identification: SVT at 168 bpm, ST segment depression

Figure 10-46

Ventricular rhythm:	irregular
Ventricular rate:	<20-60
Atrial rhythm:	regular
Atrial rate:	60
PRI:	0.16 sec
QRS:	0.16 sec
QT:	0.44 sec

Identification: Second-degree AV block type II at <20-60 bpm, ST segment elevation

Figure 10-47

Ventricular rhythm:	None
Ventricular rate:	None
Atrial rhythm:	Irregular
Atrial rate:	Varies, approximately 40
PRI:	None
QRS:	None
QT:	None

Identification: P-wave asystole

Figure 10-48

Ventricular rhythm:	regular except for the event
Ventricular rate:	90
Atrial rhythm:	regular except for the event
Atrial rate:	90
PRI:	0.16 sec
QRS:	0.10 sec
QT:	WNL

Identification: Sinus rhythm at 90 bpm with a PJC (seventh beat is the PJC)

Figure 10-49

Ventricular rhythm:	regular
Ventricular rate:	86
Atrial rhythm:	regular
Atrial rate:	86
PRI:	0.28 sec
QRS:	0.06 sec
QT:	UTD

Identification: Sinus rhythm at 86 bpm with a first-degree AV block, ST segment elevation

Figure 10-50

Ventricular rhythm:	regular
Ventricular rate:	44
Atrial rhythm:	regular
Atrial rate:	44
PRI:	0.16 sec
QRS:	0.06 sec
QT:	WNL

Identification: Sinus bradycardia at 44 bpm, ST segment depression; note the small upright U waves following each T wave

Figure 10-51

Ventricular rhythm:	regular
Ventricular rate:	56
Atrial rhythm:	regular
Atrial rate:	107
PRI:	0.16 sec
QRS:	0.08 sec
QT:	WNL

Identification: Second-degree AV block, 2:1 conduction, probably type I at 56 bpm

Figure 10-52

Ventricular rhythm:	irregular
Ventricular rate:	47-107
Atrial rhythm:	UTD
Atrial rate:	UTD
PRI:	UTD
QRS:	0.08 sec
QT:	0.32 sec

Identification: Atrial fibrillation at 47-107 bpm with a PVC, ST segment elevation

Figure 10-53

Atrial pacing?	Yes
Ventricular pacing?	Yes
Paced interval:	80

Identification: Normal functioning AV sequential pacemaker at 80 bpm

Figure 10-54

Ventricular rhythm: regular except for the events
Ventricular rate: 88 (sinus beats)
Atrial rhythm: regular except for the events
Atrial rate: 88 (sinus beats)
PRI: 0.20 sec (sinus beats)
QRS: 0.08 sec (sinus beats)
QT: 0.40 sec (sinus beats)

Identification: Sinus rhythm at 88 bpm with a PVC and run of VT, ST segment depression, inverted T waves

Figure 10-55

Ventricular rhythm: regular
Ventricular rate: 58
Atrial rhythm: regular
Atrial rate: 115
PRI: 0.16 sec
QRS: 0.16 sec
QT: WNL

Identification: Second-degree AV block, 2:1 conduction, probably type II at 58 bpm

Figure 10-56

Ventricular rhythm: regular
Ventricular rate: 80
Atrial rhythm: regular
Atrial rate: 80
PRI: 0.16 sec
QRS: 0.04 sec
QT: UTD

Identification: Sinus rhythm at 80 bpm, ST segment elevation

Figure 10-57

Ventricular rhythm: regular
Ventricular rate: 160
Atrial rhythm: regular
Atrial rate: 160
PRI: 0.10 sec
QRS: 0.04 sec
QT: UTD, rate >100 bpm

Identification: Sinus tachycardia at 160 bpm

Figure 10-58

Atrial pacing?   No
Ventricular pacing?   Yes
Paced interval: 71

Identification: Pacemaker malfunction (failure to sense); underlying rhythm is a sinus rhythm at 88 bpm with a PVC; note the pacer spikes in the T waves of the second and eighth beats from the left

Figure 10-59

Ventricular rhythm: irregular
Ventricular rate: 96-214
Atrial rhythm: irregular
Atrial rate: 96-214
PRI: 0.16 sec (sinus beats)
QRS: 0.08 sec
QT: 0.28 sec

Identification: Sinus rhythm at 96 bpm with a PAC precipitating a run of PSVT at 214 bpm, back to a sinus rhythm at 96 bpm

Figure 10-60

Ventricular rhythm: regular except for the events (PVCs)
Ventricular rate: 92 (sinus beats)
Atrial rhythm: regular except for the events (PVCs)
Atrial rate: 92 (sinus beats)
PRI: 0.20 sec (sinus beats)
QRS: 0.06 sec (sinus beats)
QT: 0.32 sec (sinus beats)

Identification: Sinus rhythm at 92 bpm with frequent uniform R-on-T PVCs

a wave: Atrial-paced event; the atrial stimulus or the point in the intrinsic atrial depolarization (P wave) at which atrial sensing occurs; analogous to the P wave of intrinsic waveforms

AA interval: Interval between two consecutive atrial stimuli, with or without an interceding ventricular event; analogous to the P-P interval of intrinsic waveforms

AV interval: In dual-chamber pacing, the length of time between an atrial-sensed or atrial-paced event and the delivery of a ventricular pacing stimulus; analogous to the PR interval of intrinsic waveforms

aberrant: Abnormal

absolute refractory period: Corresponds with the onset of the QRS complex to approximately the peak of the T wave; cardiac cells cannot be stimulated to conduct an electrical impulse, no matter how strong the stimulus

accelerated idioventricular rhythm (AIVR): Dysrhythmia originating in the ventricles with a rate between 41 and 100 beats/min

accelerated junctional rhythm: Dysrhythmia originating in the AV junction with a rate between 61 and 100 beats/min

accessory pathway: Extra muscle bundle consisting of working myocardial tissue that forms a connection between the atria and ventricles outside the normal conduction system

action potential: Reflection of the difference in the concentration of ions across a cell membrane at any given time

acute coronary syndromes: Term used to refer to patients presenting with ischemic chest pain; acute coronary syndromes consist of three major syndromes: unstable angina, non-ST-segment elevation MI, and ST-segment elevation MI

adrenergic: Having the characteristics of the sympathetic division of the autonomic nervous system

afterload: Pressure or resistance against which the ventricles must pump to eject blood

agonal rhythm: Dysrhythmia similar in appearance to an idioventricular rhythm but occurring at a rate of less than 20 beats/min; dying heart

amplitude: Height (voltage) of a waveform on the ECG

angina: Chest pain of sudden onset that may occur because the increased oxygen demand of the heart temporarily exceeds the blood supply

aortic valve: Semilunar valve located between the left ventricle and aorta

apex of the heart: Lower portion of the heart, tip of the ventricles (approximately the level of the fifth left intercostal space); points leftward, downward, and forward

arrhythmia: Term often used interchangeably with *dysrhythmia*; any disturbance or abnormality in a normal rhythmic pattern; any cardiac rhythm other than a sinus rhythm

artifact: Distortion of an ECG tracing by electrical activity that is noncardiac in origin (e.g., electrical interference, poor electrical conduction, patient movement)

asynchronous pacemaker: Fixed-rate pacemaker that continuously discharges at a preset rate regardless of the patient's intrinsic activity

asystole: Absence of cardiac electrical activity viewed as a straight (isoelectric) line on the ECG

atria: Two upper chambers of the heart (singular, *atrium*)

atrial kick: Blood pushed into the ventricles because of atrial contraction

atrial pacing: Pacing system with a lead attached to the right atrium, designed to correct abnormalities in the SA node (sick sinus syndrome)

atrial tachycardia: Three or more sequential premature atrial complexes (PACs) occurring at a rate of more than 100 beats/min

atrioventricular (AV) valve: Valve located between each atrium and ventricle; the tricuspid separates the right atrium from the right ventricle, the mitral (bicuspid) separates the left atrium from the left ventricle

augmented lead: Leads aVR, aVL, and aVF; these leads record the difference in electrical potential at one location relative to zero potential rather than relative to the electrical potential of another extremity, as in the bipolar leads

automatic interval: Period, expressed in milliseconds, between two consecutively paced events in the same cardiac chamber without an intervening sensed event (e.g., AA interval, VV interval); also known as the *demand interval, basic interval,* or *pacing interval.*

automaticity: Ability of cardiac pacemaker cells to spontaneously initiate an electrical impulse without being stimulated from another source (such as a nerve)

AV dissociation: Any dysrhythmia in which the atria and ventricles beat independently (e.g., ventricular tachycardia, complete AV block)

AV junction: AV node and the bundle of His

AV node: Specialized cells located in the lower portion of the right atrium; delays the electrical impulse in order to allow the atria to contract and complete filling of the ventricles

AV sequential pacemaker: Type of dual-chamber pacemaker that stimulates first the atrium, then the ventricle, mimicking normal cardiac physiology

axis: Imaginary line joining the positive and negative electrodes of a lead

base of the heart: Top of the heart located at approximately the level of the second intercostal space

baseline: Straight line recorded on ECG graph paper when no electrical activity is detected

base rate: Rate at which the pulse generator of a pacemaker paces when no intrinsic activity is detected; expressed in pulses/min (ppm)

bifascicular block: Block in two divisions of the bundle branches; although this term may be used to describe a block in both the anterior and posterior branches of the left bundle branch, it is more commonly used to describe a combination of a right bundle branch block and either a left anterior fascicular block (LAFB) or a left posterior fascicular block (LPFB)

bigeminy: Dysrhythmia in which every other beat is a premature ectopic beat

biphasic: Waveform that is partly positive and partly negative

bipolar limb lead: ECG lead consisting of a positive and negative electrode; a pacing lead with two electrical poles that are external from the pulse generator; the negative pole is located at the extreme distal tip of the pacing lead; the positive pole is located several millimeters proximal to the negative electrode; the stimulating pulse is delivered through the negative electrode

blocked PAC (nonconducted PAC): Premature atrial complex that is not followed by a QRS complex

blood pressure: Force exerted by the circulating blood volume on the walls of the arteries; blood pressure is equal to cardiac output times peripheral resistance

bpm: Beats/min; the abbreviation bpm usually refers to an intrinsic heart rate, while pulses/min (ppm) usually refers to a paced rate

bradycardia: Heart rate slower than 60 beats/min (*brady,* slow)

bundle branch block (BBB): Abnormal conduction of an electrical impulse through either the right or left bundle branches

bundle of His: Cardiac fibers located in the upper portion of the interventricular septum; connects the AV node with the two bundle branches

burst: Three or more sequential ectopic beats; also referred to as a "salvo" or "run"

bypass tract: Term used when one end of an accessory pathway is attached to normal conductive tissue

calibration: Regulation of an ECG machine's stylus sensitivity so that a 1 mV electrical signal will produce a deflection measuring exactly 10 mm

capacitor: Device that can store an electrical charge

capture: Ability of a pacing stimulus to successfully depolarize the cardiac chamber that is being paced; with one-to-one capture, each pacing stimulus results in depolarization of the appropriate chamber

cardiac arrest: Clinical death characterized by cessation of pulse and respiration

cardiac cycle: Period from the beginning of one heart beat to the beginning of the next one; normally consisting of PQRST waves, complexes, and intervals

cardiac index: Measure of a patient's cardiac output per square meter of body surface area (BSA)

cardiac output: Amount of blood pumped into the aorta each minute by the heart

carotid sinus pressure: Type of vagal maneuver in which pressure is applied to the carotid sinus for a brief period to slow conduction through the AV node

catecholamines: Natural chemicals produced by the body that have sympathetic actions; epinephrine, norepinephrine, dopamine

cholinergic: Having the characteristics of the parasympathetic division of the autonomic nervous system

chordae tendineae: Thin strands of fibrous connective tissue that extend from the AV valves to the papillary muscles that prevent the AV valves from bulging back into the atria during ventricular systole (contraction)

chronotropism: Refers to a change in heart rate; a positive chronotropic effect refers to an increase in heart rate; a negative chronotropic effect refers to a decrease in heart rate

circumflex artery: Division of the left coronary artery

coarse ventricular fibrillation: Ventricular fibrillation with fibrillatory waves greater than 3 mm in height

compensatory pause: Pause is termed *compensatory* (or *complete*) if the normal beat following a premature complex occurs when expected

complex: Several waveforms

conductivity: Ability of a cardiac cell to receive an electrical stimulus and conduct that impulse to an adjacent cardiac cell

contractility: Ability of cardiac cells to shorten, causing cardiac muscle contraction in response to an electrical stimulus

coronary sinus: Outlet that drains five coronary veins into the right atrium

couplet: Two consecutive premature complexes

coupling interval: Interval between an ectopic beat and the preceding beat of the underlying rhythm

cycle length: Term used for the period between any one type of event and the next

event of the same type, usually expressed in milliseconds

defibrillation: Therapeutic use of electric current to terminate lethal cardiac dysrhythmias

delta wave: Slurring of the beginning portion of the QRS complex, caused by preexcitation

demand interval: Period, expressed in milliseconds, between two consecutively paced events in the same cardiac chamber without an intervening sensed event (e.g., AA interval, VV interval); also known as the *basic interval* or *pacing interval*

demand pacemaker: Synchronous pacemaker that discharges only when the patient's heart rate drops below the preset rate for the pacemaker

depolarization: Movement of ions across a cell membrane, causing the inside of the cell to become more positive; an electrical event expected to result in contraction

dextrocardia: Location of the heart in the right thorax because of a congenital defect or displacement by disease

diastole: Phase of the cardiac cycle in which the atria and ventricles relax between contractions and blood enters these chambers; when the term is used without reference to a specific chamber of the heart, the term implies ventricular diastole

dilatation: Increase in the diameter of a chamber of the heart caused by volume overload

diphasic: Waveform that is partly positive and partly negative

dual-chamber pacemaker: Pacemaker that stimulates the atrium and ventricle

dyspnea: Shortness of breath or difficulty breathing

dysrhythmia: Any disturbance or abnormality in a normal rhythmic pattern; any cardiac rhythm other than a sinus rhythm

ectopic: Impulse(s) originating from a source other than the sinoatrial node

electrical axis: Direction (or angle in degrees) in which the main vector of depolarization is pointed

electrodes: Adhesive pads that contain a conductive gel, applied at specific locations on the patient's chest wall and extremities and connected by means of cables to an electrocardiograph

electrolyte: Element or compound that, when melted or dissolved in water or another solvent, breaks into ions (atoms able to carry an electric charge)

endocardium: Innermost layer of the heart that lines the inside of the myocardium and covers the heart valves

enhanced automaticity: Abnormal condition in which cardiac cells not normally associated with the property of automaticity begin to depolarize spontaneously or when escape pacemaker sites increase their firing rate beyond that considered normal

enlargement: Term that implies the presence of dilatation or hypertrophy or both

epicardium: Also known as the visceral pericardium; the external layer of the heart wall that covers the heart muscle

escape: Term used when the sinus node slows down or fails to initiate depolarization and a lower pacemaker site spontaneously produces electrical impulses, assuming responsibility for pacing the heart

escape interval: Time measured between a sensed cardiac event and the next pacemaker output

excitability: Ability of cardiac muscle cells to respond to an outside stimulus

extrasystole: Premature complex

extreme right axis deviation: Current flow in the direction opposite of normal (−91 to −179 degrees)

f waves: Fibrillation waves; irregularly shaped atrial waves associated with atrial fibrillation; occurring at a rate of 400 to 600 beats/min

F waves: Flutter waves; atrial waves associated with atrial flutter; usually shaped like the teeth of a saw or a picket fence

fascicle: Small bundle of nerve fibers

fine ventricular fibrillation: Ventricular fibrillation with fibrillatory waves less than 3 mm in height

fixed-rate pacemaker: Asynchronous pacemaker that continuously discharges at a preset rate regardless of the patient's heart rate

fusion beat: Beat that occurs because of simultaneous activation of one cardiac chamber by two sites (foci); in pacing, the ECG waveform that results when an intrinsic depolarization and a pacing stimulus occur simultaneously and both contribute to depolarization of that cardiac chamber

great vessels: Pulmonary arteries, pulmonary veins, aorta, superior, and inferior vena cavae

ground electrode: Third ECG electrode (the first and second are the positive and negative electrodes), which minimizes electrical activity from other sources

His-Purkinje system: Portion of the conduction system consisting of the bundle of His, bundle branches, and Purkinje fibers

hypertrophy: Increase in the thickness of a heart chamber because of chronic pressure overload

incomplete compensatory pause: Pause is termed *incomplete* (or *noncompensatory*) if the normal beat following the premature complex occurs before it was expected

indeterminate axis deviation: Current flow in the direction opposite of normal (−91 to −179 degrees)

infarction: Necrosis of tissue because of an inadequate blood supply

inherent: Natural, intrinsic

inhibition: Pacemaker response in which the output pulse is suppressed (inhibited) when an intrinsic event is sensed

inotropic effect: Refers to a change in myocardial contractility

interpolated PVC: PVC that occurs between two normal QRS complexes and that does not interrupt the underlying rhythm

interval: Waveform and a segment; in pacing, the period, measured in milliseconds, between any two designated cardiac events

intrinsic rate: Rate at which a pacemaker of the heart normally generates impulses

ion: Electrically charged particle

ischemia: Decreased supply of oxygenated blood to a body part or organ

isoelectric line: Absence of electrical activity observed on the ECG as a straight line

J point: Point where the QRS complex and ST segment meet

junctional escape rhythm: Dysrhythmia originating in the AV junction that occurs when the sinoatrial node fails to pace the heart or AV conduction fails; characterized by a rhythmic rate of 40 to 60 beats/min

junctional tachycardia: Dysrhythmia originating in the AV junction with a ventricular response greater than 100 beats/min

KVO: Abbreviation meaning "keep the vein open"; also known as *TKO*, "to keep open"

LBBB: Left bundle branch block

lead: Electrical connection attached to the body to record electrical activity

left anterior descending artery: Division of the left coronary artery

left axis deviation: Current flow to the left of normal (−1 to −90 degrees)

Lown-Ganong-Levine syndrome (LGL): Type of preexcitation syndrome in which part or all of the AV conduction system is bypassed by an abnormal AV connection from the atrial muscle to the bundle of His; characterized by a short PR interval (usually less than 0.12 sec) and a normal QRS duration

mean axis: Average direction of a mean vector; the mean axis is only identified in the frontal plane

mean P vector: Average magnitude and direction of both right and left atrial depolarization

mean vector: Average of depolarization waves in one portion of the heart

mean QRS vector: Average magnitude and direction of both right and left ventricular depolarization

mediastinum: Located in the middle of the thoracic cavity; contains the heart, great vessels, trachea, and esophagus, among other structures; extends from the sternum to the vertebral column

membrane potential: Difference in electrical charge across the cell membrane

milliampere (mA): Unit of measure of electrical current needed to elicit depolarization of the myocardium

monofascicular block: Block in only one of the fascicles of the bundle branches

monomorphic: Having the same shape

multiformed atrial rhythm: Cardiac dysrhythmia that occurs because of impulses originating from various sites, including the sinoatrial node, the atria, and/or the AV junction; requires at least three different P waves, seen in the same lead, for proper diagnosis

mV: Abbreviation for millivolt

myocardial cells: Working cells of the myocardium that contain contractile filaments and form the muscular layer of the atrial walls and the thicker muscular layer of the ventricular walls

myocardial infarction (MI): Necrosis of some mass of the heart muscle caused by an inadequate blood supply

myocardium: Middle and thickest layer of the heart; contains the cardiac muscle fibers that cause contraction of the heart and contains the conduction system and blood supply

myofibril: Slender striated strand of muscle tissue

nodal: Term formerly used for junctional beats or rhythms

no man's land (extreme right axis deviation): Current flow in the direction opposite of normal (−91 to −179 degrees)

noncompensatory pause: Pause is termed *noncompensatory* (or *incomplete*) if the normal beat following the premature complex occurs before it was expected

nonconducted PAC (blocked PAC): Premature atrial complex that is not followed by a QRS complex

nontransmural infarction: Myocardial infarction that is classified as either **subendocardial,** involving the endocardium and the myocardium, or **subepicardial,** involving the myocardium and the epicardium

output: Electrical stimulus delivered by a pacemaker's pulse generator, usually defined in terms of pulse amplitude (volts) and pulse width (milliseconds)

overdrive pacing: Pacing the heart at a rate faster than the rate of the tachycardia

PAC: Abbreviation for premature atrial complex

pacemaker: Artificial pulse generator that delivers an electrical current to the heart to stimulate depolarization

pacemaker cells: Specialized cells of the heart's electrical conduction system, capable of spontaneously generating and conducting electrical impulses

pacemaker generator (pulse generator): Power source that houses the battery and controls for regulating a pacemaker

pacemaker spike: Vertical line on the ECG that indicates the pacemaker has discharged

pacemaker syndrome: Adverse clinical signs and symptoms that limit a patient's everyday functioning, occurring in the setting of an electrically normal pacing system; pacemaker syndrome is most commonly associated with a loss of AV synchrony (e.g., VVI pacing) but may also occur because of an inappropriate AV interval or inappropriate rate modulation

pacing interval: Period, expressed in milliseconds, between two consecutively paced events in the same cardiac chamber without an intervening sensed event (e.g., AA interval, VV interval); also known as the *demand interval* or *basic interval*

pacing system analyzer (PSA): External testing and measuring device capable of pacing the heart during pacemaker implantation and used to determine appropriate pulse generator settings for the individual patient (e.g., *pacing threshold, lead impedance, pulse amplitude*)

paired beats: Two consecutive premature complexes

papillary muscles: Projections of myocardium found on the ventricular walls; during ventricular contraction the papillary muscles contract, pulling on the chordae tendineae, preventing inversion of the AV valves into the atria

parameter: Value that can be measured and sometimes changed, either indirectly or directly; in pacing, parameter refers to a value that influences the function of the pacemaker (e.g., sensitivity, amplitude, mode)

paroxysmal: Term used to describe the sudden onset or cessation of a dysrhythmia

paroxysmal atrial tachycardia (PAT): Atrial tachycardia that starts or ends suddenly

Paroxysmal supraventricular tachycardia (PSVT): Term used to describe supraventricular tachycardia that starts and ends suddenly

pericardium: Protective sac that surrounds the heart

peripheral resistance: Resistance to the flow of blood determined by blood vessel diameter and the tone of the vascular musculature

PJC: Premature junctional complex

polarized state: Period of time following repolarization of a myocardial cell (also called the *resting state*) when the outside of the cell is positive and the interior of the cell is negative

polymorphic: Varying in shape

ppm: Abbreviation for pulses/min; ppm usually refers to a paced rate, while beats/min (bpm) refers to an intrinsic heart rate

preexcitation: Term used to describe rhythms that originate from above the ventricles but in which the impulse travels via a pathway other than the AV node and bundle of His; thus the supraventricular impulse excites the ventricles earlier than normal

preload: Force exerted by the blood on the walls of the ventricles at the end of diastole

premature complex: Early beat occurring before the next expected beat

PR interval: P wave plus the PR segment; reflects depolarization of the right and left atria (P wave) and the spread of the impulse through the AV node, bundle of His, right and left bundle branches, and the Purkinje fibers (PR segment)

prophylaxis: Preventive treatment

pulse generator: Power source that houses the battery and controls for regulating a pacemaker

pulseless electrical activity (PEA): Organized electrical activity observed on a cardiac monitor (other than VT or VF) without the patient having a palpable pulse

Purkinje fibers: Elaborate web of fibers distributed throughout the ventricular myocardium

PVC: Premature ventricular complex

P wave: The first wave in the cardiac cycle; represents atrial depolarization and the spread of the electrical impulse throughout the right and left atria

QRS complex: Several waveforms (Q wave, R wave, and S wave) that represent the spread of an electrical impulse through the ventricles (ventricular depolarization)

quadrigeminy: Dysrhythmia in which every fourth beat is a premature ectopic beat

R wave: On an EGG, the first positive deflection in the QRS complex, representing ventricular depolarization; in pacing, R wave refers to the entire QRS complex, denoting an intrinsic ventricular event

rate modulation: Ability of a pacemaker to increase the pacing rate in response to physical activity or metabolic demand; some type of physiologic sensor is used by the pacemaker to determine the need for an increased pacing rate; also known as *rate adaptation* or *rate response*

RBBB: Right bundle branch block

reentry: Propagation of an impulse through tissue already activated by that same impulse

refractoriness: Term used to describe the extent to which a cell is able to respond to a stimulus

relative refractory period: Corresponds with the downslope of the T wave; cardiac cells can be stimulated to depolarize if the stimulus is strong enough

repolarization: Movement of ions across a cell membrane in which the inside of the cell is restored to its negative charge

retrograde: Moving backward; moving in the opposite direction to that which is considered normal

right axis deviation: Current flow to the right of normal (+90 to +180 degrees)

run: Three or more sequential ectopic beats; also referred to as a "salvo" or "burst"

RV interval: Period from the intrinsic ventricular event and the ventricular-paced event that follows; the pacemaker's escape interval

salvo: Three or more sequential ectopic beats; also referred to as a "run" or "burst"

sarcolemma: Membrane that covers smooth, striated, and cardiac muscle fibers

sarcomere: Smallest functional unit of a myofibril

sarcoplasm: Semi-fluid cytoplasm of muscle cells

sarcoplasmic reticulum: Network of tubules and sacs that plays an important role in muscle contraction and relaxation by releasing and storing calcium ions

segment: Line between waveforms; named by the waveform that precedes or follows it

semilunar valves: Valves shaped like half moons that separate the ventricles from the aorta and pulmonary artery

sensing: Ability of a pacemaker to recognize and respond to intrinsic electrical activity

septum: Partition

sick sinus syndrome: Term used to describe a sinus node dysfunction that may be manifested as severe sinus bradycardia, sinus arrest or sinus block, or bradycardia-tachycardia syndrome

sinoatrial node: Normal pacemaker of the heart that normally discharges at a rhythmic rate of 60 to 100 beats/min

sinus arrhythmia: Dysrhythmia originating in the sinoatrial node that occurs when the SA node discharges irregularly; sinus arrhythmia is a normal phenomenon associated with the phases of respiration and changes in intrathoracic pressure

sinus bradycardia: Dysrhythmia originating in the sinoatrial node with a ventricular response of less than 60 beats/min

sinus tachycardia: Dysrhythmia originating in the sinoatrial node with a ventricular response between 101 and 180 beats/min

splanchnic: Pertaining to internal organs; visceral

ST segment: Portion of the ECG representing the end of ventricular depolarization (end of the R wave) and the beginning of ventricular repolarization (T wave)

stroke volume: Amount of blood ejected by either ventricle during one contraction; can be calculated as cardiac output divided by heart rate

subendocardial infarction: Myocardial infarction involving the endocardium and myocardium

subepicardial infarction: Myocardial infarction involving the myocardium and epicardium

sulcus: Groove

supraventricular: Originating from a site above the bundle branches, such as the sinoatrial node, atria, or AV junction

syncope: Fainting; usually resulting from cardiac or neurologic conditions, including seizure disorders, vasodepressor syncope (the simple faint), and cardiac dysrhythmias

syncytium: Unit of combined cells

systole: Contraction of the heart (usually referring to ventricular contraction) during which blood is propelled into the pulmonary artery and aorta; when the term is used without reference to a specific chamber of the heart, the term implies ventricular systole

tachycardia: Heart rate greater than 100 beats/min (*tachy*, fast)

threshold: Membrane potential at which the cell membrane will depolarize and generate an action potential

TKO: Abbreviation meaning "to keep open"; also known as KVO, "keep the vein open"

torsades de pointes (TdP): Type of polymorphic VT associated with a prolonged QT interval; the QRS changes in shape, amplitude, and width and appears to "twist" around the isoelectric line, resembling a spindle

transmural infarction: Myocardial infarction in which the entire thickness of the ventricular wall (endocardium to epicardium) is involved

trifascicular block: Block in the three primary divisions of the bundle branches (i.e., right bundle branch, left anterior fascicle, and left posterior fascicle)

trigeminy: Dysrhythmia in which every third beat is a premature ectopic beat

T wave: Waveform that follows the QRS complex and represents ventricular repolarization

unipolar lead: Lead that consists of a single positive electrode and a reference point; a pacing lead with a single electrical pole at the distal tip of the pacing lead (negative pole) through which the stimulating pulse is delivered; in a permanent pacemaker with a unipolar lead, the positive pole is the pulse generator case

VA interval: In dual-chamber pacing, the interval between a sensed- or ventricular-paced event and the next atrial-paced event

VV interval: Interval between two ventricular-paced events

V wave: Ventricular-paced event; the ventricular stimulus or the point in the intrinsic ventricular depolarization (R wave) during which ventricular sensing occurs

vagal maneuver: Methods used to stimulate the vagus nerve in an attempt to slow conduction through the AV node, resulting in slowing of the heart rate

vector: Quantity having direction and magnitude, usually depicted by a straight arrow whose length represents magnitude and whose head represents direction

venous return: Amount of blood flowing into the right atrium each minute from the systemic circulation

ventricle: Either of the two lower chambers of the heart

ventricular activation time (VAT): Interval it takes for depolarization of the interventricular septum, right ventricle, and most of the left ventricle; VAT is measured on the ECG from the beginning of the QRS complex to the onset of the peak of the R wave

ventricular pacing: Pacing system with a lead attached in the right ventricle

ventricular tachycardia (VT): Dysrhythmia originating in the ventricles with a ventricular response greater than 100 beats/min

wandering atrial pacemaker (multiformed atrial rhythm): Cardiac dysrhythmia that occurs because of impulses originating from various sites, including the sinoatrial node, the atria, and/or the AV junction; requires at least three different P waves, seen in the same lead, for proper diagnosis.

waveform: Movement away from the baseline in either a positive or negative direction

Wolff-Parkinson-White syndrome: Type of preexcitation syndrome, characterized by a slurred upstroke of the QRS complex (delta wave) and wide QRS

CREDITS

CHAPTER 1

Figures 1-1, 1-2: Thibodeau G, Patton K: *Anatomy and physiology,* ed 4, St Louis, 1999, Mosby.
Figure 1-3: Cannobio M: *Cardiovascular disorders, Mosby's clinical nursing series,* St Louis, 1990, Mosby.
Figure 1-4: Thibodeau G, Patton K: *Anatomy and physiology,* ed 4, St Louis, 1999, Mosby.
Figure 1-5: *Managing major diseases, cardiac disorders,* vol 2, ed 2, St Louis, 1999, Mosby.
Figures 1-6, 1-7: Thibodeau G, Patton K: *Anatomy and physiology,* ed 4, St Louis, 1999, Mosby.
Figures 1-8, 1-9: Cannobio M: *Cardiovascular disorders, Mosby's clinical nursing series,* St Louis, 1990, Mosby.
Figure 1-10: Thibodeau G, Patton K: *Anatomy and physiology,* ed 4, St Louis, 1999, Mosby.
Figure 1-11: Herlihy B, Maebius N: *The human body in health and illness,* Philadelphia, 2000, WB Saunders.
Figure 1-12: Cannobio M: *Cardiovascular disorders, Mosby's clinical nursing series,* St Louis, 1990, Mosby.
Figures 1-13, 1-15: Thibodeau G, Patton K: *Anatomy and physiology,* ed 4, St Louis, 1999, Mosby.

CHAPTER 2

Figure 2-1: Thibodeau G, Patton K: *Anatomy and physiology,* ed 4, St Louis, 1999, Mosby.
Figures 2-2, 2-3, 2-4: Herlihy B, Maebius N: *The human body in health and illness,* Philadelphia, 2000, WB Saunders.
Figure 2-5: Huszar R: *Basic dysrhythmias: interpretation and management,* ed 2, St Louis, 1994, Mosby.
Figures 2-6, 2-7, 2-8: Cannobio M: *Cardiovascular disorders, Mosby's clinical nursing series,* St Louis, 1990, Mosby.
Figure 2-9: Thelan L, Urden L, Lough M, et al: *Critical care nursing: diagnosis and management,* ed 2, St Louis, 1998, Mosby.
Figure 2-10: Crawford M, Spence M: *Commonsense approach to coronary care,* ed 6, St Louis, 1995, Mosby.
Figure 2-11: Guyton A, Hall J: *Textbook of medical physiology,* ed 9, Philadelphia, 1996, WB Saunders.
Figure 2-12: Touboul P, Waldo A: *Atrial arrhythmias: current concepts and management,* St Louis, 1990, Mosby.
Figure 2-14: Clochesy J, Breu C, Cardin S, et al: *Critical care nursing,* ed 2, Philadelphia, 1996, WB Saunders.
Figure 2-15: Guyton A, Hall J: *Textbook of medical physiology,* ed 9, Philadelphia, 1996, WB Saunders.
Figure 2-16: Marriot H, Conover M: *Advanced concepts in arrhythmias,* ed 3, St Louis, 1998, Mosby.
Figure 2-17: Guyton A, Hall J: *Textbook of medical physiology,* ed 9, Philadelphia, 1996, WB Saunders.
Figure 2-18: Aehlert B: *ACLS quick review study guide,* St Louis, 1994, Mosby.
Figures 2-19, 2-20: Phalen T: *The 12-lead ECG in acute myocardial infarction,* St Louis, 1996, Mosby.
Figure 2-21: Thelan L, Urden L, Lough M, et al: *Critical care nursing: diagnosis and management,* ed 2, St Louis, 1998, Mosby.
Figures 2-22, 2-23: Goldberger A: *Clinical electrocardiography: a simplified approach,* ed 6, St Louis, 1999, Mosby.
Figure 2-24: Methodist Hospital: *Basic electrocardiography: a modular approach,* St Louis, 1986, Mosby.
Figures 2-25, 2-26, 2-27: Aehlert B: *ACLS quick review study guide,* St Louis, 1994, Mosby.
Figure 2-28: Phillips R, Feeney M: *The cardiac rhythms: a systematic approach to interpretation,* ed 3, St Louis, 1990, WB Saunders.
Figures 2-29, 2-30: Thelan L, Urden L, Lough M, et al: *Critical care nursing: diagnosis and management,* ed 2, St Louis, 1998, Mosby.
Figure 2-31: Grauer K: *A practical guide to ECG interpretation,* ed 2, St Louis, 1998, Mosby.
Figure 2-32: Clochesy J, Breu C, Cardin S, et al: *Critical care nursing,* ed 2, Philadelphia, 1996, WB Saunders.
Figure 2-33: Lounsbury P, Frye S: *Cardiac rhythm disorders,* ed 2, St Louis, 1992, Mosby.
Figure 2-35: Goldberger A: *Clinical electrocardiography: a simplified approach,* ed 6, St Louis, 1999, Mosby.
Figure 2-36: Thibodeau G, Patton K: *Anatomy and physiology,* ed 4, St Louis, 1999, Mosby.
Figure 2-37: Goldberger A: *Clinical electrocardiography: a simplified approach,* ed 6, St Louis, 1999, Mosby.
Figures 2-41, 2-42: Thibodeau G, Patton K: *Anatomy and physiology,* ed 4, St Louis, 1999, Mosby.
Figure 2-43: Goldberger A: *Clinical electrocardiography: a simplified approach,* ed 6, St Louis, 1999, Mosby.
Figure 2-44: Thibodeau G, Patton K: *Anatomy and physiology,* ed 4, St Louis, 1999, Mosby.
Figure 2-45: Thelan L, Urden L, Lough M, et al: *Critical care nursing: diagnosis and management,* ed 2, St Louis, 1998, Mosby.
Figure 2-46: Grauer K: *A practical guide to ECG interpretation,* ed 2, St Louis, 1998, Mosby.
Figure 2-47: Goldberger A: *Clinical electrocardiography: a simplified approach,* ed 6, St Louis, 1999, Mosby.
Figure 2-48: Thibodeau G, Patton K: *Anatomy and physiology,* ed 4, St Louis, 1999, Mosby.
Figure 2-50: Goldberger A: *Clinical electrocardiography: a simplified approach,* ed 6, St Louis, 1999, Mosby.
Figure 2-51: Chou T: *Electrocardiography in clinical practice: adult and pediatric,* ed 4, Philadelphia, 1996, WB Saunders.
Figures 2-52, 2-53: Thibodeau G, Patton K: *Anatomy and physiology,* ed 4, St Louis, 1999, Mosby.

Figures 2-54, 2-55, 2-56: Sanders M: *Mosby's paramedic textbook*, St Louis, 1994, Mosby.

Figure 2-57: Thelan L, Urden L, Lough M, et al: *Critical care nursing: diagnosis and management*, ed 2, St Louis, 1998, Mosby.

Figure 2-58: Crawford M, Spence M: *Commonsense approach to coronary care*, ed 6, St Louis, 1995, Mosby.

CHAPTER 4

Figure 4-1: Crawford M, Spence M: *Commonsense approach to coronary care*, ed 6, St Louis, 1995, Mosby.

Figure 4-3: Kinney M, Packa D, Andreoli K, et al: *Andreoli's comprehensive cardiac care*, ed 8, St Louis, 1995, Mosby.

Figure 4-5: Goldberger A: *Clinical electrocardiography: a simplified approach*, ed 6, St Louis, 1999, Mosby.

Figure 4-7: Thelan L, Urden L, Lough M, et al: *Critical care nursing: diagnosis and management*, ed 2, St Louis, 1998, Mosby.

Figure 4-9: Goldman L, Braunwald E: *Primary cardiology*, Philadelphia, 1998, WB Saunders.

Figure 4-10: Conover M: *Understanding electrocardiography*, ed 7, St Louis, 1996, Mosby.

Figure 4-11: Sanders M: *Mosby's paramedic textbook*, St Louis, 1994, Mosby.

Figure 4-12: Crawford M, Spence M: *Commonsense approach to coronary care*, ed 6, St Louis, 1995, Mosby.

Figure 4-13: Chou T: *Electrocardiography in clinical practice: adult and pediatric*, ed 4, Philadelphia, 1996, WB Saunders.

Figure 4-16: Goldberger A: *Clinical electrocardiography: a simplified approach*, ed 6, St Louis, 1999, Mosby.

CHAPTER 6

Figure 6-1: Kinney M, Packa D, Andreoli K, et al: *Andreoli's comprehensive cardiac care*, ed 8, St Louis, 1995, Mosby.

Figure 6-7: Chou T: *Electrocardiography in clinical practice: adult and pediatric*, ed 4, Philadelphia, 1996, WB Saunders.

CHAPTER 9

Figure 9-1: Thibodeau G, Patton K: *Anatomy and physiology*, ed 4, St Louis, 1999, Mosby.

Figures 9-2, 9-3: Goldberger A: *Clinical electrocardiography: a simplified approach*, ed 6, St Louis, 1999, Mosby.

Figure 9-4: Methodist Hospital: *Basic electrocardiography: a modular approach*, St Louis, 1986, Mosby.

Figure 9-5: Thelan L, Urden L, Lough M, et al: *Critical care nursing: diagnosis and management*, ed 2, St Louis, 1998, Mosby.

Figure 9-6: Grauer K: *A practical guide to ECG interpretation*, ed 2, St Louis, 1998, Mosby.

Figure 9-7: Chou T: *Electrocardiography in clinical practice: adult and pediatric*, ed 4, Philadelphia, 1996, WB Saunders.

Figures 9-8, 9-9: Thelan L, Urden L, Lough M, et al: *Critical care nursing: diagnosis and management*, ed 2, St Louis, 1998, Mosby.

Figure 9-10: Grauer K: *A practical guide to ECG interpretation*, ed 2, St Louis, 1998, Mosby.

Figure 9-11: Phalen T: *The 12-lead ECG in acute myocardial infarction*, St Louis, 1996, Mosby.

Figure 9-12: Clochesy J, Breu C, Cardin S, et al: *Critical care nursing*, ed 2, Philadelphia, 1996, WB Saunders.

Figure 9-13: Lounsbury P, Frye S: *Cardiac rhythm disorders*, ed 2, St Louis, 1992, Mosby.

Figure 9-14: Conover M: *Understanding electrocardiography*, ed 7, St Louis, 1996, Mosby.

Figure 9-15: Kahn M: *Rapid ECG interpretation*, Philadelphia, 1997, WB Saunders.

Figure 9-16: Phalen T: *The 12-lead ECG in acute myocardial infarction*, St Louis, 1996, Mosby.

Figure 9-17: Goldberger A: *Clinical electrocardiography: a simplified approach*, ed 6, St Louis, 1999, Mosby.

Figure 9-18: Phalen T: *The 12-lead ECG in acute myocardial infarction*, St Louis, 1996, Mosby.

Figure 9-19: Kinney M, Packa D, Andreoli K, et al: *Andreoli's comprehensive cardiac care*, ed 8, St Louis, 1995, Mosby.

Figure 9-20: Phalen T: *The 12-lead ECG in acute myocardial infarction*, St Louis, 1996, Mosby.

Figure 9-21: Kinney M, Packa D, Andreoli K, et al: *Andreoli's comprehensive cardiac care*, ed 8, St Louis, 1995, Mosby.

Figure 9-22: Phalen T: *The 12-lead ECG in acute myocardial infarction*, St Louis, 1996, Mosby.

Figure 9-23: Kinney M, Packa D, Andreoli K, et al: *Andreoli's comprehensive cardiac care*, ed 8, St Louis, 1995, Mosby.

Figure 9-24: Phalen T: *The 12-lead ECG in acute myocardial infarction*, St Louis, 1996, Mosby.

Figure 9-25: Thelan L, Urden L, Lough M, et al: *Critical care nursing: diagnosis and management*, ed 2, St Louis, 1998, Mosby.

Figures 9-26, 9-27, 9-28, 9-29: Phalen T: *The 12-lead ECG in acute myocardial infarction*, St Louis, 1996, Mosby.

Figure 9-30: Goldberger A: *Clinical electrocardiography: a simplified approach*, ed 6, St Louis, 1999, Mosby.

Figure 9-31: Chou T: *Electrocardiography in clinical practice: adult and pediatric*, ed 4, Philadelphia, 1996, WB Saunders.

Figures 9-32, 9-33, 9-34: Johnson R, Swartz M: *A simplified approach to electrocardiography*, St Louis, 1986, Mosby.

Figure 9-35: Kinney M, Packa D, Andreoli K, et al: *Andreoli's comprehensive cardiac care*, ed 8, St Louis, 1995, Mosby.

CHAPTER 10

Figure 10-4: Goldberger A: *Clinical electrocardiography: a simplified approach*, ed 6, St Louis, 1999, Mosby.

INDEX

b denotes box, *f* denotes figure, *t* denotes table.